Breeds and Health Management of DOGS

Breeds and Health Management of DOGS

M.C. Sharma BVSc & AH, MVSc, PhD (Vety. Medicine), FNAAS, FNAVS, FISVM, FIAAVR, F Mobs.
Joint Director, Extension Education, Indian Veterinary Research Institute, Izatnagar, Bareilly (UP)
Former Principal Scientist and National Fellow (ICAR),
Division of Medicine, Indian Veterinary Research Institute, Izatnagar, Bareilly (UP)
Former Professor and Head, Department of Veterinary Epidemiology and Preventive Medicine
Joint Director (Veterinary Extension), GBPUAT, Pantnagar
Former ITEC Expert to Government of Vietnam
Former ITEC Expert and Project Leader to Government of Mauritius

N.N. Pathak BSc, BVSc & AH, MVSc, PhD, FNAVS, FANA, FMobs
Member of American Academy of Veterinary Nutrition
Member, Governing Council of National Academy of Veterinary Sciences
Former Director, Central Institute for Research on Buffaloes, Hissar
Former Head and Director, Centre for Advance Studies, Animal Nutrition Division,
Indian Veterinary Research Institute, Izatnagar, Bareilly (UP)
Former ITEC expert and Project Leader to Government of Vietnam

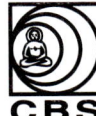

CBS Publishers & Distributors

New Delhi • Bangalore • Pune

Breeds and
Health Management of
DOGS

© 2008, Authors and Publisher

First Edition 2008

ISBN: 978-81-239-1636-1

Published by :
Satish Kumar Jain for CBS Publishers & Distributors,
4819/XI Prahlad Street, 24 Ansari Road,
Daryaganj, New Delhi 110002, India.
E-mail : cbspubs@vsnl.com
Website : www.cbspd.com

Production Director : Vinod K. Jain

Branch Office :
Seema House, 2975, 17th Cross, K.R. Road,
Bansankari 2nd Stage, Bangalore - 560070
Fax : 080-26771680 • E-mail : cbsbng@dataone.in

Printed at :
Swastik Packagings, Delhi-92

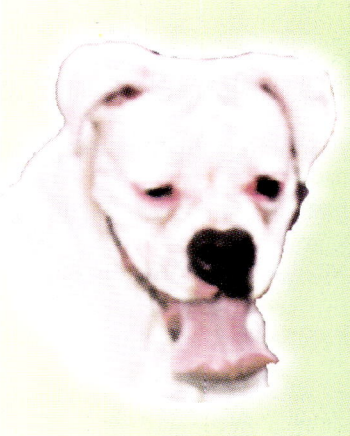

Foreword

It is believed that the ancestors of dog appeared on the earth about twenty million years ago and probably it was first animal to be domesticated by the man along with horses because these two species started to live in the near vicinity of human settlements. Because of its active habits, retrieving nature, courage, loyalty and obedience the dogs were evolved to perform diversified functions. Modern dogs of more than four hundred breeds are mostly developed in the European and American societies and many of them were induced in India from time to time.

A large number of exotic breeds of dog were brought during the last century when kennel breeding was started for commercial purpose. At present one or more dog breeding kennels are operating in almost all big cities and towns in India due to increasing demand of pedigreed dogs as a most suitable pet animal. Ranging from less than one kilogram to almost one hundred kilogram body weight, dogs have been found to suit all kinds of accommodation of the urban families. Due to the development of small families and employment of almost all eligible members of the urban families, the need of pet dogs has also increased.

Today dogs are being kept to perform the duties of companion, guard, guide and protector of households in urban areas besides their age-old duties of the assistance in the management of flocks and herds of domesticated farm animals and hunting the games. In addition to common duties, a few breeds have been employed for performing highly important specialised job of searching, seizing and guarding in many services responsible for security, maintenance of peace, identification of culprits, and protection of territory.

Organising of dog shows in India is quite old but for very long time it was limited to a small circle. During the past three–four decades its dimension has increased and now a larger number of owners are participating and many wish to participate, while a large number of owners do not have even the minimum knowledge about the breeds, behaviour and disposition of their pet dogs. A good number of illustrated books on dog breeds, behaviour and other traits of foreign publishers are available in the market but they are expensive, scanty and most of them do not contain informations on all important aspects of dog keeping, and owners are often required to procure several books. In most of the books on dog rearing, major positions, being important aspects of dog husbandry, are bound to be repeated. In this book authors have made good attempt to compile almost all the important information on various aspects of dog rearing. They have also provided a good illustration of important breeds of dog besides separate illustrative information on the characteristics, behaviour and utility of so far recognised and established Indian breeds of dog. The authors deserve appreciation for producing such an illustrative and informative book that will be a useful reference not only for the professionals but also for the common nonprofessional dog owners, besides the students, teachers and researchers of the veterinary profession.

Mangala Rai
Secretary
Government of India (DARE)
and
Director General
Indian Council of Agricultural Research
Krishi Bhavan,
New Delhi-110 001

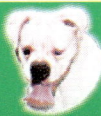

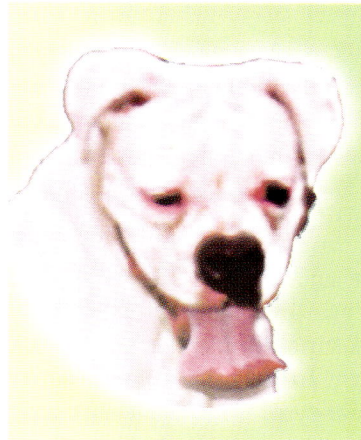

Preface

In recent years a few books, including the two, viz. *A Hand Book of Dog Keeping* and *Dogs—Breeding, Nutrition, Diagnosis and Health Management* by the authors have been published and are available in the market. Indeed, there was continued demand from the students and dog lovers for a comprehensive book in a concise volume.

The popularity of our earlier book *Dogs—Breeding, Nutrition, Diagnosis and Health Management* published in 1993 and reprinted in almost every third year is a clear indication of increasing interest in the scientific management of pet dogs and increasing dimension of canine practitioners in the veterinary practice. In the busy and stressful urban life people are finding some relaxation in the company of the pets, and dog is becoming a most popular companion in today's competitive and stressful life. Besides companionship, the dimension of working dogs in various services is also increasing at a fast rate. Now well organised kennels have been established by various departments or organizations responsible for the maintenance of law and order in the country, protection of borders of the country, detection of narcotics, inflammable materials, explosives and other watch and guard works. Dogs are men's best friends. They are loyal and responsive to their owners' moods. In today's fast track world, they provide solace, relief and peace in a man's life. Their significant presence in home keeps all the family members active and happy.

India is a paradise of about 25 million dogs of different shapes, sizes and behaviour distributed from Kanyakumari to high Himalayan ranges. Larger populations of Indian dogs are stray animals, found in groups of different sizes throughout the country. Since most of the species of domesticated animals enjoy sentimental protection of Indian people, it is difficult for any organization to reduce the population of dogs by stamping. It is well known to even common people in India that dog-bite terminates mostly fatal due to rabies, still a majority of people will not support any attempt of elimination of dogs from the society. Although rearing of the dogs as a controlled pet is less common in suburban and rural areas, yet almost every household daily offers some food to dogs living in their

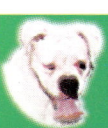

locality. Thus, maintenance of groups of community dogs on the food provided by the families of that area is quite common throughout India.

Campaign for the protection of even stray dogs by anti rabies vaccination is organised from time to time by different government and non-government organizations, but it is not easy to provide coverage of such a large population. Therefore, it is important to educate people on different phase of the life of dogs along with the merits and demerits of the stray, community, pet and working dogs for humans. To provide comprehensive information on various aspects of dog life the book entitled *Breeds and Health Management of Dogs* has been prepared. The book has been organised in seven chapters covering all important aspects of dog's life cycle. Starting with a brief introduction, detailed information on important and popular breeds, select management practices, foods and feeding of dogs, diseases of dogs, common systemic diseases, infectious diseases and common poisons are given with details in chapters five to seven respectively. Information has also been provided on zoonotic diseases because in the presence of a large number of free-living community dogs it is important for the public to have detailed knowledge of the diseases communicable from dogs to humans and *vice versa* so that they will be able to take necessary preventive measures for protection.

The fancy aspect of dog-keeping is the organization of dog shows. In India, although organization of dog shows is quite old, in the pre-Independence period it was generally limited to the royals and their organization was mostly on the line of practices followed in European countries. However, with the increase in the number of dog owners, breeding kennels and good veterinary care there has been good proliferation in the establishment of kennel clubs throughout the country resulting in the increase in the number and frequency of dog shows not only in cosmopolitan cities but even spread to small towns. Under such a changed situation there was a demand for an illustrated book on dogs covering almost all important aspects of dog management under Indian scenario. Honouring the wishes of dog lovers, students and teachers of veterinary sciences, we have made an attempt to put forward a comprehensive and a well illustrated book.

In the preparation of this book we have received help from different corners and it is our duty to put a word of gratitude for their help. The assistance rendered by Dr. Rupasi Tiwari, Senior Scientist–Officer-incharge, ATIC, Dr. P.K. Sharma, veterinary practitioner at Lucknow, Dr. Chinmay Joshi, Dr. Gunjan Das, Dr. Pankaj Kumar, Shri Kundan Singh, Shri Deepak Kumar Sheel, Shri J.P. Singh and Shri Gaurav Singh is cordially acknowledged.

Mahesh Chandra Sharma
Nityanand Pathak

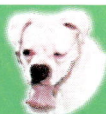

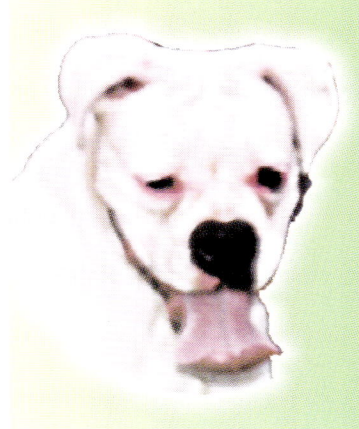

Contents

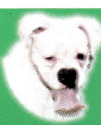

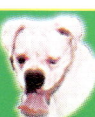

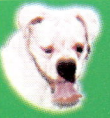

4. FOODS AND FEEDING OF DOGS

123-135

5. DISEASES OF DOGS

136-181

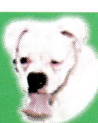

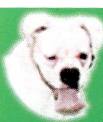

6. INFECTIOUS DISEASES

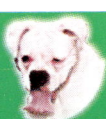

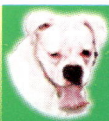

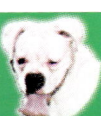

7. COMMON POISONS

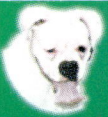

APPENDICES   245-287

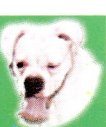

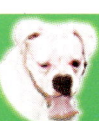

Breeds and Health Management of DOGS

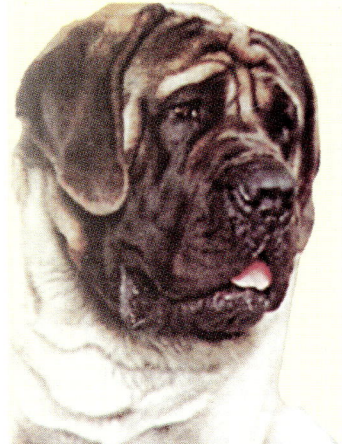

Introduction

Today's pedigreed dog breeds have descended down from the illustrious and sophisticated families of Maharajas, Rajas, Nawabs and big business houses to common families. The reasons are the need of a suitable companion for the old person as well as young children of small families in towns and families engaged in farm animal keeping and other farming in the rural areas. Although dog keeping is not new but the methods have significantly changed. About four-five decades ago most of the people did not bother for the breed, type, feeding and management of the dogs. The dogs are integral member of almost all nomadic and tribal groups of India and they are adopted in a manner to move from place to place along with the family and their domestic animals and birds. In rural areas, earlier dogs were reared unchained as a yard dog and house dog. But there have been great changes in dog keeping and due to increasing demand of pedigreed dogs of some recognized exotic and indigenous breeds many dog breeding kennels have been established in almost all big cities and towns of the India. Most of the commercial dog breeders are non-technical for the production of healthy puppies

to fetch good price. Dog keepers also require some basic informations on the important aspects of breeding, feeding, maintenance of health and other managemental practices in a concise form.

Most of the informations on various aspects of management have already been provided in our earlier book entitled "Dogs: Breeding, Nutrition, Diagnosis and Health Management" by M.C. Sharma, N.N. Pathak and P.N. Bhat published by CBS in 1993. The book has shown its worth as evident from its reprinting almost every alternate year. Although informations on dog breeds have been provided in the book but that is not adequate for the purpose of dog show and selection of a breed for keeping to meet different requirements.

In addition to information about the physical characteristics and distinguishing traits the dog breeders also require informations on the practical aspects of food selection, food processing and daily dietary requirements of different kinds of dogs specially during gestation and nursing period in bitches and also for the stud dogs used for breeding. On the other hand, dog keepers need informations on the diet preparation and feeding of weaned puppies, growing pups and adult dogs. The other important aspects of dog husbandry are the exercise, brief training at least for obedience and performance of the job for which it is kept, viz., companionship of lonely person in the house, guarding of the house, guide for the handicapped persons, herding the flock and other activities.

To meet the requirements of dog breeders, dog owners, specialists of the show, dog show organisers, veterinarians and other related personnels with the kennel activities this book has been organized in a manner to provide important informations of more than one hundred exotic and Indian breeds. Efforts have been made to provide original photographs of most of the breeds. A chart of foods suitable for feeding the dogs along with nutritional requirements for different categories of dogs have been presented in tabular form.

Details about the infectious and the non-infectious diseases of dog have been described in this book apart from all the managemental and nutritional practices. Infectious diseases such as bacterial, viral, fungal, parasitic and non-infectious diseases like deficiency and metabolic diseases, common poisoning cases which the pet dogs come across and their causes, treatment and prevention have also been dealt in detail. Several systemic diseases involving the systems, viz., gastrointestinal system, respiratory system, cardiovascular system, nervous system, musculoskeleton system and urogenital system have been elaborated along with their causes, treatment and prevention. These aspects have been covered with reasonable details to facilitate proper application by the technical persons. Adequate indications and guidelines have been provided at different places for need-based

consultation of veterinarians; particularly the dog specialists, if available. Most important among the health management practices are the deworming and vaccination. Regarding the vaccination and deworming, every detail have been given in the Appendix and under the parasitic diseases.

There are certain aspects of routine management and others of one time action in life span of the dog, which require education of the new dog owners and trainees. Important routine management practices are exercise, outing for defaecation and urination as per schedule, feeding, watering and grooming. The grooming of a dog is one of the most tedious jobs when coat is long and wiry. Any relaxation in grooming of long haired, double coated and wiry haired dogs may result in mat formation and roping. Such changes in body coat create problems in brushing and combing and often require removal of mats and cords when few in number but complete saving becomes necessary when mats and cords are many and soiled. These conditions provide hiding places for ectoparasite. Tick infestation is frequently encountered during summer and rainy season in long haired dogs. The ears, face, neck, both aspects of shoulders, toe space and other parts of the body with prominent cutaneous circulation are the main sites of attachment for the blood sucking ticks. The other managemental activities are bathing, nail cutting, docking, hair dressing, spaying and castration etc.

Although this book has been organized in the shape of a well illustrated atlas containing one or more original photographs of the important dog breeds, the other gestures differentiating it from the other available publications are the informations provided on important aspects of dogs rearing.

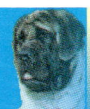

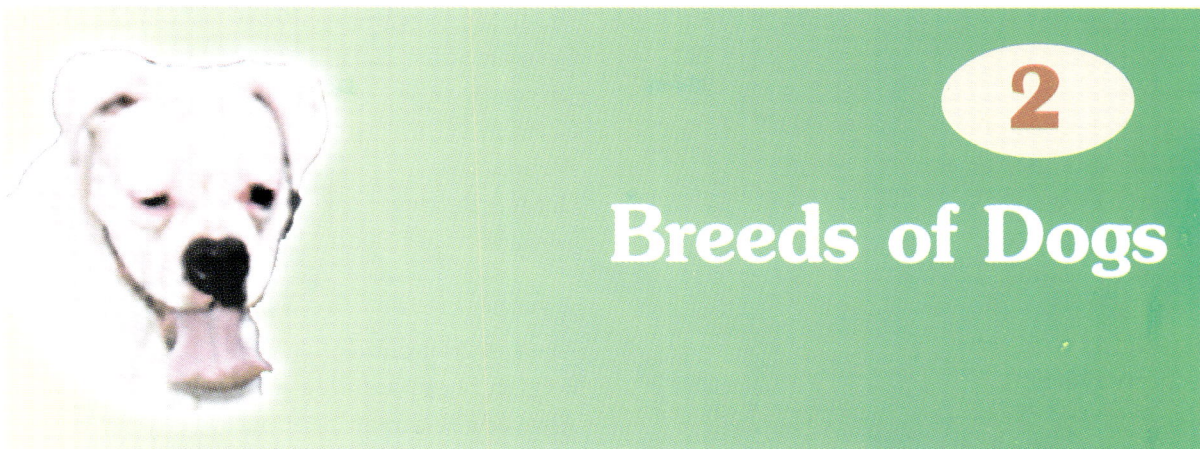

Breeds of Dogs

Since the beginning of civilization, dogs have been selected and bred for different purposes like companionship, sports, protection against strangers and hunting. Dogs of small breeds are good companions, hounds are loved by hunters while shephered dogs are maintained for pulling sledge carts on the snow-covered ground of Tundra. In recent years, they are being used in several new fields such as in police, military, railways, prisons, blind homes to watch and search for missing, deserted or absconding persons, and also to guide blind persons.

Dogs were domesticated in prehistoric period but wild, feral and street dogs are still found in every country.

Wild dog: Varieties available today are the Dingoes of Australia, Pariah of South and West Asia and wild dogs of India.

Feral dogs: Feral dogs are domesticated breeds that have returned to their wild habitat and have also regained their original habits.

Pet dogs: Pet dogs are mostly pedigreed animals maintained under controlled management.

CLASSIFICATION OF DOGS

Zoological Classification

Dogs belong to the Class Mammalia, subclass Metatheria, Order Carnivora, Family Canidae, and Genus *Canis*.

Modern breeds suited for maintaining as pet dogs are classified according to the British or American Kennel Club's classification. A widely accepted well-defined classification of Indian domestic dogs is not available. Most of the Indian breeds of dogs are known by different names. However, a, tentative classification has been proposed to bring uniformity and easy identification.

British Classification

Dogs have been classified into the following 6 main groups on the basis of body size, morphology, behaviour, place of breeding (origin) and utility:

1. Non-sporting Breeds (Utility Group)

Boston Terrier
Chow Chow
Bulldog

Dalmatian
Canaan Dog
French Bulldog
Giant Schnauzer
Poodle (Standard)
Iceland Dog
Poodle (Miniature)
Japanese Akita
Poodle (Toy)
Keeshond
Schipperke
Leonberger
Schnauzer
Lhasa Apso
Shih Tzu
Mexican Hairless
Tibetan Spaniel
Miniature Schnauzer
Tibetan Terrier

2. Gun dogs

American Cocker Spaniel
Gordon Setter
Chesapeake Bay Retriever
Hungarian Vizsla
Clumber Spaniel
Irish Setter
Cocker Spaniel
Irish Water Spaniel
Curly Coated Retriever
Italian Spinone
English Setter
Labrador Retriever
English Springer Spaniel
Large Munsterlander
Field Spaniel
Pointer
Flat Coated Retriever
Pointing Wire-Haired Griffon
German Longhair Pointer

Small Munsterlander
German Short Hair Pointer
Sussex Spaniel
German Wire Hair Pointer
Weimaraner
Golden Retriever
Selsh Springer Spaniel

3. Non-sporting Breeds (Working Group)

Alaskan Malamute
Belgian Shepherd Dog (Groenendal)
Alsatians (German Shepherd)
Belgian Shepherd Dog (Tervueren)
Anatolian (Karabash) Dog
Bernese Mountain Dog
Australian Kelpie
Bouvier De Flandre
Bearded Collie
Boxer
Beauceron
Briard
Bullmastiff
Pembroke Welsh Corgi
Cardigan Welsh Corgi
Polish Sheep Dog
Great Dane
Pyreneam Mountain Dog
Hungarian Kuvasz
Rottweiler
Hungarian Puli
St. Bernard
Husky
Samoyed
Maremma Italian Sheep Dog
Shetland Sheep Dog
Mastiff
Siberian Husky
New Found Land
Smooth Collie

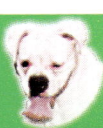

Norwegian Buhund
Tibetan Mastiff
Old English Sheepdog

4. Terrier Breeds

Airedale Terrier
Miniature Bull Terrier
Australian Terrier
Norfolk Terrier
Bedlington Terrier
Norwich Terrier
Border Terrier
Scottish Terrier
Bull Terrier
Sealyham Terrier
Cairn Terrier
Skye Terrier
Dandie Dinmont Terrier
Smooth Fox Terrier
Glen of Imaal Terrier
Soft-Coated Wheaten Terrier
Irish Terrier
Staffordshire White Terrier
Kerry Blue Terrier
Welsh Terrier
Lakeland Terrier
West Highland White Terrier
Manchester Terrier
Wire Fox Terrier

5. Hound Breeds

Basenji
Borzoi
Basset Hound
Dachsbracke
Basset Griffon Vendeen
Dachshund (Long Haired)
Beagle
Dachshund (Miniature long haired)
Bloodhound

Dachshund (Smooth haired)
Dachshund (Miniature smooth haired)
Irish Wolfhound
Dachshund (Wire haired)
Otterhound
Pharaoh Hound
Dachshund (Miniature wire haired)
Portuguese Warren Hound
Deerhound
Rhodesian Ridgeback
Elkhound
Saluki
Finnish Spitz
Swedish Foxhound
Foxhound
Swiss Laufhund (Jura)
Greyhound
Ibizan Hound

6. Toy Breeds

Affenpinscher
Lowchen
Bichon Frise
Maltese
Cavalier King Charles Spaniel
Miniature Pinscher
Chihuahua (Long coat)
Papillon
Chihuahua (Smooth coat)
Pekingese
Chinese Crested Dog
Pomeranian
English Toy Terrier (Black and Tan)
Pug
Griffon Bruxellosis
Silky Terrier
Italian Greyhound
Yorkshire Terrier
Japanese chin
King Charles Spaniel

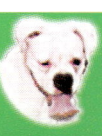

AMERICAN CLASSIFICATION

It is different from the British classification that it gives more emphasis on the type of the dogs.

1. Non Sporting Breeds

Boston Terrier
French Bulldog
Bulldog
Keeshond
Chow Chow
Lhasa Apso
Dalmatian
Poodle (miniature)
Schipperke

2. Working Breeds

Akita
New Found Land
Alaskan Malamute
Old English Sheep Dog
Belgian Malinois
Puli
Belgian Sheep Dog
Rottweiler
Belgian Tervuren
St. Bernard
Bernese Mountain Dog
Samoyed
Bouvier Des Flandres
Schnauzer (Giant)
Boxer
Schnauzer (Standard)
Briard
Shetland Sheepdog
Bull Mastiff
Siberian Husky
Collie

3. Sporting Breeds

Griffon (Wire haired pointing)

Pointer German (Wire haired)
Pointer
Retriever (Chesapeake Bay)
Pointer (German short haired)
Retriever (Curly coated)
Retriever (Flat coated)
Spaniel (Cocker)
Retriever (Gloden)
Spaniel (English Cocker)
Retriever (Labrador)
Spaniel (English Springer)
Setter (English)
Spaniel (Field)
Setter (Gordon)
Spaniel (Irish water)
Setter (Irish)
Spaniel (Sussex)
Spaniel (American water)
Spaniel (Welsh springer)
Spaniel (Brittani)
Vizsla
Spaniel (Clumber)
Weimaraner

4. Terrier Breeds

Airedale Terrier
Lakeland Terrier
Great Dane
Dobermann Pinscher
Great Pyreness
German Shepherd Dog
Komondor
Kuvasz
Welsh Corgi (Cardigan)
Mastiff
Welsh Corgi (Pembroke)
Australian Terrier
Manchester Terrier
Bedlington Terrier

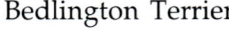
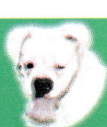

Norwich Terrier
Border Terrier
Schnauzer (Miniature) Terrier
Bull Terrier
Scottish Terrier
Cairn Terrier
Sealyham Terrier
Dandie Dinmont Terrier
Skye Terrier
Fox Terrier
Staffordshire White Terrier
Irish Terrier
Welsh Terrier
Kerry Blue Terrier
West Highland White Terrier

5. Toy Breeds

Affenpinscher
Pinscher Miniature
Bichon Frise
Pomeranian
Chihuahua
Poodle (Toy)
English Toy Spaniel
Pug
Griffon (Brussels)
Shih Tzu
Italian Greyhound
Silky Terrier
Japanese Spaniel
Toy Manchester Terrier
Maltese
Yorkshire Terrier

6. Hound Breeds

Afgan Hound
Foxhound (American)
Basenji
Foxhound (English)

Basset Hound
Greyhound
Beagle
Terrier
Blood Hound
Norwegian Elkhound
Borzoi (or Russian wolfhound)
Otterhound
Coonhound (Black and tan)
Rhodesian Ridgeback
Dachshund
Saluki
Deerhound (Scottish)
Shippet
Wolfhound (Irish)

INDIAN CLASSIFICATION

In India, selection of dogs is based on their utility. Nomadic and settle tribes like Banjara, Tharu, Bhatu, Cole, Bhil and Mundia. Farmers use dog for guarding their livestock and fields. For urban families, dog is a companion and a symbol of social status. Looking into this huge variations in the functions, owner and environment of the Indian dog, it can be classified as:

House dogs: These are kept as pet animals inside the house, loose or tied and taken out of the house only for urination and defaecation and certain amount of exercise. These types of breed are usually exotic like Alsatian, Pomeranian, Labrador, Terriers etc. selected local breeds are also kept as house dogs.

House yard dogs: These are kept by the villagers as guard dogs. These have freedom of movement both indoor and outdoor. These are selected breeds which are sometime cross between local Indian breed and exotic breeds.

Yard dogs: These are kept by farmers to guard the standing crops, vegetables and fruits and are always kept outside and offered meals two-

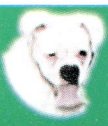

three times a day. These are exclusively the local breeds.

Nomad: These are kept by nomadic tribes to guard their camps and to assist in hunting. These dogs adapt easily to the changing environment and do not have affinity to any place except their owner.

Mongrels: These are stray dogs which like to remain near the food sources like slaughter houses, meat shops, restaurants and garbage dumps. They are found in large numbers in rural as well as urban areas. As they are in habit of stealing the food either from kitchen or shops, hence these are the nuisance in these areas.

Non-sporting (Working group)

1. Akita
2. Alaskan Malamute
3. Belgian Malinois
4. Belgian Sheep Dog
5. Belgian Tervuren
6. Bernese Mountain Dog
7. Bouvier Des Flandres
8. Boxer
9. Briard
10. Bull Mastif
11. Collie
12. Doberman Pinscher
13. German Shepherd/Alsatian
14. Great Dane
15. Komondor
16. Kuvasz
17. Maremma Sheep Dog
18. Mastiff
19. New Found Land
20. Rottweiler
21. St. Bernard
22. Samoyed
23. Schnauzer Giant
24. Schnauzer Standard
25. Schnauzer Miniature
26. Siberian Husky
27. Tibetan Mastiff
28. Welsh Corgi

AKITA

It is also known as Akita Inuc and belongs to one of the three breeds of apparently similar configuration and are distinguished from each other on the basis of some very specific differences. They appear like a cousin of Chinese Chowchow but different, as they do not possess blue tongue and mouth tissue besides some other differences in coat size. The Akita is largest of the group of three Japanese breeds and falls under the group of heavy dogs. This breed was evolved for hunting deer and also bear. It has been found very good guard. The animal is intelligent, large and active. The breed is gaining popularity.

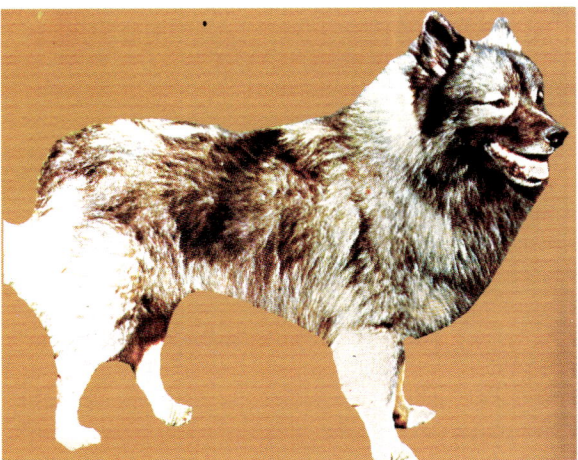

Fig. 1 Akita

Head and Face: It is massive and broad with prominent central furrow on fore head and well developed stop. The length of muzzle is medium and face as well as skull is smooth. Nasal bone is straight and nose is black.

Mouth: The level bite strong teeth are present in flesh marked gums. The long tongue is pinkish.

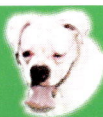

Ears: The erect ears are short with broad base and pointed tips, and facing forward.

Eyes: These are small and bright with tight lids. Expose hew is a disqualification.

Neck: Medium size muscular and strong neck is well fused with the shoulders and brisket and carried high with moderate arching in alert manner.

Body: It is well muscled, round, compact and straight dorsally with less sloping from chest to loin. The chest is deep and spacious with well-sprung ribs and brisket is prominent.

Tail: Usually double curved fox like tail is carried over the back and in some animals it may be slightly tilted on sides.

Forequarters: Strong and muscular close set shoulders slope moderately to continue with upper arm. The legs are boned and straight while pasterns are medium and supple.

Hindquarters: The croup is almost at the level of shoulders. Hips and thighs are compact and powerful. Hind-legs are moderately angled with almost straight shannons.

Feet: These are round, broad and well padded with close set and arched toes.

Coat: It is double coated animal decorated with fine, dense and woolly under coat covered with outer coat of coarse hairs of medium size. Coat colour is variable and there is little scope of discard but for the white which should be less than one-third of entire body. White markings generally appear on face, collar, forelegs, hind feet and tip of the tail. Commonly face and ears are darker than the body.

Size and Weight: The height at withers ranges between 63 and 67 cm approximately. The body weight of dogs is 39 to 50 kg and that of bitches is 34 to 44 kg approximately.

ALASKAN MALAMUTE

Famous as cart horse of the Arctic region the Alaskan Malamute is considered one of the powerful breed amongst the known sledge dogs. It is a large breed of working dogs of a charming, active, alert and intelligent disposition. It is decorated with unusual coat colour and markings. This is a loyal and devoted companion and had served people in very difficult areas of arctic region where other means of transport were not available till the development of modern electromechanical power driven vehicles.

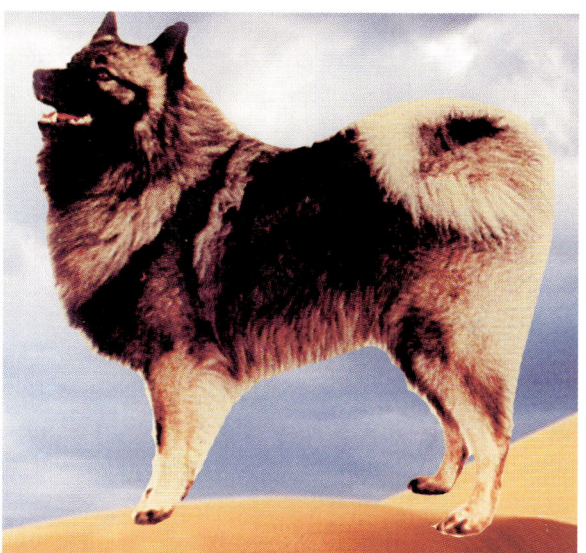

Fig. 2 Alaskan Malamute

The dog is friendly and playful but aggressive with stranger dogs. The animal is heavily boned and strong for transporting heavy loads. The animals fit well in a square framework.

Head and Face: The head is broad and strong with prominent fore head. The occiput is broad due to placement of ears on either side of the skull and moderately round, which gradually becomes flattened and slightly depressed at the

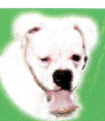

stop. The muzzle is large which becomes slightly narrower towards the oral opening. Nose is black or black with flesh mark and brown in red and white in white dogs.

Mouth: The jaws are broad and strong and large teeth are embedded in strong black gums. The teeth on both the jaws are arranged in a complete scissor bite.

Ears: The short, triangular and erect ears are a little rounded at the tip. These are placed apart and forward with wide occiput. The ears may be dropped on the skull at certain occasions while working.

Eyes: The eyes are set obliquely with outer canthus higher than the inner canthus. These are relatively large and as usual almond shaped. Colour is brown but dark eyes are preferred over light colour.

Neck: It is moderately arched, short and strong, and covered with fairly long coat. A white band of collar is present in most of the animals.

Body: The body is compact, strong and powerful with broad and deep chest. Back is straight with light slope over the croup. Well muscled loins are reasonably long and flexible which facilitate tireless working and powerful drive of posterior limbs.

Tail: The tail is in line with the dorsal line and set over the croup as loose coil.

Forequarters: Well muscled shoulders are very strong and moderately sloping. Heavily boned forelegs are covered with strong muscles. The legs are almost straight and short pasterns are very strong.

Hindquarters: The hindlimbs are well covered with strong muscles upto thigh which provide strength. These are moderately bent at stifle. Hock joints are well developed and strong which are further extended almost straight from behind and these possess great propelling powers.

Feet: The compact feet are large with close set and moderately arched toes. Thick pads are covered with coarse skin. The dark sickle shaped short nails are very strong which prevent from sliping while trotting or galloping.

Coat: Outer guard coat is fairly long and coarse and possesses different markings of variable colour. Coat colour may be wolf-like gray and white, black and white, silvery white, red and white or white. The ventral aspect of body is mostly white. Face may be decorated with different kinds of markings. The neck and chest may also possess markings.

Size and Weight: The dogs and bitches look different with later having characteristic feminine look. The dogs measure 63 to 71 cm at withers while bitches may be 58 to 66 cm. Body weight of adult of both sexes ranges between 38 to 57 kg depending on the height and females are relatively lighter than the males of corresponding litter.

BELGIAN MALINOIS

There are many theories about the evolution of this breed. It is a variety of Belgian sheep dog but another group believes its origins from the Central European sheep dogs or guard dogs. This breed closely resembles German Shepherd phenotypically but smaller in size due to which its good qualities like agility, excellent temperament for guarding and great ability for training are overlooked.

Head and Face: The head is long and skull is flat at the occiput. The muzzle is strong and shallow stop is present at the junction of skull and nasal bone and length on either side of stop is almost equal.

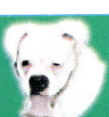

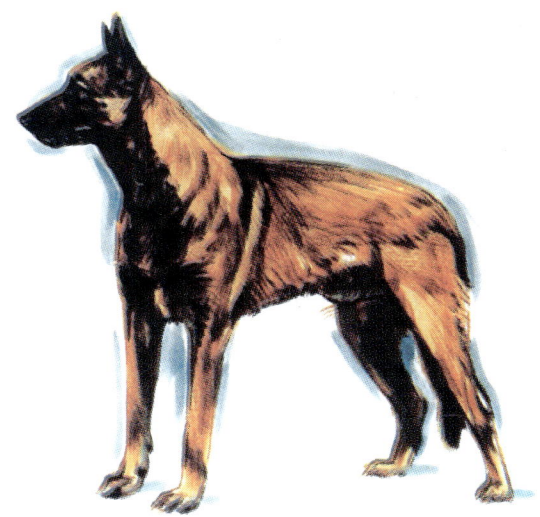

Fig. 3 Belgian Malinois

Hindquarters: These are well muscled and properly angled and kept pushed back while standing. The pasterns are medium and straight.

Feet: These are round with arched toes and padded sole.

Coat: Medium length coat cover the body. The tail is bushy and posterior of hind legs is fringed. The coat is much dense around the neck upto throat. The common colours are tawny or flecked with black. Ears and face should be black.

Size and Weight: Height at withers may be 50 to 65 cm and body weight 22 to 28 kg. As in most breeds the bitches are smaller and lighter than the males.

BELGIAN SHEEP DOG

Ancient Belgian sheep dogs were bred for performance for herding the sheep flocks and protecting them from wolves. Due to ecological changes and advancements, their utility has considerably declined. Utility of this breed was diversified during first World War. The breed is also known as Groenendaels. Except for the whole black colour, light bone and longer back the dog resembles much with the German Shepherd.

Head and Face: Prominent and alert in look, the head is moderately flat and muzzle is somewhat pointed. Nose is black and stop is present in the middle of head and face. Frosting on the muzzle and chin is quite common.

Mouth: The lips are level and teeth are either level or scissors bite.

Ears: Medium size triangular erect ears are set close on the skull with V-shaped presentation and facing forward.

Eyes: Almond shaped and medium size eyes are bright and dark brown.

Mouth: It is broad and level. Prominent teeth are embedded in thick and black or flesh marked gums and arranged scissors bite.

Ears: Pricked and triangular ears face forward.

Eyes: Almond shaped moderately big eyes are set close at the level of stop. Eyes are distinct by a darker rim.

Neck: It is broad and massive at shoulders and sloping upwards, moderately arched, muscular and carried up in alert disposition.

Body: The body is a little longer than the height. Deep chest with well sprung ribs reaches upto the level of elbow. Dorsal line from withers to rump is almost straight with moderately sloping croup. Muscular brisket is strong.

Tail: Medium size curved tail has heavy brush and reaches upto hocks.

Forequarters: Compact shoulders continue down with straight forelegs and supple pasterns.

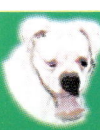

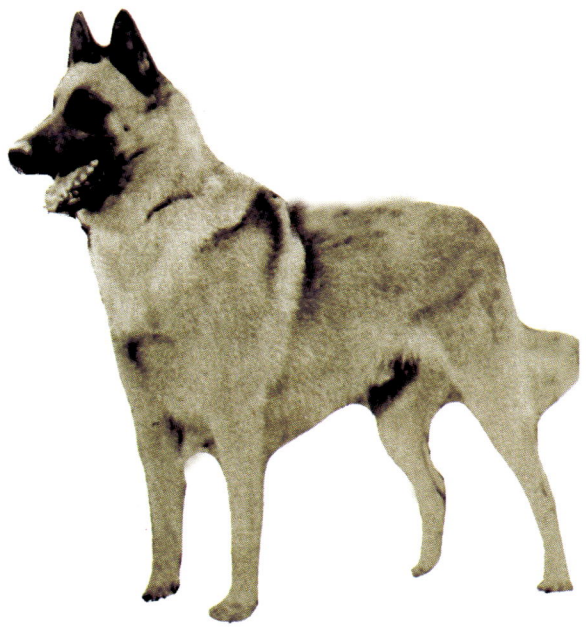

Fig. 4 Belgian Sheep Dog

Neck: Well muscled neck full of dense mane is moderately arched and carried elegantly.

Body: The well muscled and compact body moderately slopes from wither to rump. Deep chest reaching up to elbow forms a small curve.

Tail: Moderately long tail reaches upto the hock and carried up while at work but without any curving.

Forequarters: Well muscled and strong shoulders slope obliquely to upper arm. The forearms are lightly boned and straight with supple pastern.

Hindquarters: The hips down the croup are sloping and hindlimbs are angled to support fast running.

Feet: These are round, arched, close set and well padded.

Coat: The body is covered with long and dense coat of black colour. However, small strips or small patches of white hairs on the fore chest and on the tips of the hind toes, but not on fore toes, these strips or patches are permissible.

Size and Weight: The height of dogs at withers is 60 to 65 cm (may be allowed in competition between 56 and 69 cm) and that of bitches is 55 to 60 cm (may be permitted in range of 51 and 64 cm). Body weights of both sexes range between 20 and 30 kg, and females of same litter are lighter than the males.

BELGIAN TERVUREN

Belgian Tervuren is less known Belgian sheepdog in most of the countries outside Belgium. However, Belgian Tervuren has gained rapid popularity after its recognition in the United State during the middle of the twentieth century. It is a medium size active and dependable guard dog.

Head and Face: The head is almost flat, stop is shallow and muzzle is strong with straight bridge of nose. Nose is black.

Mouth: It is level with level or scissors bite teeth.

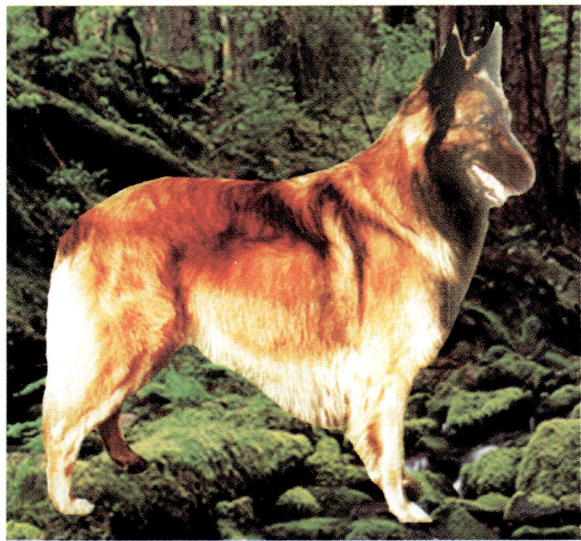

Fig. 5 Belgian Tervuren

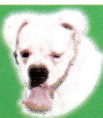

Ears: Pricked ears are set high on the skull and face forward. Tips are pointed.

Eyes: Prominent and dark eyes are set at the level of stop.

Neck: Muscular, strong, arched, and elegant neck is covered with mane. These may be collar markings.

Body: Muscular and compact body is round and slightly arched in loin region. Moderately sloping croups blends with hips and tail. The chest is deep and sloping towards loin.

Tail: Bushy tail reaches upto hocks and usually carried high while working.

Forequarters: Sloping shoulders join with muscled arms which extend down in boned forelegs. Pasterns are less supple.

Hindquarters: The croup is almost at the level of withers. Hips and thighs are strong. Hindlegs are properly angled. Pasterns are straight.

Feet: These are round with close set and well arched toes and padded sole. The toes are moderately feathered.

Coat: Medium length coat is mostly fawn to russel mahogany colour and black shaded tips. The chest is covered with a mixture of black with grey. The ears and face mask are generally black or dark mahogany, and tips of the tail is mostly black. A little white marking is permitted on the chest and tip of the toes.

Size and Weight: Height of adult dogs at withers is 56 to 69 cm and that of bitches 51 to 64 cm.

BERNESE MOUNTAIN DOG

This is a less known breed of strong, cheerful, gentle and feathered dog. It is a medium size dog of jet-black colour with bright tan markings.

Head and Face: The head is broad, massive and prominent with well defined stop. The muzzle is short and large.

Mouth: The upper lip is level and lower lip is serrated. Strong teeth are embedded in thick gums.

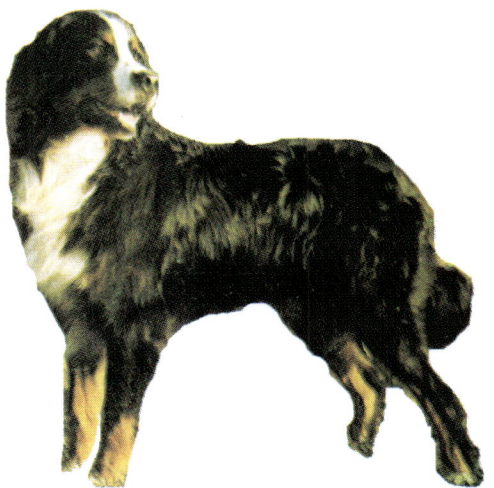

Fig. 6 Bernese Mountain Dog

Ears: These are medium V-shaped and low set. The leather hangs close to cheek.

Eyes: These are dark and bright.

Neck: It is muscular, powerful, feathered and moderately arched.

Body: The body is muscular, compact and strong with deep chest, well sprung ribs, less sloping waist and slightly arched loin.

Tail: Low set tail is heavily feathered.

Forequarters: The muscled shoulders are powerful and densely feathered. The forelegs are boned and straight. The pasterns are short.

Hindquarters: The hips and thighs are muscled and feathered with moderately angled strong hind legs.

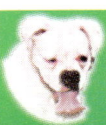

Feet: These are semicircular, wide with well arched toes and padded soles. These are moderately furred.

Coat: The coat is dense and medium size. The colour is jet black with all the legs tan marked. There is spots above forelegs, on dorsal eyebrow and chest. The feet and tip of tail are white. There is star on chest and blaze on forehead.

Size and Weight: The height at withers may be between 52.5 and 68 cm. Body weight is proportionate to body size as in large framed dogs.

BOUVIER DES FLANDRES

It is a Belgian breed of working dog known for its endurance, active habits and usefulness as guard.

Head and Face: The skull is level at top and a little longer than the muzzle. The stop is very shallow but eyebrows are deeply arched. The muzzle is broad and nasal bridge is prominent. Nose is black.

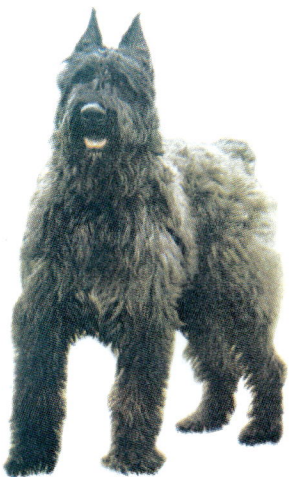

Fig. 7 Bouvier Des Flandres

Mouth: The lips are dry and tight, and teeth are arranged scissors bite. There is a prominent and profuse beard.

Ears: High set ears are given triangular shape through proper cropping.

Eyes: These are almost oval, bright and brown but black eyes are also accepted.

Neck: It is short, massive and broad at the shoulders with moderate arching.

Body: It is muscular, compact and more or less square in shape. The chest is deep with wide rib cage which slopes less towards the loin. The rump is broad with very little posterior sloping.

Tail: It is docked with about 10 cm stump, which is carried high.

Forequarters: Muscular shoulders are well blended with neck and chest. The forelegs are boned, medium, straight and feathered.

Hindquarters: The powerful posterior limbs are moderately angulated and almost straight down the hocks. These are profusely feathered.

Feet: These are round, short and deeply padded with arched toes and black nails. The feet are covered with soft hairs.

Coat: Double body coat is formed of short, dense and woolly under coat covered with rough and wiry outer coat. Coat colour may vary from fawn to black or may be pepper and salt, grey or brindle. A white spot on chest may be accepted but tan are disqualification.

Size and Weight: The height at withers ranges between 59.5 and 70 cm, and bitches should not be less than 58 cm.

BOXER

This breed was evolved in Germany during the nineteenth century. A moderate animal of strong built it is well known for loyalty, amiable

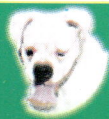

behaviour and protectiveness. These are easily adapted and can mix freely with other dogs. It is liked by people due to its active, inquisitive and extrovert habits. This breed is considered to be originated from the bull fighting dogs. It is a very good companion and guard breed.

Head and Face: Head is round and smooth with convex forehead, clearly depressed stop and much short nasal bone joining backwards pulled black nose. Lower jaw projects beyond the upper jaw. Strong and flewed upper jaws overlapps the side of lower jaw but not the anterior upwards turned portion.

Mouth: The mouth is short and pulled. Breadth of muzzle is more than the length. Teeth and tongue are not visible for most of the time as mouth is kept close. Strong teeth are embedded in thick black gums.

Ears: The ears are set a little high on the skull. These are projected slightly side way and then hang like flaps. Length is medium and remains almost at the level of stop. Cropping of ears is quite common.

Eyes: Relatively smaller eyes are dark, bright and obliquely set with inner conthus narrower at the level of stop. Area around the eyes is darker than the other parts.

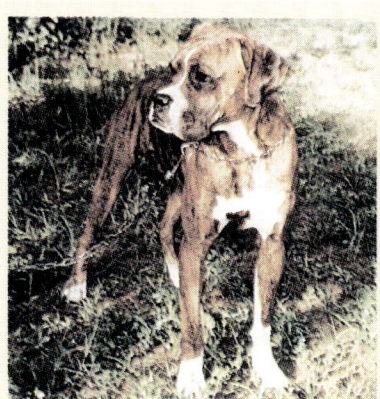

Fig. 8a Boxer Brindle with White Marking on Face, Brisket and Feet

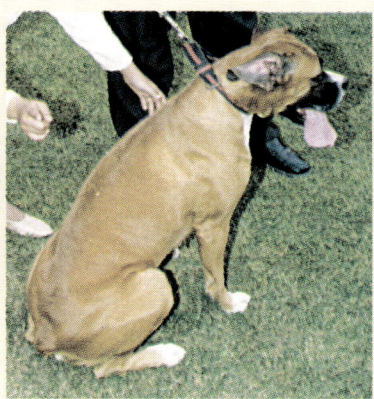

Fig. 8b Boxer Brown with Owner

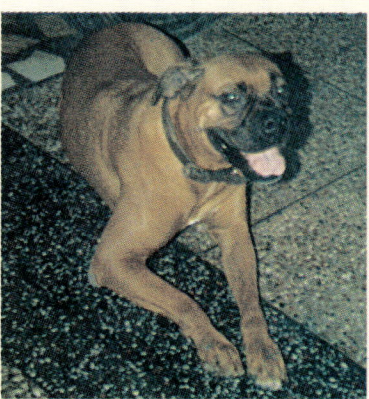

Fig. 8c Boxer Fawn

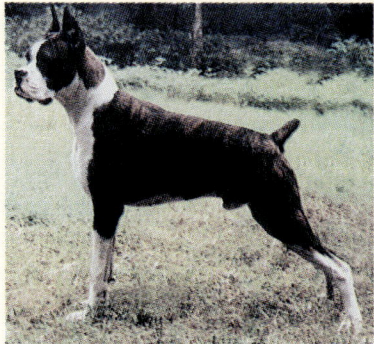

Fig. 8d Boxer Brindle with White Marking on Face, Brisket and Feet

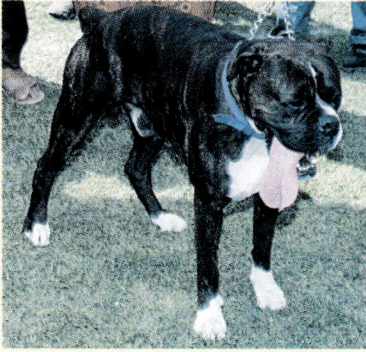

Fig. 8e Boxer Brindle with White Brisket and Feet.

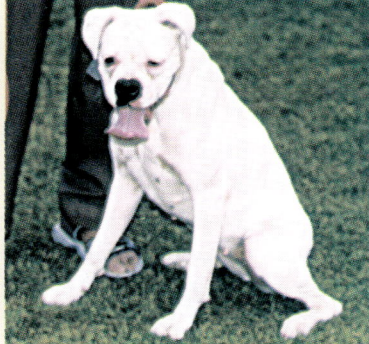

Fig. 8f Boxer-White but not Albino

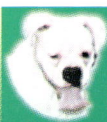

Neck: It is moderately long, strong, muscular, smooth and slightly arched to continue with occiput. Skin of the neck is loose on the ventral aspect which folds or stretches on turning the head.

Body: Body is well muscled, strong and flexible. Back line is straight and sloping on croup is small. Chest is deep with well sprung ribs and waist region is moderately tapering. Brisket is well muscled and very strong. Skin over the body is loose set.

Tail: Medium size tail is placed high. Docking is popular for the breed living behind a 4-5 cm long stump.

Forequarters: Covered with well developed muscles from shoulders to arms and made of thick bones. The forequarters are very strong. Legs are held perpendicular on the ground. Pasterns are long, straight and flexible.

Hindquarters: Hips and thighs are covered with well developed muscles mostly without the sign of fattyness. Hindlimbs are well boned and suitably angled at joints to facilitate thrust while running.

Feet: Feet are lighter in colour than the body, circular and well arched. Feet pad is thick and coarse, and nails are dark.

Coat: Body coat is very short, fine and smooth. Colour is various shades of red, fawn and brindle. White marking may be present. Lower parts of limbs are usually lighter in colour than the body.

Size and Weight: Height at withers of dogs is 55 to 64 cm and bitches 53 to 59 cm; and weight is 30 to 34 and 24 to 25 kg respectively.

BRIARD

It is a dog of Asian origin introduced in Europe by Asian invaders before the middle ages. It has been mentioned differently by different people as cattle dog or sheep dog, but it gained fame as a French Army dog during World War I for carrying small ammunitions, first aid box and also for locating wounded troops etc. It has been standardized recently during the middle of the twentieth century.

Head and Face: The head is long and massive and strong muzzle is almost equal to skull. The stop is deep and nose is black.

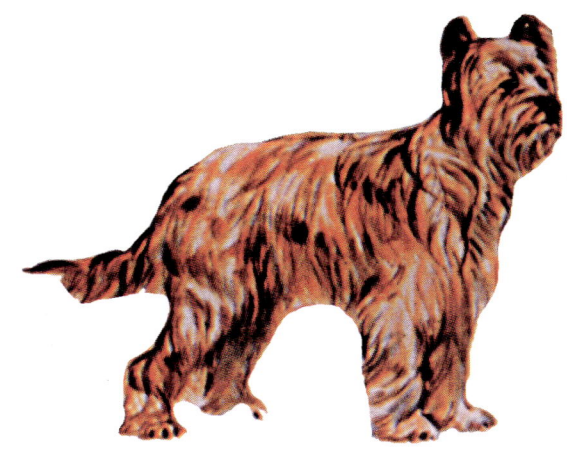

Fig. 9 Briard

Mouth: The mouth is short and lips are smooth. The teeth are arranged even bite.

Ears: Medium size ears are semi erect. If cropped, the ears are carried erect.

Eyes: These are small, bright and black.

Neck: It is moderately long, plumed and slightly arched.

Body: The body is short with straight dorsal line, sloping hips and deep chest is broad due to well sprung ribs. The rib cage gradually slopes posteriorly.

Tail: The thickly feathered hanging tail is crooked at tip at the level of hocks.

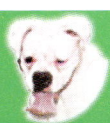

Forequarters: The limbs are plumed from top to bottom and forelegs are straight.

Hindquarters: The hips are slightly sloping, thighs are strong and well angulated at stifles but slight set under hock due to deflated metatarsals. Each hind leg contains two dew claws.

Feet: These are small and feathered.

Coat: It is long, stiff, slightly wavy and strong but never curled. The hairs on head, face and ears are heavy and long. Colour may be all solid like black, light grey and tawny. There may be also combination of two colours.

Size and Weight: The height of dogs at weathers is 57.5 to 67.5 cm, and that of bitches is 55 to 64 cm.

BULL MASTIFF

This breed has been developed by inter breeding Mastif and Bulldog in England in a way to retain the proportionate morphology of both the breeds. A highly spirited animal is fearless, amiable, friendly, loyal, powerful and devoted. These are good guards and gentle companion.

Head and Face: The large head is massive, square and wrinkled. Muzzle is wide and nose is broad. Oral end including nose is black. The head and face are perfect blend of Mastif and Bulldog.

Mouth: The dogs keep their mouth closed and normally do not exhibit teeth and tongue which makes their look square. The mouth is broad and down the stop is shorter than upper part. Upper jaw is flewed.

Ears: These are V-Shaped and placed posteriorly on either end of skull. The length is medium drooping to the level of eyes.

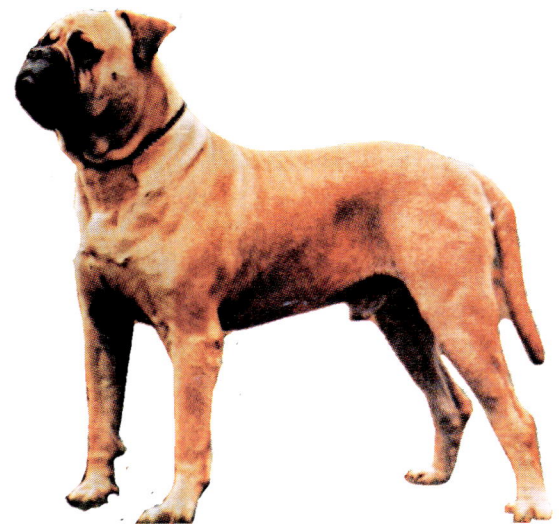

Fig. 10 Bull Mastiff

Eyes: These are dark hazel with dark rim and almost in line with the stop.

Neck: It is short, muscular, massive, fine, smooth and slightly arched.

Body: Body is muscular, compact and heavy with deep chest and well sprung ribs. Brisket is broad and strong. The body moderately slopes towards the waist. Dorsal line is smooth and straight but sloping at the croup.

Tail: It is thick at the root and tapers to the tip. It may be carried either straight or somewhat curved at the distal end.

Forequarters: Strong well developed shoulders slope moderately forward then angled backward upper arm. Forearms are boned, strong and straight. Pasterns are supple.

Hindquarters: Massive well developed and smooth buttocks and thigh and angled lower limbs. Pasterns are flexible.

Feet: These are round and toes are arched. Sole is thickly padded. Nails are sharp and curved with pointed tips.

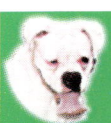

Coat: Coat is fine, dense, smooth but hard to touch. Colour is pure brindle, or red with usually lighter shoulder and extremities.

Size and Weight: Height of dogs at withers is 63 to 69 cm and that of bitches is 61 to 66 cm, and corresponding body weight is 50 to 60 kg and 40 to 55 kg.

COLLIE

The Collie or Scotch Collie dog has two varieties, one is rough coated and another smooth coated originated from Scotland. These are medium size working dogs, which are intelligent and very efficient for managing sheep flocks on pastures and grassland. These are also used in Australia and some other countries for the same purpose.

Head and Face: The head is medium size with slightly raised forehead than the nasal bone and distinguished at very shallow stop. Muzzle is smooth and nose is black. Front of head and face are clean.

Mouth: The lips are sharply defined, smooth and without flew. Strong teeth are arranged scissors bite in black gums.

Ears: These are medium size and half bent and set low on either side of occiput living behind wide space between the base of the two ears. These are covered with dense coat in hairy type and smooth in others.

Eyes: Almond shaped obliquely set eyes are brown and smaller but bright.

Neck: It is long, moderately arched and frilled in hairy type.

Body: It is long and moderately arched behind saddle in the loin region. Chest is deep with well sprung ribs and body gradually slopes backward to continue with narrow waist.

Tail: Long and bushy tail is due to plumes and carried low.

Forequarters: These are well muscled, bony and strong with straight forelimbs and flexible pasterns.

Hindquarters: The croup is almost arched and hindlimbs are angled.

Feet: These are rounded and covered with coat.

Coat: Body is covered with double coat and hairy type outer coat is long and coarse. The coat colour is variable and black and tan, blue merle or sable are common. There may be white blaze.

Size and Weight: Height at withers is 50-60 cm and body weight is 20-30 kg. As usual bitches in same litter are lighter than the male dogs.

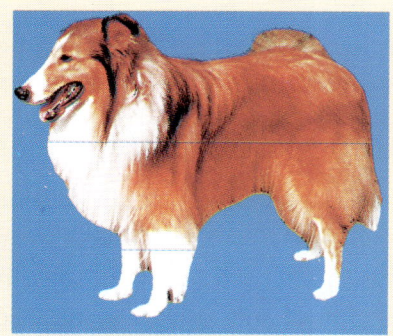

Fig. 11a Collie –Smooth Coated

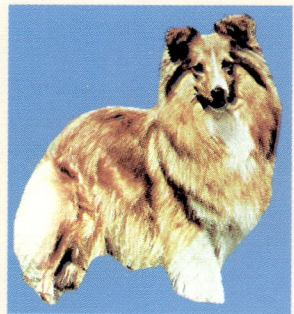

Fig. 11b Collie–Rough Coated

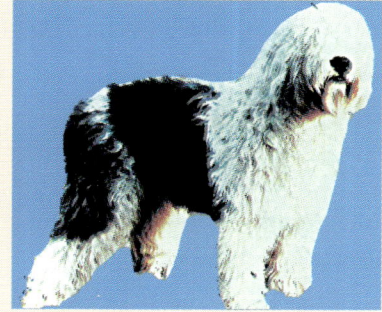

Fig. 11c Collie–Bearded

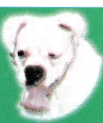

DOBERMAN PINSCHER

It is commonly called Doberman and it was developed in Apolda in Germany during the terminal decades of nineteenth century. This has been evolved through a complex cross breeding programme involving Pinscher, Weimeraner and Vorste hound breeds. It is also believed that this breed contains some blood of Rottweiler and Terrier breeds.

It is an elegant, slim, compact, powerful and loyal dog excellent for guard and search by scent. This breed is extensively trained and used in different services for guarding, searching and protecting due to its loyalty and courageous nature.

Head and Face: Head is long, clean cut, sharp and fine with prominent fore head, defined stop and strong nose bridge. Muzzle is clean and strong.

Mouth: Mouth is long with level sharp lips. Teeth are very strong. Levelled in scissors bite and embedded in black or black with flesh gums.

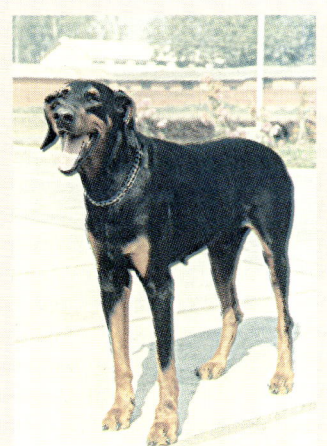

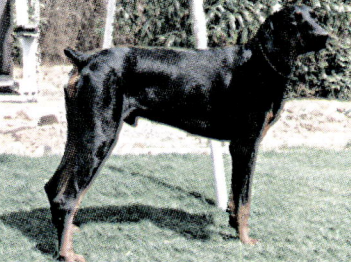

Fig. 12b Doberman Pinscher– Male

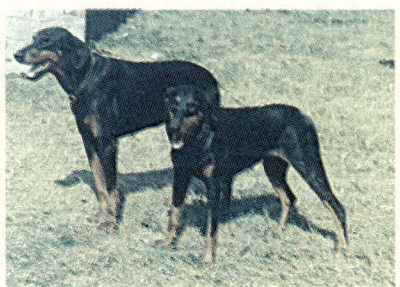

Fig. 12c Doberman Pinscher–Pair

Fig. 12a Doberman Pinscher –Female

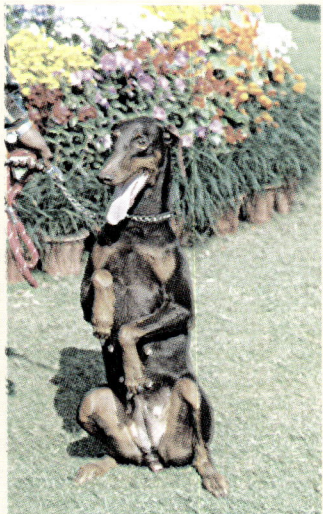

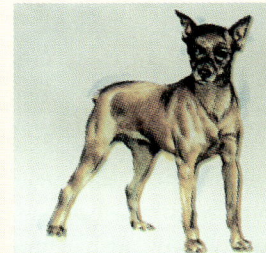

Fig. 12f Miniature Pinscher –Brownish

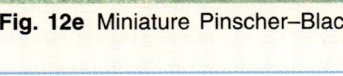

Fig. 12e Miniature Pinscher–Black

Fig. 12d Doberman Pinscher–Brown & Sitting

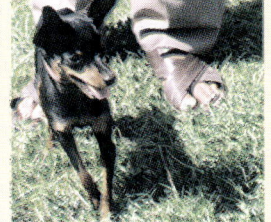

Fig. 12g Miniature Pinscher–Black

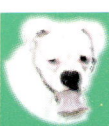

Ears: Erect ears are scoop like and triangular with pointed tip and set high on the head in line with the occiput. These are turned forward and sideward and moderately arched.

Eyes: Dark, big and shining eyes are set oblique slightly above the level of stop.

Neck: It is long, fine, smooth and powerful and held high in attentive position.

Body: It is well muscled and compact with deep chest, strong brisket and moderately narrower waist. Croup is sloping down the hips. Dorsal line is straight.

Tail: It is docked short in early life living behind a little stump.

Forequarters: The shoulders are close set, fine and smooth and long limbs are bony and straight. Pasterns are straight and flexible. A dewclaw may be present which is generally cut off in early life.

Hindquarters: These are well muscled, smooth and powerful and almost straight below the hocks.

Feet: These are rounded and sole is made of thick pad covered with cornified skin. Toes are distinct, arched and knotty.

Coat: Coat is short, dense and coarse and its colour may be whole black, tan or dark brown. There may be tan or blue with red marking but these are not liked.

Size and Weight: Height at withers ranges from 65-75 cm and body weight 25-35 Kg. Bitches are mostly lighter that the dogs.

GERMAN SHEPHERD/ALSATIAN

The inherent instinct of guard and protect and very effective response to command has made it a most wanted breed among the few popular dogs. The animal is very intelligent and can be trained for performing variety of diversified works. The high adaptability and utility of this breed have made its distribution cosmopolitan and favourite of all classes of families longing for an useful pet for guarding and companionship. It is one of the most obedient, loyal, energetic and protective breed. It has drive to play with other dogs and children, requires heavy exercise and non-destructive. The nature is shy and exhibit some fear to changed circumstances but adaptation is quick. The males are largely, more powerful and less delicate than the females. This multipurpose breed can be trained for performing multifarious activities.

Head and Face: The head is moderately broad at the occiput with prominent forehead and clear-cut stop at the level of lower lids of eyes. It continues into long tapering muzzle. Tip of the nose is slightly circular, glossy and strong and colour of nose is black except in white and light coloured rare specimens it may be lighter. Moderately long ears are placed on the either side of skull.

Mouth: Normally, mouth remains open exhibiting slightly protruding tongue and lower teeth. Teeth are strong and arranged in scissors bite and upper gum alongwith teeth is covered with overlapping flew. Colour of gum and flew is black in gray, roan and black alsatians.

Ears: Moderately long erect ears are broad at the base and tapering to pointed tip. Wide distance between the tips provides V-shaped appearance. Inner surface of the ear is mostly bare whereas outer surface alongwith margin is covered with short coat. Erect and front facing ears provide majestic and alert look of the animal.

Eyes: The almond shaped eyes are mostly black and placed obliquely at the level of stop.

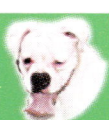

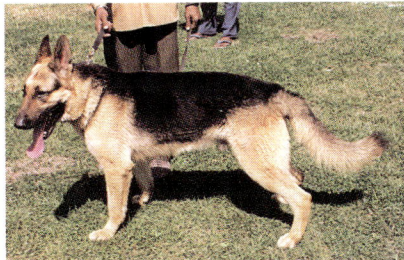

Fig. 13a German Shepherd/ Alsatian –Standard

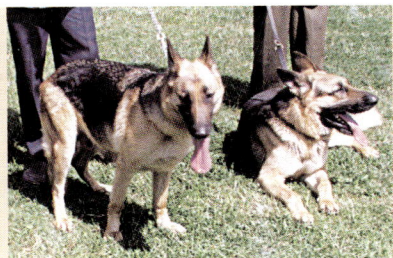

Fig. 13b German Shepherd –Ready for Action

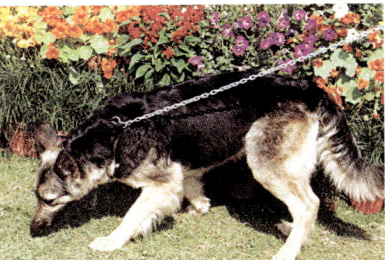

Fig. 13c German Shepherd –Sniffing Act

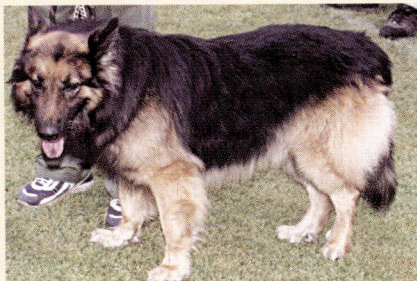

Fig. 13d German Shepherd –At Display

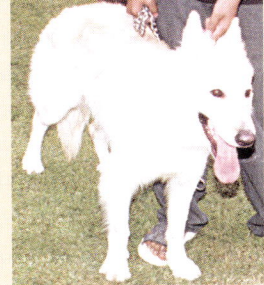

Fig. 13e German Shepherd –White but not Albino

Neck: A slightly arched and long neck is carried erect on the strong shoulders. It is covered with well-grown mane and provides alert look of an active animal, ready to receive command of the master. Neck is very strong and stretched forward during chasing a prey.

Body: A little greater body length than the height provides a beautifully balanced shape. A slightly elevated shoulder than the croup presents an elegant gait. The back is straight, strong and muscular which gradually slopes downwards from the croup. The chest is broad and deep with well sprung ribs but it never extends below elbow joint. This helps in friction free movements during work. Loin region is narrower than the chest and belly is moderately drawn in the males. In females two rows of prominent teats appear from the pectoral to pelvic region.

Tail: The long tail is fairly straight and bushy extending below the hock joint and often hangs in J shape at rest but lifted in line with the back while running.

Forequarters: The shoulder bones are close set obliquely with the chest and are covered with strong muscles. Forelegs are longer than the depth of the chest and carried straight giving alert expression. Pastern is supple.

Hindquarters: Covered with well developed muscles broad hindquarters are strong. It is almost straight upto hock joint, drawn out to stifle joint and then straight depicting a balanced gait.

Feet: The feet are rounded and toes are arched but uneven due to prominent joints of digits. The toes are arranged in semicircles and bear strong, curved and sharp pointed dark nails. Foot pads are well cushioned and covered with hard cornified skin.

Coats: Greater number of animals are a

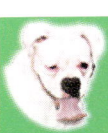

mixture of black and tan or black and gold. Single coloured black or white dogs are also found. However, white coloured coat is unwanted and in some countries it is a disqualification for show. Majority of animals bear widely acceptable short coat. Long coated animals are also liked by many people due to elegance of feathery mane, tail and fringe on hind limbs. Long coat requires more care and considered unsuitable for movement in dense and bushy forests for hunting. Undercoat is close set to the body.

Size and Weight: There are distinct sex differences. The males are larger, more powerful and less delicate than the females. The males are more territorial, whereas females are gentle and easier to train. However, females are more playful with other dogs and mostly compromise with the males and strangers, due to this behavior males are preferred as service dogs.

Height of males is 60-66 cms at withers and that of females is 55-61 cm and weight of corresponding sexes is 34-45 kg and 30-40 kg.

GREAT DANE

It is an ancient German breed considered to be existed about 2000 B.C. and since then has been refined to modern large sized dog of majestic look, powerful body and active disposition. The dog is very intelligent and like to feel as a member of the family. These are patient but may turn aggressive when instructed. Growth rate of this breed is very high but its life is short. It is an excellent hunting dog. It is light on feet and moves with a long free stride.

Head and Face: Head is long, elegant and smooth and muzzle is long and fine. Stop is clear. Nose is black and there may be flesh markings.

Mouth: It is broad with flewed upper lip and levelled oral opening. Teeth are large, sharp and strong.

Ears: These are medium, pointed and half dropped on sides.

Eyes: These are usually dark and more or less round and often an inverted semilunar dark spot is present on the upper lid towards the stop.

Neck: A long crested and smooth neck flows into the withers. It is moderately arched and held high giving attentive look.

Body: It is square in outline, compact and smooth with deep chest and undershot shallow brisket. Dorsal line is loin straight and croup is sloping. Slightly arched loin is narrower than the rib cage and belly is pulled up displaying skin fold on either side.

Tail: The medium length tail is thick at the root and gradually tapering to the tip. It is straight and reaches below the hock joint.

Forequarters: Shoulders are close set to chest, fine, smooth and powerful. Limbs are boned, strong, long and perpendicular. Pasterns are straight but flexible.

Hindquarters: Fine and smooth hips gradually slope down to hock joints. All joints are moderately angled. Pasterns are flexible.

Feet: These are fine and smooth with arched toes and padded sole.

Coat: Short coat is close, fine and glossy. Coat colour may range from whole colour deep orange to light buff, fawn, brindle, light grey

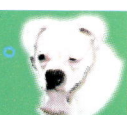

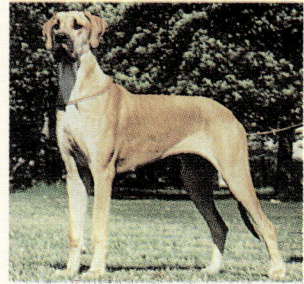

Fig. 14a Great Dane–Brown

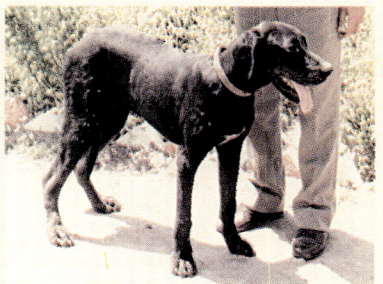

Fig. 14b Great Dane–Blackish Brown Female (Brindle)

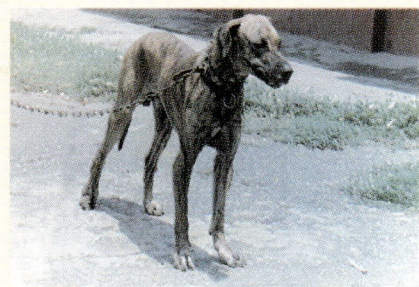

Fig. 14c Great Dane–Blackish Brown (Brindle) Male

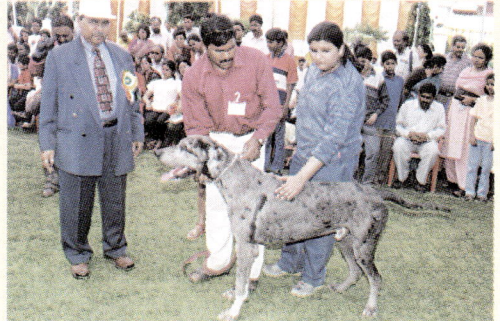

Fig. 14d Great Dane–On Show

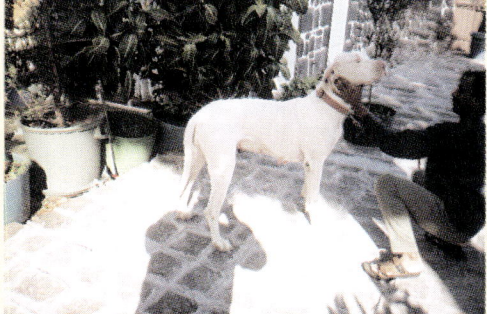

Fig. 14e Great Dane–Albino

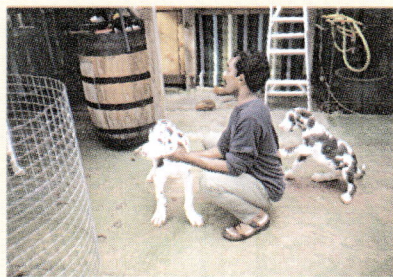

Fig. 14f Great Dane–Pups

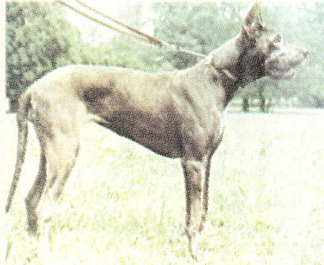

Fig. 14g Great Dane–With Erect Ears

to steel blue, slaty or white with black, brown or blue patches.

Size and Weight: Dogs are larger than the bitches. Height at withers of dogs is more than 76 cm and for bitches more than 71 cm. Body weight of dogs is minimum 54 kg and that of bitches is minimum 45 kg.

COMODOR

The origin of dog is considered to be the central part of Asia and it was developed as one of the largest breed of Hungarian dogs. The special quality is its utility as a guardian of the sheep flock and also for protecting the cattle. Long and profuse body coat with cord formation and matting provides better protection against

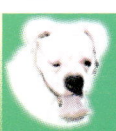

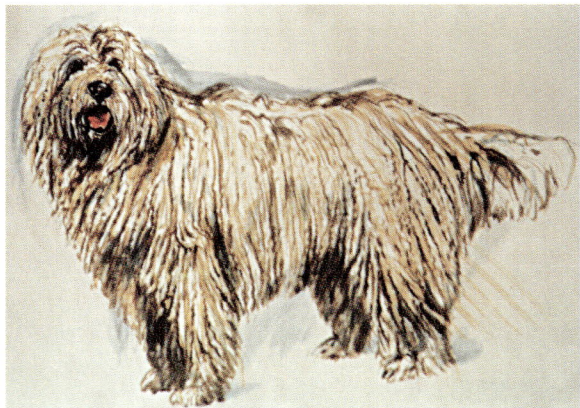

Fig. 15 Komodor

harsh weather and require much less care for dressing. Bathing and swimming do not disturb coat matting.

Head and Face: The head is round and muzzle is short. The head and face are profusely covered with corded long hairs. The nose is mostly black but may be slaty.

Mouth: It is short with even lips and strong teeth.

Ears: The ears are low set, drooping and heavily furred.

Eyes: These are brown. Other colours are disqualification.

Neck: Medium size heavily feathered neck is slightly arched.

Body: The body length is a little more than the height at withers. The chest is deep and broad and belly is little tucked up.

Tail: The hanging feathered bushy tail appears as a continuation of spines and reaches upto the hock. Curling is not required.

Forequarters: The straight forelegs are covered with dense corded feathering.

Hindquarters: These are strong and almost

straight with moderate angulation for efficient propulsion.

Feet: These are close set, arched, powerful and feathered.

Coat: The body is covered with long and profuse coat which is highly corded and matted except the relatively shorter hairs on face. Cording and matting provides protection and these are not disturbed. Only white coat colour is permissible and curling is disqualification.

Size and Weight: The height at withers ranges from 63 to 78 cm and taller animals are preferred.

KUVASZ

It is a tall, white breed of working dogs developed in Tibet for guarding. However, another group believe that it was brought by Kurds in Europe and originally it was a sheep dog for taking care of the flocks. The name has perhaps originated from the Turkish word kawasz means 'protector'. Due to their large size and strength the dogs were extensively used for herding cattle and flocking sheep and also for hunting specially the wild boar. It is a pure

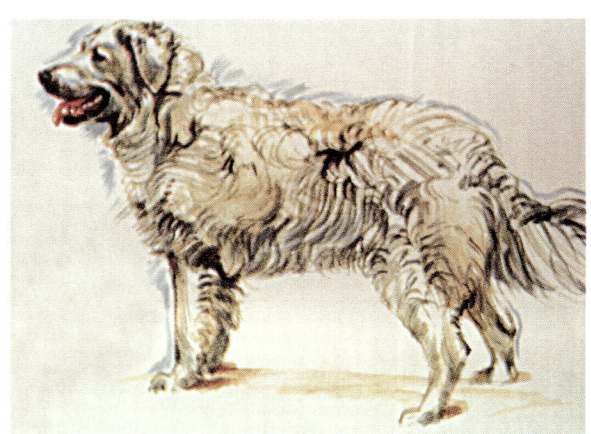

Fig. 16 Kuvasz

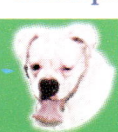

white and handsome animal of affectionate and active habits.

Head and Face: The rounded head continues with nose bridge through a shallow stop. The muzzle is short, broad and rounded dorsally. Nose is wide and black.

Mouth: Lips are level and teeth are strong.

Ears: Small size triangular, drooping and low set ears had broad base and rounded tip.

Eyes: Medium size eyes are dark and bright.

Neck: Heavily muscled and moderately arched neck is well blended with the shoulders. It is covered with heavy mane.

Body: Length of body is almost equal to height. The back is straight and drooping down the croup. It is well muscled, compact and rounded. Chest is deep with well sprung ribs. Loin is less narrow.

Tail: Heavily feathered long tail hangs down the hocks.

Forequarters: Well muscled slopy shoulders are very strong and blend with arms to continue as bony and perpendicular forelimbs. Pasterns are straight.

Hindquarters: Hips and thighs are well muscled with moderate angulation of joints and straight down the hock joint.

Feet: Feet are rounded with moderately close set and arched toes. Soles are well padded.

Coat: It is a double coated animal with fine, dense and woolly under coat covered with pure white, fine and glossy outer coat of medium length. Other colours are not accepted.

Size and Weight: The height at withers ranges between 70 and 76 cm, and body weight between 50 and 55 kg. As usual, females are lighter than the males.

MAREMMA SHEEP DOG

This is a member of large breed and best among the all Italian sheep dog varieties. It is also known as Maremmani and the Abruzzi sheep dog. Many consider it closely related with the Kuvasz of Hungary, others believe it to be originated from central Asia.

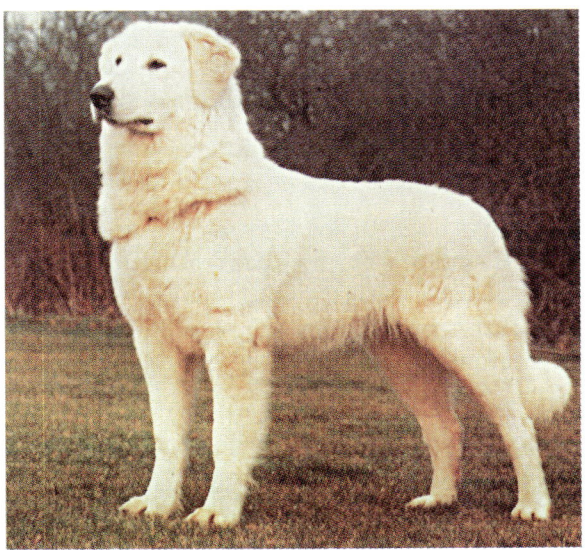

Fig. 17 Maremma Sheep Dog

Head and Face: The skull is moderately convex in contour form, stop is shallow and nasal bone is straight. The nose is black or flesh marked. Muzzle is broad and conical.

Mouth: Lips are black and level. Teeth are strong and arranged scissor bite or level also.

Ears: Medium size ears are set wide apart on the occiput and drooping.

Eyes: Almond shaped small eyes are dark brown.

Neck: Strong and massive neck is covered with fluffy mane. It is moderately arched, long and forward.

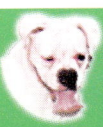

Body: Moderately muscular body is sloppy from withers to root of the tail. The chest is moderately deep and waist is sloping with moderately tucked up belly.

Tail: Heavily feathered tail forms a plume.

Forequarters: The shoulders are broad and sloping and moderately boned forelegs are straight. The pasterns are also almost straight with less flexibility.

Hindquarters: The hips down the croup are sloppy and hindlegs are kept pushed back.

Feet: These are moderately round with long and somewhat arched toes and padded sole.

Coat: The body is covered with long coat but head is smooth. The legs are feathered and tail is heavily feathered. Coat colour is white but may turn a little lemon yellow on ears in some aged animals.

Size and Weight: Average height of males at withers is about 64 cm and body weight 30 kg. The bitches of same litter are generally smaller and lighter than the dogs.

MASTIFF

Ancestory of Mastiff dogs is ancient which has been refined through breeding from an Asiatic hunting dog. It has been mentioned for its performances and usefulness in Persian, Roman and early English literatures. It has been also depicted on the bas relics of Assyrian region. Modern Mastiff is a large sized, massive, symmetrical and powerful dog which looks very ferocious.

Head and Face: The head is broad, square and prominent with sharp stop and straight nose bridge of moderate length. Muzzle is small and black shaded. Nose is black with wide nares. There may be few wrinkles on the face.

Mouth: It is short and wide with black lips and strong gums holding the teeth. Upper lip is slightly pendant. Jaws are well developed and powerful.

Ears: Base of ears is wide, convex and set high on the skull. These are V-shaped, half bent and darker in colour.

Eyes: These are small at the level of stop and brown with a dark rim in other than black dogs.

Neck: It is short, muscular, stout, heavy and slightly arched.

Body: It is full, massive, fine and smooth with straight dorsal line, deep chest with well sprung ribs and strong, muscular brisket. Sloping from chest to loin is less. There is very little sloping over the croup. A few skin folds may be seen over the withers in some specimens.

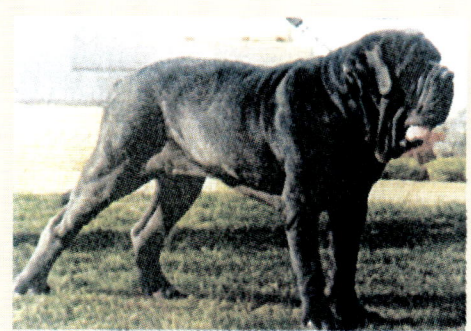
Fig. 18a Mastiff

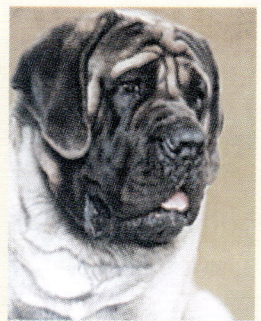
Fig. 18b Mastiff–Face

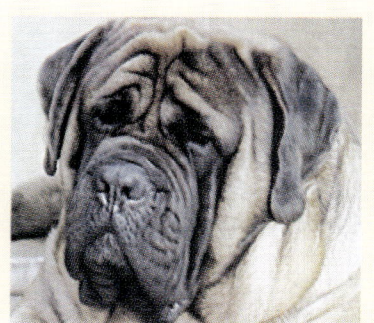
Fig. 18c Mastiff–Ears

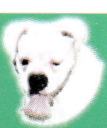

Tail: It is long and smooth and may be docked in some countries. It may be carried straight or may hang in the relaxing dogs.

Forequarters: Strong and highly muscular shoulders slope moderately. Massive upper arm is clearly differentiated from the lower legs at elbow. Forelegs are boned, strong and held perpendicular. Pasterns are straight.

Hindquarters: Hips and thighs are compact and powerful and second thighs with moderate angles are placed backwards. Rear pasterns are strong and straight.

Feet: Feet are rounded with padded sole and toes are moderately arched.

Coat: It is close, short, smooth and glossy. Its colour may be whole apricot, dark fawn, silver fawn or brindle.

Size and Weight: Height of males at withers is 63-71 cm and in females 58-66 cm; while body weights are 25-34 kg and 20-30 kg respectively.

NEW FOUND LAND

This breed was standardized in England during the mid of nineteenth century as a heavy bear dog. It is useful for hunting in water and saving from drowning. In arctic region its performance in sledge pulling was satisfactory. It is a heavy animal of endurance.

Head and Face: The head is massive, skull is flat, stop is distinct and free from wrinkles. The muzzle is shorter than the skull, deep and square in shape.

Mouth: It is small with rudimentary flew and level teeth.

Ears: Small, triangular, drooping and low set ears lie close on either side of the head.

Eyes: Obliquely set eyes are small and brown.

Neck: Broad and medium size neck is covered

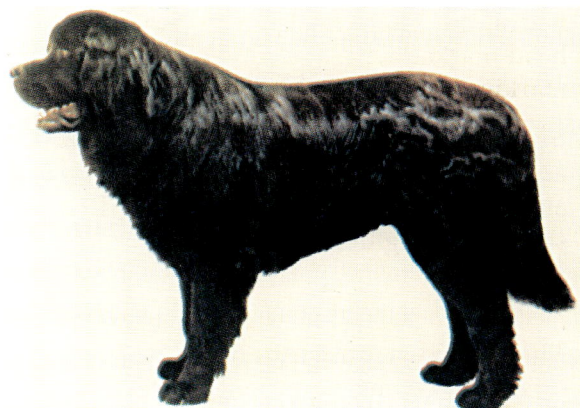

Fig. 19 New Found Land

with fluffy mane. It is well blended with shoulders and brisket.

Body: The length and height of dogs is almost equal whereas bitches are a little longer than the height. Dorsal line is straight with slightly raised croup. The chest is broad and deep and sloping towards loin is moderate.

Tail: Fully furred tail is broad and hanging to reach below the hocks.

Forequarters: The muscular shoulders are broad dorsally and close set with chest. The arms are powerful and forelegs are boned. Pasterns are short and supple.

Hindquarters: The hips and thighs are massive and hindlegs are less angled with almost straight and boned sannons.

Feet: These are elongated and cat like with well padded sole.

Coat: The body coat is double. The under coat is fine, dense and woolly. Moderately long outer coat is water resistant. The hairs are straight. The coat colour is usually dull black but there may be shades of bronze or white on the toes, chest and sometimes on limbs. In some cases saddle marking is present. Other solid colours are though accepted but black or bronze

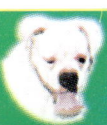

is desired. There is also a variety with black head marked with a narrow blaze. Only white markings are acceptable.

Size and Weight: The average height of dogs at withers is about 70 cm and body weight is about 70 kg. The bitches of same litter are shorter and lighter.

ROTTWEILER

This breed a descendent of drover dogs originally belong to ancient Rome. The breed has been refined in Germany as highly intelligent, **rugged** and dependable working dog. The **animals** are large and sturdy.

Head and Face: Head is large and compact with massive face, straight nasal bone, shallow stop and black nose.

Mouth: Muzzle is well developed, lips are levelled and teeth are arranged scissors bite.

Ears: These are triangular in shape and set apart in line with the prominent occiput. These are half bent.

Eyes: These are dark, expressive and alert.

Neck: Moderately long and arched massive neck is fused well with shoulders. It is carried high in attentive form.

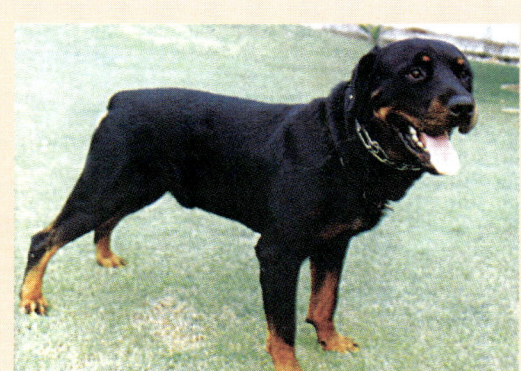

Fig. 20a Rottweiler–Male

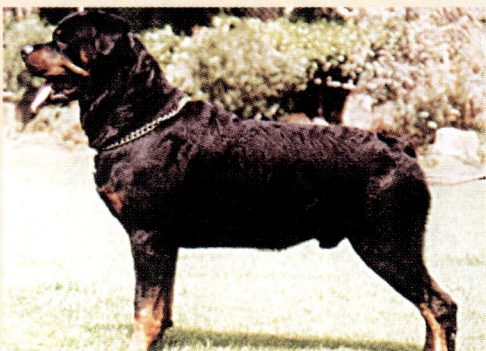

Fig. 20b Rottweiler–Male

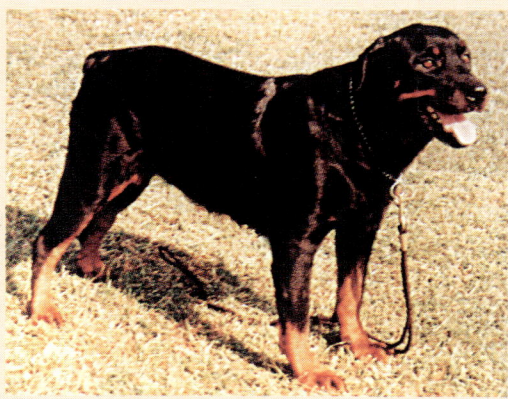

Fig. 20c Rottweiler–Female

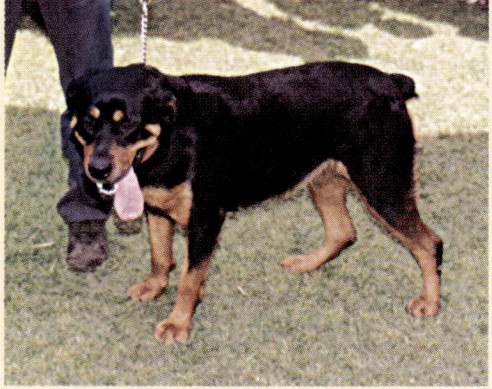

Fig. 20d Rottweiler–Female

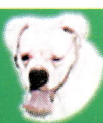

Body: It is muscular, broad and strong with deep chest and well sprung ribs. The brisket is prominent and dorsal line is hard.

Tail: It is docked short living behind a stump of 3-4 cm.

Forequarters: The shoulders are close set, moderately sloping forward and strong. Fore limbs are thick boned, straight and strong. Strong pasterns are relatively short, straight and flexible.

Hindquarters: Compact hips are well developed and sloping to hock joints. Hind limbs are properly angled and boned. Pasterns are almost straight.

Feet: These are round with close set and moderately arched toes and padded sole.

Coat: Body is covered with double coat. Outer coat is short, flat and coarse. Coat colour is black with tan markings on extremities, muzzle, eyes, chest and beneath the tail.

Size and Weight: Height at withers of males is 61-68 cm and body weight 45-50 kg. The females are 56-63 cm high and body weight 45-50 kg.

SAINT BERNARD

This is largest breed of domesticated dogs of the modern age. It is believed to be evolved from the Tibetan Mastiff in Switzerland about a thousand years ago. The massive size dog is heavily muscular, compact, robust and powerful. The shape and size of dog is fearful and people unaware with the behaviour of this breed are scared, whereas the animal is benevolent, intelligent and trustworthy. It is a breed of steady and courageous dogs that helped monks and other people during travelling through difficult terrain of Alps mountain. Now-a-days its number is decreasing due to heavy size and need of extensive exercise. It is becoming difficult to maintain in busy modern living in multistorey short apartments of limited space.

Head and Face: The head is large and broad and face is short and wide. Fore head and muzzle are demarcated by a clear and deep stop and circumference of head is more than its length from nose to occiput. Nose bridge is short and straight. Nose is flesh colour or black and nostrils are wide. The skin is mildly wrinkled. The muzzle is short and square while cheeks are flat deep.

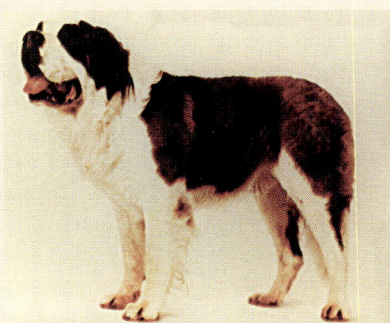

Fig. 21a St. Bernard–Adult

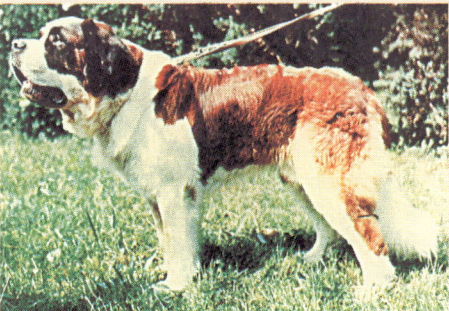

Fig. 21b St. Bernard–Adult

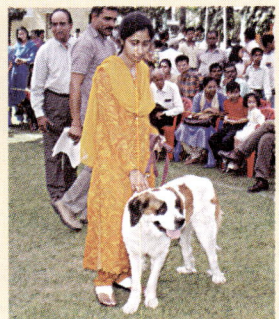

Fig. 21c St. Bernard –Young with Owner

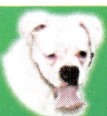

Mouth: The mouth is short with almost triangular oral opening and upper lip is heavily flewed like large flap overlapping the lower jaw.

Ears: These are medium sized and flaps on either side of the skull. The base of ears is very wide and tip is blunt.

Eyes: Large and somewhat round and bright eyes are placed at the level of stop distantly from each other.

Neck: Medium size massive neck is strong. It is slightly arched and much broader at the base where it blends well with the shoulders and brisket.

Body: It is well muscled, compact with well sprung ribs. The circumference of loin is only moderately less than the front part of the body. The back is straight with very little slope over the croup.

Tail: Long tail is fully feathered with shallow upward turning of the distal end.

Forequarters: The shoulders are well blended with the chest and dorsally at level with the dorsal line of back. Leg bones are thick and strong. The pastern is short, strong and supple.

Hindquarters: The hips are moderately developed but not bulging and hind legs are well angled to facilitate running.

Feet: These are broad, heavy and well arched. The sole is well padded and covered with cornified coarse skin. The nails are very strong.

Coat: Body coat may be either short haired or long haired. Whereas long haired coat is wavy but not curled. The coat colour may be mahogany brindle, red brindle or orange colour with prominent white markings on muzzle, blaze, collar, chest, feet, forelegs and lower part of the tail.

Size and Weight: The height of dogs at withers is 65-70 cm and that of bitches is 62-65 cm. The body weights of corresponding sexes are 70-90 kg and 65-75 kg respectively. In some exceptional cases body weight may reach almost upto 100 kg.

SAMOYED

The breed was evolved by Samoyed tribe of hunters and fisherman of Siberia. Unlike other tribal groups of the area the samoyed tribe reared reindeer for milk and draught but not for meat and they evolved their dogs for herding of reindeer and guarding. However, samoyed has been used for pulling sledge. This is a strong, active, disciplined, graceful and intelligent dog of glamorous look. This is an animal of medium shape and size with moderately strong skeletal frame. A high degree of disease tolerance has been seen in the breed. However, incidence of hip dysplacia is recorded sometimes which is considered hereditary but does not pose serious problem for the breeder. The animal is peace loving, gentle, loyal and obedient dog, which is a very good companion and watch dog in urban households and at farm houses.

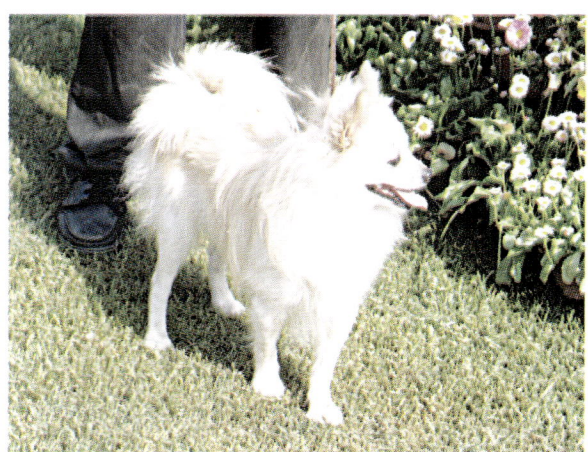

Fig. 22a Samoyed

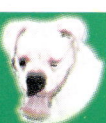

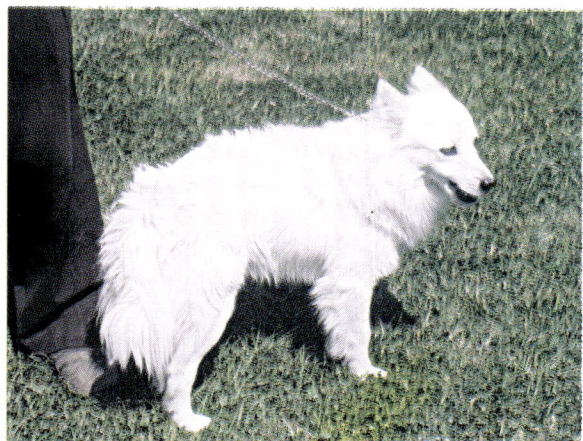

Fig. 22b Samoyed

Head and Face: Wedge shaped head is powerful. It is broad and flat above the stop. The muzzle is medium and face is slightly tapering to end at nose. Jaws are strong and lips are black. Black nose is preferred but it may be brown, flesh-coloured or mixed colour. Coat on the head and face is much shorter except some light fringe at the base of ears posteriorly in continuation with mane.

Mouth: The animals usually keep their mouth open with protruding wet and pink tongue. Gum is black or lighter and strong teeth are well embedded in the gums. Upper teeth are arranged in scissors bite manner just overlapping the lower row.

Ears: Pricked and medium size ears are a little rounded at the tip and face forward providing an attractive look. These are placed well apart in line with the occiput and appear almost parallel. Outer surface is covered with a short and dense coat but fibers are scanty on the inner surface.

Eyes: The eyes are almond shaped and mostly dark brown but may be lighter also. Eyelids are black. Alert disposition gives intelligent expression.

Neck: Medium sized neck is moderately arched and covered with fine and fluffy well developed mane.

Body: Back is medium and broad and properly covered with strong muscles. The chest is broad and deep with well sprung ribs. Loin is somewhat narrower. Back is slightly longer in proportion to height in females, probably for providing more room for the developing foetii during gestation.

Tail: Long and bushy tail carried rolled over the back in an alert dog but mostly remains hanging during rest of the time.

Forequarters: Shoulders are smooth and slope downwards. Forelegs are strong and straight.

Hindquarters: Croup is broad and hips are well developed to continue with angulated stifles.

Feet: Pastern is moderately long, feet is almost flat with loose set toes and inward curled pointed nails. Sole is well cushioned and covered with hard and rough cornified skin.

Coat: The body is well insulated with thick cover of dense, wooly, soft and short undercoat. The outer coat is made of long growing and standing coarse hairs. Under surface of tail and posterior aspect of thigh are fringed. The outer coat is lustrous and bright but in white animal on inter breeding for 3-4 generation it looses luster and turns dull. For maintaining glossy shine white animals should be mated to cream or yellow for the revival of coat luster.

Pure white colour is preferred but off white, yellow and creamy shades are acceptable.

Size and Weight: Males are, as usual, taller than the females. Height at withers of male is 50 to 60 cm and that of females is 45-54 cms. Body weight ranges between 22 to 30 kg.

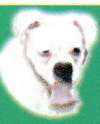

SCHNAUZER GIANT

This breed has originated from the highlands of south Bavaria. The dog was bred for services in police and military. Now it is a popular working dog in Germany and also in some other country.

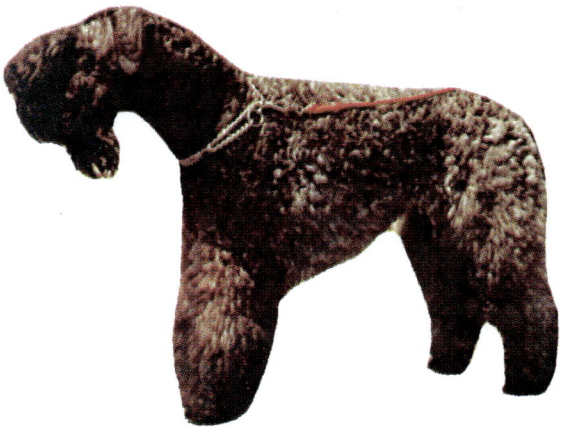

Fig. 23 Schnauzer Giant

Head and Face: The head is almost rectangular and about one third of the length of the back. The muzzle is broad, stop is shallow and chin is decorated with prominently thick beard.

Mouth: Level and teeth are scissors bite.

Ears: Uncropped ears are V-shaped and cropped are erect.

Eyes: These are bright and dark.

Neck: Heavily muscled and well blended with shoulders, the neck is moderately long, arched and strong.

Body: It is almost square, compact and round with deep chest and moderately sloping waist. Dorsal line is straight or slightly arched posteriorly.

Tail: Stump of dock is present. Docking is done at the third coccigeal vertebra.

Forequarters: Moderately sloping shoulders blend with strong arms to continue down in perpendicular forelegs. Pasterns are almost straight.

Hindquarters: Slope at the croup is left much less and limbs are proportionately angled and mostly kept pushed back in standing position.

Feet: These are small, less arched but thickly padded.

Coat: The dog displays a good beard. The coat is rough, wiry and dense of moderate length. Coat colour is mostly black but may be pepper and salt or black and tan also.

SCHNAUZER STANDARD

This medium size breed is shorter than the Schnauzer Giant but larger than the Schnauzer Miniature. Probably this breed was evolved earlier than the two other breeds of the family. The breed came in prominence in Germany during the last quarter of the nineteenth century and spread to other European countries and United States of America by the first quarter of the twentieth century.

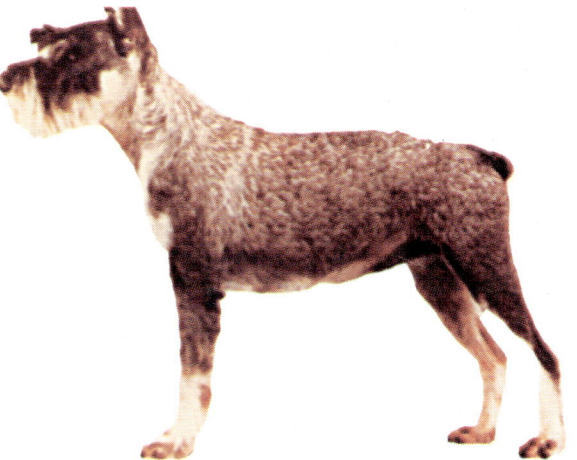

Fig. 24a Schnauzer–Standard

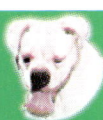

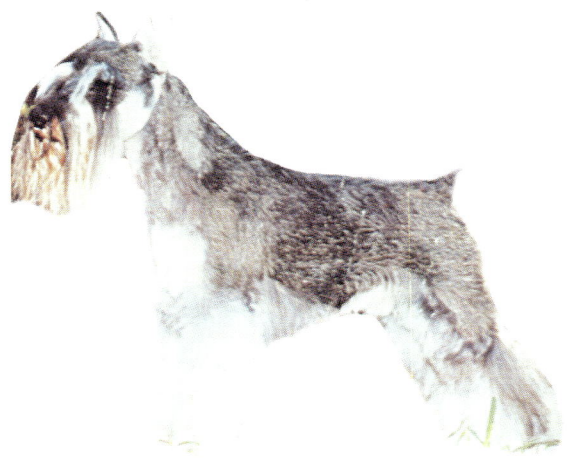

Fig. 24b Schnauzer–Standard

Head and Face: The head is long and rectangular and slightly narrow between ears and eyes. The muzzle is barrel like and length of head including face is almost half of the body. The stop is shallow.

Mouth: It is elongated and covered with black and tan hairs. Mouth can be only recognized when dog is opening the mouth otherwise it is covered with hairs.

Ears: The cropped ears are erect, and intact ears are small and V shaped.

Eyes: Dark and bright with fading grey or silver white colouration over the eyebrows.

Neck: It is moderately long, well muscled and strong with mane of moderate length.

Body: The compact body is almost square and chest is deep and wide but slope at croup is little.

Tail: It is docked to live behind a stump not below 2.5 cm and more than 5 cm in length.

Forequarters: The shoulders are close set with chest and strong. The forelegs are boned and straight with less supple pasterns.

Hindquarters: The hips are compact, thighs are broad and stifles are well angled for running

Feet: These are small, less arched and thickly padded.

Coat: It is rough coated animal with pepper and salt, silver grey to steel grey or pure black colour. Occasionally fawn or tan colour dogs are also found and accepted in the show. Fading of colour particularly in grey shades under the throat, brisket, across the chest, cheeks, eyebrows, under the tail and body etc. are not uncommon and permissible.

Size and Weight: Height at withers of the dogs may be 45 to 50 cm and that of bitches 42 to 48 cm.

SCHNAUZER MINIATURE

The meaning of schnauzer in German language is a man with distinct moustache. It is a German breed and smallest among the three types. Modern clubs of United States of America and Canada and also in European countries have rigidly fixed the height of Schnauzer Miniature for show.

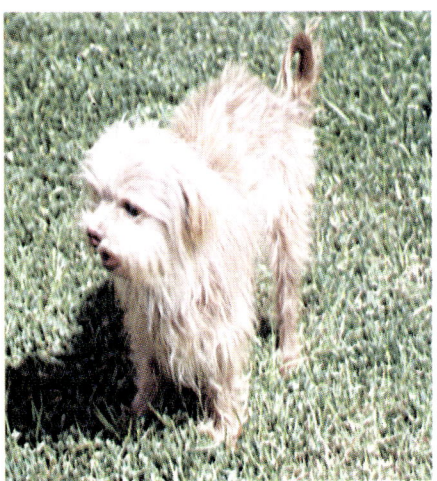

Fig. 25 Schnauzer–Miniature

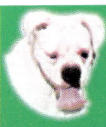

Head and Face: The head is longer than the other two varieties and also more sharp. The muzzle is broad and stop is shallow.

Mouth: Well developed dense beard on chin is characteristic.

Ears: Cropped ears are erect and uncropped are as usual V shaped.

Neck: Well muscled, strong and fused with shoulders. The length is medium with moderate arching.

Body: It is short, compact and strong with straight back, deep chest and muscled brisket.

Tail: As per breed requirement it is docked.

Forequarters: The shoulders are well blended with chest and strong. The legs are boned and straight with less supple pasterns.

Hindquarters: Hips and thighs are covered with compact muscles and hindlegs are well angled to have spring action.

Feet: Round feet are small, moderately arched, close set and padded.

Coat: The dog possesses good beard and body is covered with medium size harsh coat. Pepper and salt followed by black and silver are more liked but black are more common.

Size and Weight: At present there are two slightly different standards for the height at withers. The animals height should range between 30 and 35 cm in United States of America and Canada, whereas in European countries it should be maximum 35 cm for dogs and 32.5 cm for bitches.

SIBERIAN HUSKY

The Siberian Husky was evolved by a nomadic tribe, Chukchis as family pet and working dog. These dogs were companions, guards and

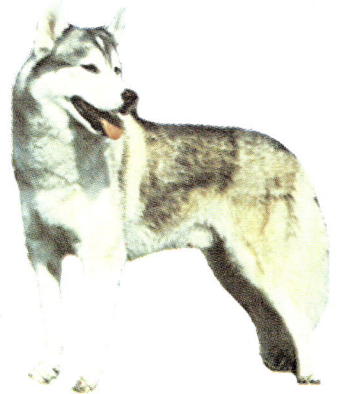

Fig. 26 Siberian Husky

sources of power for transportation. This is a good breed of gentle dogs with tremendous stamina, power and speed. Siberian Husky dogs are smaller and docile in comparison to Eskimo dogs. The dogs are medium in size with balanced movement and moderate bone. These are gentle but alert and do not react aggressively with the strangers and other dogs. These traits make them unfit for guard. Siberian Husky is an excellent companion and very good working dog due to its tractability and keenness. It possesses good traits of working sledge dogs, viz., balanced strength, satisfactory speed and endurance. The males are more muscular than the females but not bulky. Common man can be confused from Alsatian grades.

Head and Face: Head is medium in size and moderate. The top is slightly rounded and tapers slightly upto the level of Eyes. Stop clearly differentiates muzzle. Muzzle tapers gradually to amalgamate with the rounded nose. Stop is normally situated in the centre. Nose is black in black, tan and grey dogs, pinkish or flesh coloured in whole white specimen and dark tan in copper coloured animals.

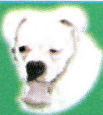

Mouth: Closely fitted lips are properly pigmented and do not develop overgrowing flews. Teeth are strong and arranged in scissors bite order.

Ears: The triangular ears are of medium length, erect, set high on the head living behind ample open occiput. Height of pina is a little more than the width of its base. The ears are slightly arched forward and pulled parallel in alert dogs. These are thick and full furred on either side.

Eyes: Almond shaped and obliquely placed eyes are moderately apart and gives a keen, friendly and often mischievous expression. There may be any shade of blue, brown or parti-colour.

Neck: The medium size neck is moderately arched and carried gracefully erect while standing. The head is slightly extended forward during trotting.

Body: The strong back is straight and levelled from withers to croup. The length is medium and shoulders are a little longer. The chest is deep, moderate and strong. Although ribs are well sprung initially but flattens downwards to give a balanced shape. The waist is narrower compact and leaner than the rib cage. Sloping of croup is quite little which is helpful for rearward thrust of the hind limbs.

Tail: Drooping fox brush like tail is fully furred and hangs almost straight from the croup. The tail is carried up over the back in loose curl or sickle shaped in attentive dogs. It does not coil tight or pushed on the sides. The hairs covering the tail are of almost uniform medium length.

Forequarters: The shoulder slopes forward moderately and then continues with the upper arm pushed slightly backward and it is never vertical with the ground. Shoulder muscles are very strong. The forelegs are straight and parallel in standing position. The elbows remain close to the body. The pasterns are a little slanted with strong and flexible joint. Length of forelimbs below elbow is a little more than the length between withers and elbow. Bones are moderate and strong.

Hindquarters: Hindlegs are moderately spaced and parallel in standing dogs when examined from rear side. Well muscled upper thighs are very strong, stifles bent properly and then straight down the well defined hock joints. Dew claws are removed, if present.

Feet: Feet are oval in shape and moderate in length. Toes are slightly webbed in between and moderately arched. Nails are sickle shaped and sharp. Feet are properly furred. Pads are thick and coated with coarse cornified skin.

Coat: Double coat of medium length covers the entire body. As usual under, coat is dense and soft. Almost all colours with or without markings are present.

Size and Weight: Height of dogs at withers is 53-60 cm and bitches 51-56 cm; and corresponding weights are 20-27 kg and 16-23 kg in two sexes.

TIBETAN MASTIFF

It is also known as Dokhiyi and a native of Tibet. Most of the Mastiff breeds are the descendents of this breed. Originally Tibetan Mastifs were black coated guard dogs with terrifying barking habits and were kept by the Tibetan nomadic tribes for protecting their animals and belongings. These Mastifs have great strength and stamina and are well adapted for living in hard conditions of high altitude mountain range.

Head and Face: The head is broad and massive with well clearly defined stop and moderate muzzle with straight nose bridge. The nose is mostly black.

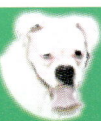

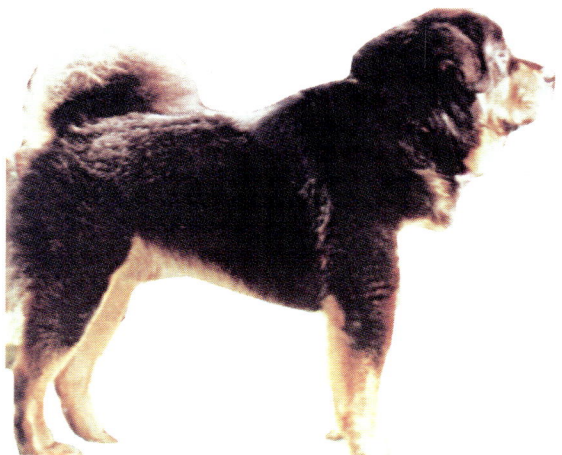

Fig. 27 Tibetan Mastiff

Mouth: The cheeks are fine and well developed scissor bite teeth are strongly set in black gums.

Ears: These are high set and bent on either side extending upto the cheeks.

Eyes: Obliquely set almond shaped eyes are placed at the level of stop.

Neck: Massive neck is moderately arched and blended with the shoulders.

Body: Body is well muscled on an almost rectangular frame of strong bones. Chest is deep with well sprung ribs.

Tail: It is carried loose curled over the back.

Forequarters: The strong shoulders are close set with the chest and extend down in massive arms and perpendicular bony legs. Pasterns are supple.

Hindquarters: Hip and thigh muscles are well developed and angulations are appropriate as per the requirements of a working dog. Pasterns are straight.

Feet: These are circular and strong with close set and arched toes, and well padded sole.

Coat: It is a double coated dog with thick and woolly under coat and moderately long and coarse outer coat. Coat colour may be black, brown, bluish grey, red and golden.

Size and Weight: The height at withers is 60-66 cm and body weight 30-35 kg.

WELSH CORGI

Corgi means a dwarf variety of dog. At present two varieties of Welsh Corgi, i.e. Cardigon and Pembroke are quite popular as a companion of pleasant disposition. It has probably evolved from the crossbreeding of Flemish dwarf dogs with native Welsh dogs in England in the early years of the twentieth century. Welsh Corgi is an active, energetic and highly spirited dog.

Head and Face: The moderately broad and flat between the ears the head appears fox like. The central furrow on skull is prominent and stop is shallow. Nose bridge is rounded and muzzle is moderately blunt. The face is bony and nose is black.

Mouth: The mouth is reasonably broad with levelled lips. Teeth are arranged in scissors bite manner but levelled are also accepted.

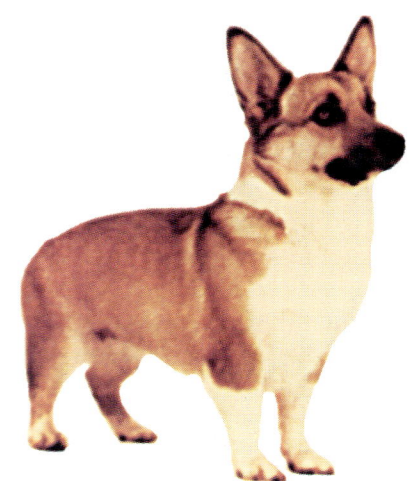

Fig. 28a Welsh Corgi

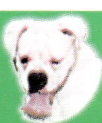

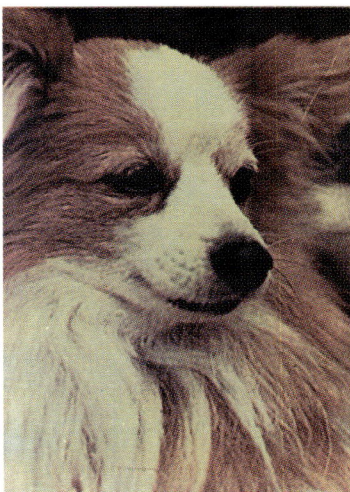

Fig. 28b Welsh Corgi–Face

Ears: Large size prominent ears are broad and low set at base, blunt pointed, pricked and somewhat forward placed on the skull. The tips of the ears are well apart and occiput is clear.

Eyes: These are medium to large in size, bright and attractive, and placed oblique at the level of shallow stop. Colour may be amber, blue, black or hazel.

Neck: The muscular neck is well formed, arched and strong. It is rounded dorsally and carried high.

Body: The body is long with rounded back and deep chest. The loin region is a little less wider than the rib region.

Tail: It is moderately long and set in line with the body.

Forequarters: The shoulders are heavily muscled and well blended with the chest. Bony strong fore limbs are very short and slightly bowed but not crooked. Pasterns are very short.

Hindquarters: These are muscular with moderately angled short hindlegs which is almost perpendicular down the hocks.

Feet: These are rounded with moderately arched and close set toes. The sole is well padded.

Coat: The body is covered with a coat of medium length, dense and somewhat coarse. The coat colour is highly variable and all combinations except pure white are acceptable. However, white flashings over chest, neck, face, feet or tip of the tail are quite common. Common coat colours are black, black brindle, red, red-brindle, sable, blue marle or tri-colour.

Size and Weight: The height at withers is 25-31 cm and weight 9-11 kg for dogs. The bitches are lighter in weight range of 8 to 10 kg.

Welsh Corgi Pembroke has few clear differences from the Cardigon variety, that are self coloured coat and also with some white markings. Tail in either rudimentary or docked.

II. Non-sporting (Utility group)

1. Bulldog
2. Chow Chow
3. Dalmatian
4. French Bulldog
5. Keeshond
6. Lhasa Apso
7. Schipperke

BULLDOG

This has been bred in Britain long back and has been recognized as the national dog of Britain. This was developed originally for bull baiting but due to changes in life style of human the uses of this dog has also changed. This has been recognized world over for stubborn determination, tenacious action and stead fastness, but at the same time it is charming and good-natured when handled nicely.

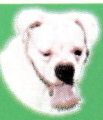

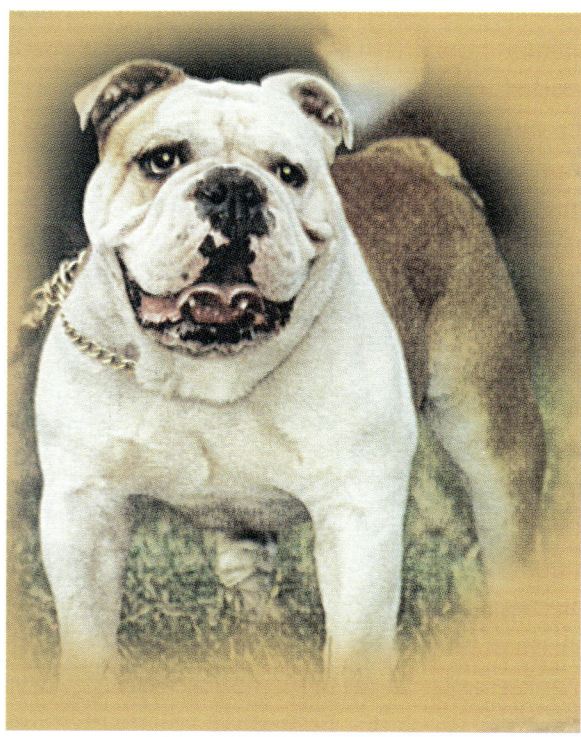

Fig. 29 Bulldog

Head and Face: The head is large and massive and extensively wrinkled face is characteristically blunt. Short muzzle with laidback moderately flat nose is specific for the breed. Occiput is flat and wide and stop is prominent. A clear furrow extends from occiput to stop.

Mouth: The jaws are broad and square and upper jaw is heavily flewed with the teeth undershot.

Ears: It possesses rose ears at either end of occiput. These are small due to compact wrinkles. Colour of ears is darker than the body coat.

Eyes: The eyes are prominent, dark and relatively less obliquely set than most of the other breeds. There is a clear semicircular shallow furrow over the upper eyelid.

Neck: The neck is short, massive and arched and it is also decorated with dewlop.

Body: The body is broad, massive with highly developed musculatures and deep chest with well sprung ribs. Waist region is only slightly narrower than the ribs cage. Brisket is massive and wide.

Tail: A short tail is carried low. It is thick at the root and tapering onwards.

Forequarters: The shoulders are tacked on and projected apart from the chest. Limbs are short, bones are thick and fore arms are straight with flexible pasterns.

Hindquarters: Hips and thighs are highly muscular, hocks are somewhat angular and limbs are short.

Feet: Feet are rounded and toes are loose set. Small nails are visible. Sole is padded and rough.

Coat: Close, dense, short, shining and smooth coat covers the body. Its colour may be various shades of red ranging from fawn to tan and also white but never black or black with tan. Face and terminal part of extremities are generally lighter colour than the body.

Size and Weight: Height at withers is 35-40 cm in dogs and 30-35 cm in bitches, where as body weights are 23-25 Kg in dogs and 20-23 Kg in bitches.

CHOW CHOW

The Chow Chow is originally a Mongolian breed evolved by a tribal group for help in hunting and guarding. It was introduced to China including Tibet and other neighbouring coun-

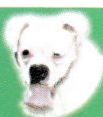

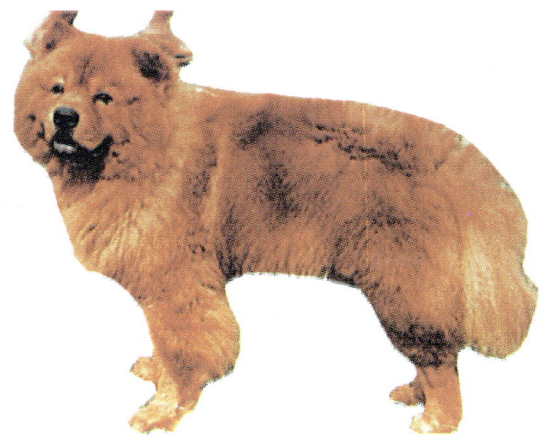

Fig. 30 Chow Chow

Ears: The ears are erect, small and triangular with rounded tip. These are stiff, facing forward and slightly bent inwards over the eyes. They are placed wide apart on either side of skull in line with the occiput. Dorsal aspect of ears is well protected with double coat which extends considerable inwards along the margin.

Eyes: Almond shaped small eyes are dark in most of the red coated dogs, black in black coated and lighter in fawn and other light coated variants.

Neck: The strong well set neck over the shoulders is of moderate length and somewhat arched. It is well covered with full grown mane similar to that of male lion.

Body: Compact body with well developed deep chest fit the square frame. The back is short, straight and strong with powerful waist. The croup is almost at the level of back.

Tail: Tight curled tail covered with plumes is set high on the back.

Forequarters: Muscular shoulders are strong and sloping downwards to shoulder joint. Forelegs of moderate length are made of strong bones and carried straight while standing.

Hindquarters: The top of hindquarter is almost in line with the back and covered with well formed hip muscles. Hindlimbs are straight down the hock which make the gait magnificent as expected for the Chow Chow.

Feet: The feet are small and well set on compact paws. The toes are close set and moderately arched and continue with curved, sharp and pointed nails.

Coat: Outer coat is formed of dense long hairs which is largely straight and fluffy. Feathering around the neck provides lion like look. Under coat is soft, dense and wooly.

tries thousands of years back. The breed was introduced into Europe and other countries during the last quarter of nineteenth century. It is a clean breed and does not emit character-istic doggy odour. Lately certain possibly he-reditary diseases have emerged in the breed which appears to be due to inbreeding system of multiplication for the maintenance of certain desired phenotypic characteristics. Chow Chow is a disciplined animal and does not like major changes in its routine activities. The dog has inherent drive for hunting and should not be let loose while going out for walk or otherwise.

The powerful energetic animals standing alert on its four straight limbs with balanced compact body look like a miniature lion.

Head and Face: The skull is broad with flat occiput but almost undefined stop. The muzzle of moderate length is broad from the level of eyes to the point, which give blocky shape to face. Nose is made of thick skin and preferably black but light colour nose is acceptable in blue and fawn specimen.

Mouth: The mouth is short and strong teeth embodied in preferably black gums are arranged in scissors bite fashion. The flews are also black.

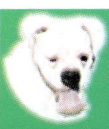

Common colour of coat is variety of whole colour and may be black, blue, red, cream, fawn or white. Markings are demerits but under coat of tail and posterior of thigh may be of lighter shade.

Size and Weight: As usual males are heavier and taller than the females. Height at withers ranges from 45 to 50 cm and body weight from 25 to 27 kg. However, reasonable variation in size and weight is accepted in this breed.

DALMATIAN

The origin of Dalmatian is considered to be Dalmasia in the earstwhile Yugoslavia and introduced into England during the last quarter of eighteenth century. Its ancestors are probably the English pointer and this was developed for hunting, guarding and herding. The animal is clean and does not emit doggy odour. It is a good companion.

Head and Face: The head is convex and face is long differentiated by clean stop. Colour of nose may be black or tan depending on the colour of body spots Occiput is wide.

Mouth: The muzzle is moderately tapering towards the oval end. The rim of jaws is sharp and smooth. Strong teeth are scissors bite and embedded in well developed gums.

Ears: These are medium to long in size set on either side of the occiput and bend like flaps. The tips are tapering and blunt.

Eyes: These are round and either black or brown depending on the colour of spots on the body.

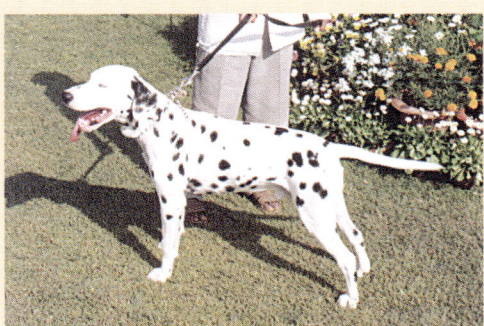

Fig. 31a Dalmatian–Standing with Erect Tail

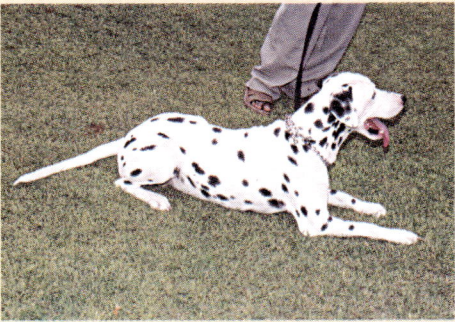

Fig. 31b Dalmatian–Sitting

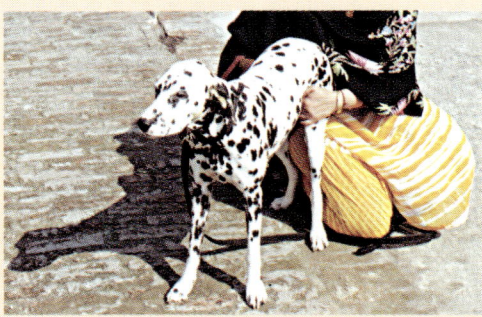

Fig. 31c Dalmatian–At Show

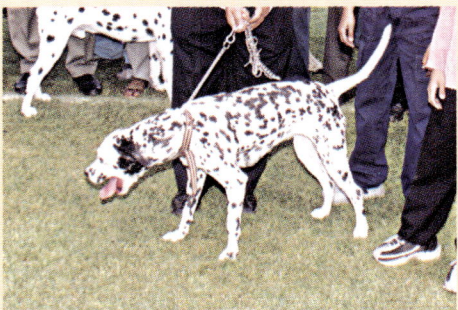

Fig. 31d Dalmatian–At Show

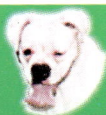

Neck: The neck is long, smooth and moderately arched. Muscles are well developed and form a shallow but clear furrow extending from throat to brisket.

Body: Well-muscled body is compact, rounded dorsally and smooth with deep chest and protruded briskets. Croup is slopping and waist is moderately narrow.

Tail: It is smooth, fine, tapering and carried straight in a shallow curvature form.

Forequarters: Shoulders are compact, fine, smooth and powerful. Limbs are much longer than the body length, perpendicular and boned. Pastern is supple.

Hindquarters: Well-muscled hips descend in strong and tight thigh further extending as properly angled hindlegs.

Feet: These are bony and arched with well-developed coarse pads.

Coat: It is short, dense, rough and shining. The colour is bright white and decorated with round to ovoid shaped black or tan colour spots scattered irregularly and may be scanty to abundant in number and never in the form of patches.

Size and Weight: Height at wither is 55 to 60 cm and weight 20 to 25 kg.

FRENCH BULLDOG

This breed was developed in France and considered to have linkage with English Bulldog but it is smaller in size. It received favour as a pet and amiable companion.

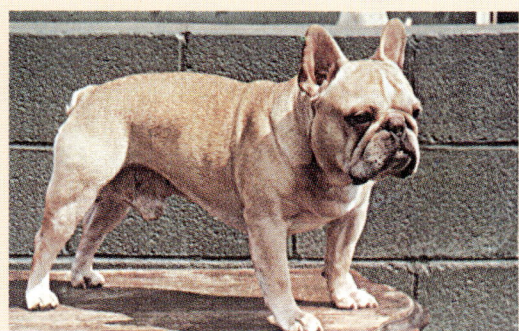

Fig. 32a French Bulldog–Whole Colour Brown

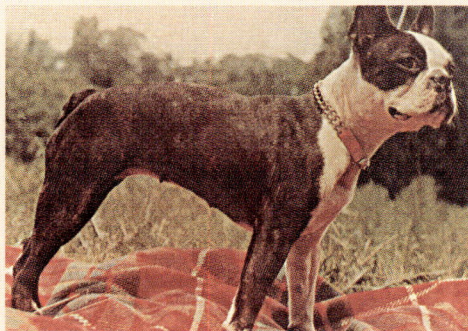

Fig. 32b French Bulldog–Brownish with Blaze Collar and Brisket

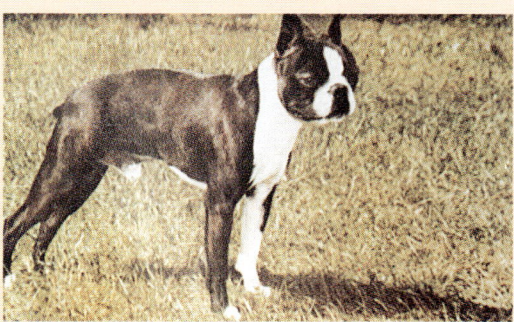

Fig. 32c French Bulldog–Brindle

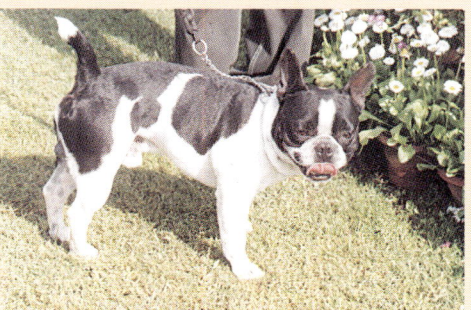

Fig. 32d French Bulldog–Pie Bald Black

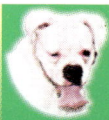

Head and Face: Head is massive, compact and square. Nose bridge is short, stop is clear and short nose is drawn backwards. Muzzle is small. Head and face are extensively wrinkled.

Mouth: It is short and wide. Lips are leveled loose and black, and canines teeth are long and strong.

Ears: Bat like triangular erect ears are broad at the base and blunt pointed at the tip and set high on the skull.

Eyes: These are slightly prominent, large and dark.

Neck: It is short, massive and wrinkled.

Body: It is short, compact and round with deep chest, broad brisket, straight back and somewhat sloping croup.

Tail: It is thick at the root and short.

Forequarter: Shoulders are well developed and upper arm is heavily muscular. Limbs are thick and short. Pasterns are flexible.

Hindquarters: Strong and powerful hind-quarters continue with short and angular limbs.

Feet: These are broad and round and prominent toes are moderately arched.

Coat: Coat is short, smooth, fine and glossy. Its colour may be fawn, brindle or pied.

Size and Weight: Height at weathers is about 30 cm and body weight is 10-13 kg, the bitches being lighter.

KEESHOND

The name of this breed remained controversial and dogs were called by different names till the finalization of Keeshond. It is a variety of spitz with square body, curled tail and pricked ears. The dog is popular as companion due to its amiable temperament, intelligence, good behaviour and affinity for children.

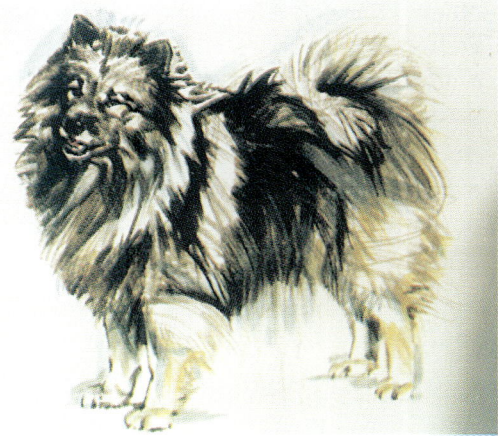

Fig. 33 Keeshond

Head and Face: It is fox like, clean and attentive. Dorsally head is wedge shaped with wide occiput and tapering muzzle. The forehead is decorated with a shallow median furrow and stop is well defined. Nose is black.

Mouth: The lips are even.

Ears: These are small, pricked, pointed at tips and set high on head. The distance between tips is much greater than between the inner border of the base.

Eyes: Large and prominent eyes are decorated with distinct colour well defined spectacles.

Neck: It is carried gracefully high and covered with dense and fluffy feathered well blended with the body. It is moderately arched which gives majestic look and makes the dog more graceful and attractive.

Body: Body length is almost equal to height. The well muscled chest is deep and broad with moderately sloping loin. There is gradual sloping of very low gradient from withers to rump and a little more on the croup.

Tail: Fluffy tail is tightly curled over the back. Its top line is covered with white plume and black tip.

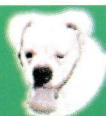

Forequarters: These are powerful with well formed bones, straight and heavily feathered above the pasterns.

Hindquarters: These are strong and feathered like forequarters except the limbs below hock joints.

Feet: These are round and broad with arched and close set toes. The soles are well padded.

Coat: The under coat is soft, light coloured and woolly whereas outer coat is long, dense, straight and coarse. Coat colour should be like that of wolf or jackal or ash grey but never whole colour black or white.

Size and Weight: Average height of dogs at withers is about 45 cm and that of bitches is about 42.5 cm.

LHASA APSO

It is a Tibetan dog and often called Apso or Tibetan Apso. The name Apso for this toy breed of dog has evolved either from the Tibetan word Apso (goat) or Abso Seng Key (barking sentinel lion). The modern Lhasa Apso is considered to be evolved from the crossbreeding with Chinese Shih Tzu. However, the two may be strains of a otherwise similar dog. It is an excellent companion but requires plenty of time for regular grooming for preventing mat formation. Many recognized Kennel clubs have classified it among terrier. These are naturally alert but tend to be watchful and slightly scared of stranger.

Head and Face: The head is densely covered with long and straight silky hairs almost

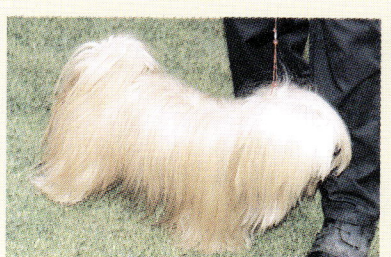
Fig. 34a Lhasa Apso–Lateral View

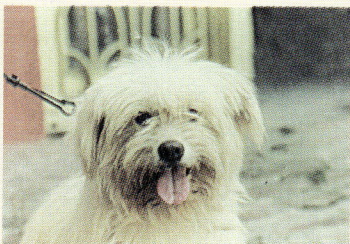
Fig. 34b Lhasa Apso–Face

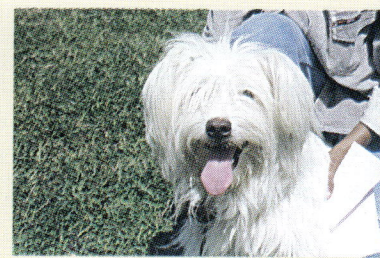
Fig. 34c Lhasa Apso–Face

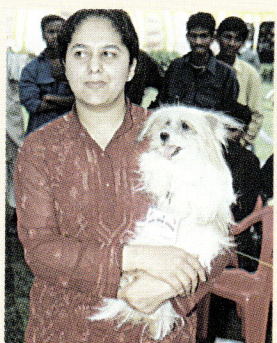
Fig. 34d Lhasa Apso –In Lap

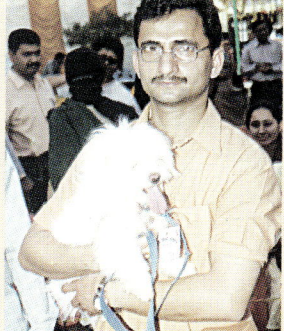
Fig. 34e Lhasa Apso –In Lap

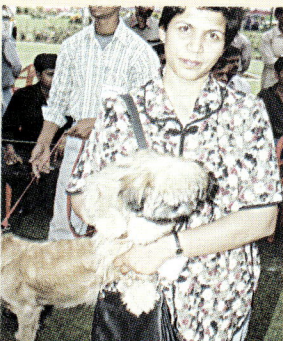
Fig. 34f Lhasa Apso –In Lap

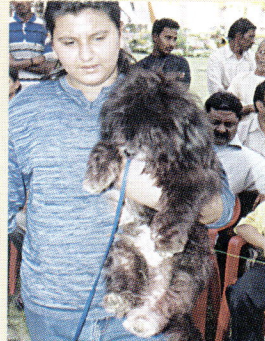
Fig. 34g Lhasa Apso –In lap

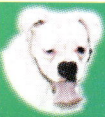

curtaining the eyes and greater part of face. The skull is narrow and slightly convex but not domed. Muzzle is medium in length. Stop defined and nose is black.

Mouth: It is small and slightly flewed with level or under shot bite.

Ears: These are pendant and highly feathered. Ears are totally covered with long hairs and can be felt only by touching.

Eyes: These are dark and bright.

Neck: It is strong, moderately arched and heavily covered with long mane, which gives lion like look.

Body: The body length is more than the height. Back is strong and moderately rounded and slightly sloping down the croup.

Tail: Heavily feathered tail is carried over the back.

Forequarters: Sloping shoulders continue down with bony short and strong cat like legs. These are densely covered with long hairs.

Hindquarters: These are strong, short and more or less straight. The legs are not visible due to dense feathering with long hairs.

Feet: Heavily feathered feet are cat like and well padded.

Coat: Entire body, except a small part of muzzle including nose, is heavily covered with very long, dense, and straight silky hairs. The coat appears parted along the spines and head. The under coat is dense, soft and woolly which is largely shaded off during the hot season. Golden or lion like colour is preferred and other common colours of coat are sandy, honey, gizzle, slate, smoke, parti-color, black, white or brown. At certain clubs, dark ear and beard tips are liked.

Size and Weight: Height at withers is 20 to 28 cm and body weight 5-7 kg.

SCHIPPERKE

This is a Belgian breed developed during fifteenth to seventeenth century. Some believe that its ancestors were a Belgian sheep dog, which are now extinct. The outline of dog is that of a Spitz.

Head and Face: Its head is fox like with well defined stop, tapering muzzle and black nose.

Mouth: The lips are fine, smooth and level with blunt pointed oral opening. The teeth are level and strong, and may be scissors bite also.

Ears: Small ears are pricked, pointed, set high and turned forward.

Eyes: These are bright and black.

Neck: It is short, massive, and slightly arched, and also decorated with a thick ruff.

Body: It is short with slightly raised at withers and loin. The chest is deep with well sprung ribs with less sloping towards waist.

Tail: The tail is docked close to body at birth.

Forequarters: The shoulders are well muscled, close set with chest and powerful. Boned fore-legs are straight. The pasterns are short and a little supple.

Hindquarters: The hindquarters are lighter than the forequarters. The stifles are properly angled.

Feet: These are round, small and padded with arched toes.

Coat: It is profuse, straight and slightly coarse. The coat is relatively longer around the neck forming a ruff and cape. The hairs on posterior part form culotte on hips. Whole black colour is characteristic but other whole colours are also acceptable.

Size and Weight: Average height at withers is about 30 cm and body weight 7 kg.

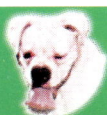

III. Gun Dogs (Sporting Breeds)

1. Clumber Spaniel
2. Cocker Spaniel (American)
3. Cocker Spaniel (English)
4. English Setter
5. Fila Brasileiro
6. Flat Coated Retriever
7. Golden Retriever
8. Gordon Setter/English Setter
9. Irish Setter
10. Irish Water Spaniel
11. Labrador Retriever
12. Pointer
13. Poodle Standard
14. Rhodesian Ridgeback
15. Sussex Spaniel
16. Tibetan Spaniel
17. Welsh Spring Spaniel

CLUMBER SPANIEL

It is a sporting and highly dignified breed of Great Britain. It is more different than the other spaniel breeds. These are massive dogs of long coat.

Head and Face: The head is broad dorsally. It is large, medium in length and almost square in overall shape. Forehead is prominent and stop is well defined. The muzzle is large. Nose is also square.

Mouth: The upper lip has well formed flew and lower lip is sharp. The mouth is well formed and teeth are level.

Ears: These are low set, large, vine leaf shaped and densely covered with straight hairs. The leathers are drooping.

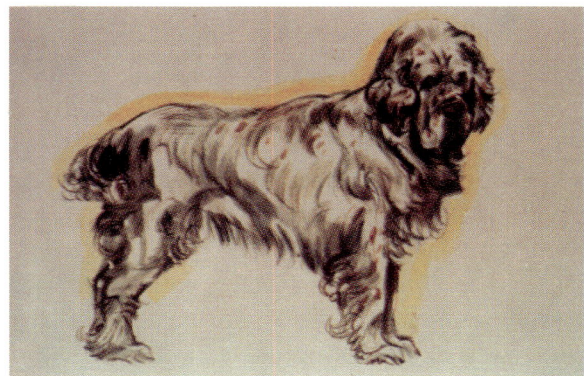

Fig. 36 Clumber Spaniel

Eyes: The eyes are set apart at the level of stop and moderately sunk. The colour is dark amber.

Neck: Well muscled massive and long neck is slightly arched and heavily feathered.

Body: It is massive, broad and long with straight and rounded dorsal line.

Tail: Low set and heavily feathered tail is carried inline with the back line.

Forequarters: Strong and muscular shoulders are sloping forward. The chest is deep and capacious with well sprung ribs. The legs are short, straight, boned and strong.

Hindquarters: Heavily muscled hindquarters are very powerful with strong loin. The stifle is well angled and hocks are low.

Feet: These are round, broad and densely covered with long hairs. The toes are moderately arched and soles are padded.

Coat: Profusely growing straight and silky coat provides ample feathering of body, legs and tail. The characteristic coat colour is white with lemon markings. Orange colour markings are unwanted but accepted.

Size and Weight: The height is moderate. Body weight of dogs is 25 to 32 kg and that of bitches is 16 to 27 kg.

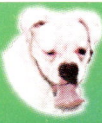

COCKER SPANIEL (AMERICAN)

Both type of Cocker Spaniels have been evolved from the Spanish Spaniel used for hunting wood cock. American Cocker Spaniel was developed later than the English Cocker Spaniel. The lighter among the two strains weighing less than 12.73 kg or 28 lb were evolved as American Cocker Spaniel. Changes were also introduced for shortening face and projecting skull through selection for several generations. The controversy on the standard characteristics of this breed continued for long and ultimately decided during the mid twentieth century. The dogs are kept neat and tidy by hair dressing and clipping on certain parts of the body.

Head and Face: The well developed skull is prominently round with sharply deep stop and prominent eye brows. The muzzle is short and somewhat square in shape with broad oral end and pronounced black nose.

Mouth: It is small and level. The teeth are arranged scissors bite.

Ears: These are set very low on either end of occiput. The drooping leather is very long and reaches upto the level of jaw.

Eyes: These are round, prominent, dark and possess well defined eye brows.

Neck: It is arched and carried elegantly high. The base of neck at shoulders is very broad which sharply slopes upwards.

Body: Although dogs in standing position appear generally uneven due to backward drawn hindlegs but actually body is square. The chest is deep with well sprung ribs and it is not possible to differentiate the depth of chest and belly due to canopy of long and dense coat reaching upto ground.

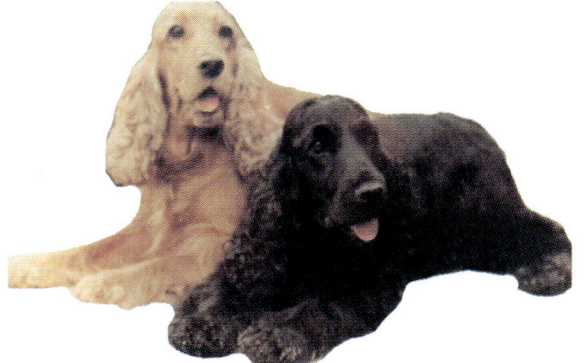

Fig. 37a Cocker Spaniel (American)–Brown, Black Whole Colour

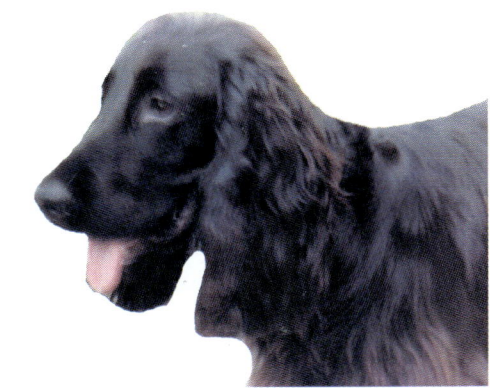

Fig. 37b Cocker Spaniel (American)–Front Part

Tail: The tail is set at the line with top line and it is docked living moderate stump and kept clear by close clipping.

Forequarters: Heavily feathered forelegs are strong and straight.

Hindquarters: The strong angulations of hind-legs at stifle joint presents sloping dorsal line.

Feet: Round and small feet are embedded in heavy feathering.

Coat: Very long coat of straight hairs forms a cover over the body from top to bottom upto the level of feet. The head is kept clean by

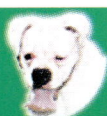

clipping. Minor trimming of feet is also made to give shape. Coat colour is paid more attention. Brown or liver colour radiant are not permitted on the black coat. However, a small white marking may be allowed on the throat and chest with deduction of marks at a show. Similarly such markings are equally penalized on other single colour coat but lighter shading of feathers may be allowed. The black and tan coloured animals must be jet black with clear tan marking which should not exceed 10 per cent. Parti-coloured animals should have at least two well defined colours. Roan colour coat is uncommon.

Size and Weight: Standard height of dogs at withers is 37.5 cm and that of bitches is 35 cm, and only 1.25 cm upward limit may be extended for both sexes. Body weight ranges from 11 to 13 kg.

COCKER SPANIEL (ENGLISH)

It is a beautiful breed of small dogs. A native of Spain it was refined to present form in England. Its flat, silky and long coat is special attraction. This is an active dog of compact body, pleasing disposition, loyal and friendly with children. It is an excellent companion.

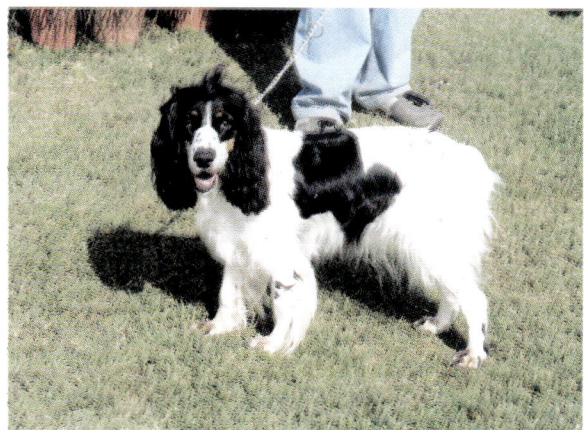

Fig. 38a Cocker Spaniel (English)—Black and White

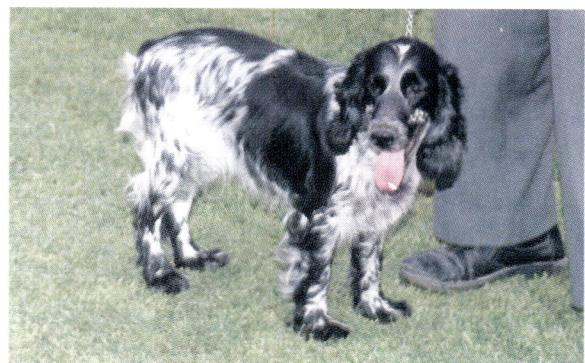

Fig. 38b Cocker Spaniel (English)—Parti-coloured Black and White

Head and Face: The head is clean, rounded and capacious with well defined stop, almost square muzzle and wide nose.

Mouth: The jaws are level and fine. The strong teeth are arranged nicely.

Ears: The ears are set low and heavily feathered.

Eyes: These are bright, gentle, hazel and brown with intelligent look.

Neck: The long and muscular neck is well blended with sloping shoulders.

Body: Compact body is powerful with deep chest and less sprung ribs giving somewhat flatten appearance. The back is short and straight but sloping at croup.

Tail: Low set full tail is carried in line with back and hangs down; though docking is practised but long stump is left behind.

Forequarters: Muscular and sloping shoulders are powerful, and well boned forelegs are straight.

Hindquarters: The hips are sloping and full. The thighs are compact and stifle is proportionately angular.

Feet: Cat like feet are round with arched toes and padded sole.

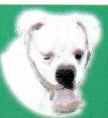

Coat: It is long, flat and silky with profuse feathering. Solid black and white, blue roan, red, strawberry roan and tri-coloured animals are also found.

Size and Weight: The height of dogs at withers is 40 to 42.5 cm and body weight 12 to 15.5 kg, and corresponding values for bitches are 37.5 to 40 cm and 11 to 14.5 kg.

ENGLISH SETTER

This beautiful feathery large size breed of dogs was recognized as a breed during the early years of the nineteenth century. This breed has been used for hundreds of years for setting wild partridge and similar other game birds. Due to its strong body, long legs, active habits and endurance, this dog is preferred for working in fields and guarding at farm houses and bungalows.

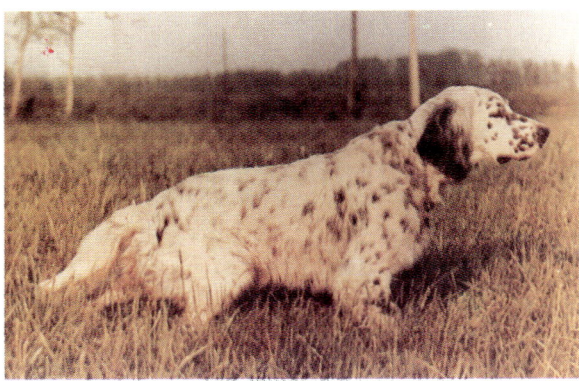

Fig. 39 English Setter

Head and Face: The head is moderately convex and forehead slopes to well defined stop. The face is long due to long nose bridge and nose is black. The skin of head and face is smooth. A shallow depression may be present above the stop on forehead.

Mouth: It is large with thick lips. Flew is clear and overlaps the lower lip. Teeth are very strong.

Ears: Long size triangular ears with rounded blunt tip and set slightly low on either side of skull hang like flaps and often reach below the jowls. These are dorsally covered with moderately long, dense and darker coat.

Eyes: These are placed on either side close to stop and in line with it. These are generally black and hazel.

Neck: Long neck is well muscled, strong and broader at shoulder end. There may be one or two skin folds on the ventral aspect of the neck.

Body: The body is compact with straight back and elevated withers. Chest is deep with well sprung ribs to provide large space for lungs. The brisket is broad and prominent. The loin is somewhat narrower and skin folds behind the naval are prominent. Croup is slightly sloping.

Tail: Well feathered medium size tail is broad at the base and tapering distally. It is mostly carried stretched in running dogs.

Forequarters: Strong shoulders are well blended with chest and muscles slope over the thick upper arm. Forearms are smooth and thick boned. Pasterns are moderate and flexible.

Hindquarters: Hindlimbs are characteristically carried pulled back. Hips and thighs are very strong due to well developed muscles. The joints are properly angled for fast running. Pasterns are long and straight.

Feet: These are thick and semicircular anteriorly. The toes are close set and moderately arched. Soles are heavily padded and covered with coarse skin.

Coat: It is moderate in length covering almost entire body except shorter on head and face. The hairs are silky and flat but may be slightly

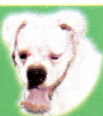

wavy in some animals. The coat colour is normally white with black, tan, lemon or liver colour spots scattered all over the body. The number, shape and size of spots is highly variable but characteristic for the breed.

Size and Weight: Height of dogs at withers is 55 to 70 cm and that of bitches is 53-65 cm. Body weight of animals ranges between 27 and 32 kg and generally bitches in the same litter are some what lighter than the males.

FILA BRASILEIRO

This breed of furious dog is a native of Brazil. These dogs are used for fighting along with soldiers in war and also to capture the run away slaves from the farms. This breed was evolved from inter breeding and selection between Blood hounds, Bulldogs and English Mastiffs for several generations. However, this breed suffered a setback and remained neglected until its revival in 1940. After the mid twentieth century its popularity increased again as a guard dog. This breed inherited the traits of many breeds and gained reputation for its dangerous behaviour.

Head and Face: Large and heavy head is like a Mastiff breed. The big skull is almost square shape which narrows at the level of distinct stop to continue as broad muzzle.

Mouth: Flew is overlapping the lower jaw. The teeth are strong and scissors bite.

Ears: Large V-shaped drooping ears reach upto the cheeks.

Eyes: Almond shaped medium Eyes are set apart obliquely with inner canthus at the level of stop.

Neck: Muscular neck is broad at base blending with the shoulders and sloping upwards with moderate arching. Jowl is prominent in this breed.

Body: It is muscular, compact and strong. The chest is deep and wide with well sprung ribs and sloping towards waist is moderate. The dorsal line is straight and sloping down the croup.

Tail: It is broad at the base and tapering at the end in a pointed tip.

Forequarters: The heavily muscular shoulders slope forward to join strong arms. Boned forelegs are perpendicular. The pasterns are small.

Hindquarters: The hips and thighs are heavily muscled and strong. The stifles and hocks are properly angulated.

Feet: These are fine and strong with close set and well arched toes and thickly padded soles.

Coat: It is short, fine, dense and coarse. Dogs of all colours are found but different shades of fawn and brindles dominate.

Size and Weight: The height of this breed at withers is about 70 to 75 cm.

FLAT COATED RETRIEVER

This breed was evolved in England from cross breeding between New Found Land and Labra-

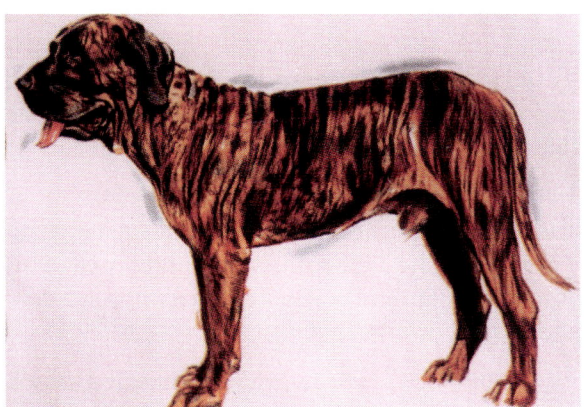

Fig. 40 Fila Brasileiro

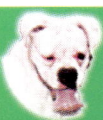

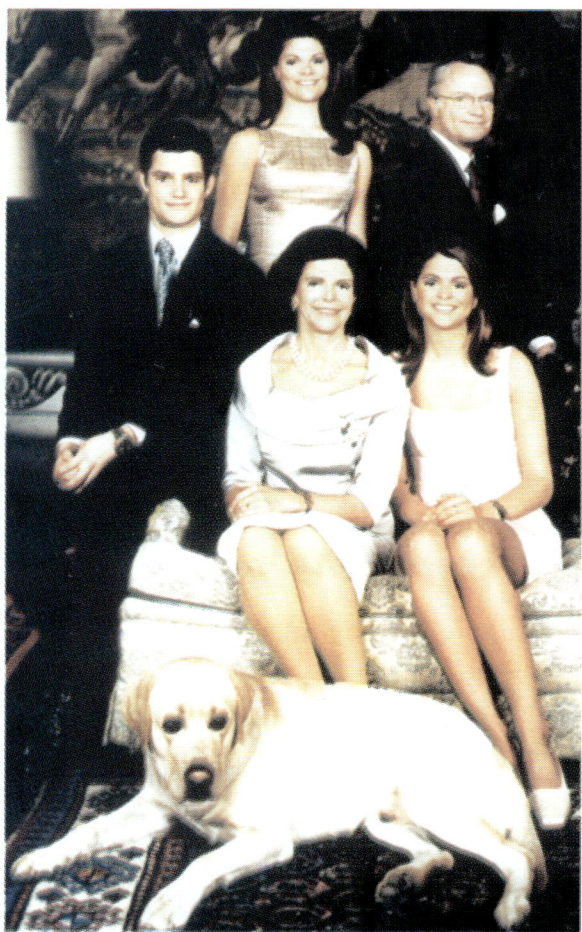

Fig. 41a Labrador Sitting with Royal Family of Sweden
(Sitting L to R): HRM Prince Phillipe, HRM Queen
Syhria, HRM Princess Madeloire
Standing (L to R): HRM Crown Princess Victoria, HRM
King Carl XVI (Rusting)

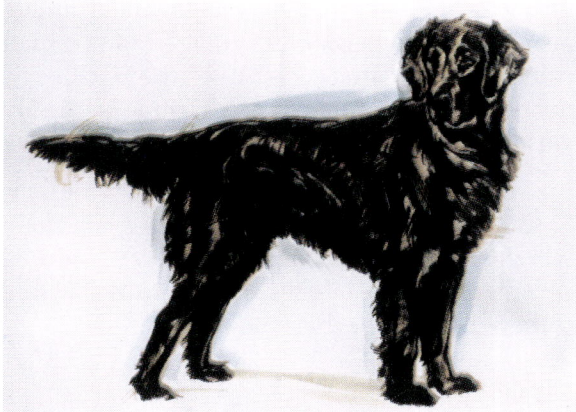

Fig. 41b Flat Coated Retriever

broad and strong nose bridge. Nose is black with clear nasal passage. Face is smooth.

Mouth: It is broad with strong teeth.

Ears: These are fringed and drooping on either side of the head.

Eyes: These are obliquely set, dark and bright.

Neck: The medium size, massive and strong neck is slightly arched and fused with the shoulders.

Body: The body is balanced, broad, massive and strong with straight dorsal line and moderately sloping croup. The chest is distinctly broader than the waist.

Tail: It is broad, long and extended backward and upward to form a shallow curvature. The tail is highly feathered from root to tip.

Forequarters: Shoulders are well developed and closely blended with chest and upper arm. Thickly boned forelegs are straight and smoother than the body. Pasterns are relatively short and moderately supple.

Hindquarters: The hips are well muscled which gradually slope down to terminate as tendons at the hock joint. Thighs are moderately pushed

dor. It possesses high working ability. These are active, lively, easy and out going dogs of medium size. Blood of the Gordon Setter of Scotland is also believed to be in the composition of Flat Coated retrievers. It is a breed of powerful dogs.

Head and Face: The head is moderately broad, clean and convex with shallow defined stop and

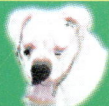

back and pasterns are straight. Limb bones are very strong.

Feet: These are moderately broad with arched toes and padded sole. The feet are covered with coat.

Coat: Body is covered with fine, dense and flat fibres. Single colour black or liver colour animals without markings are accepted for registration.

Size and Weight: Height at withers ranges from 50 to 60 cm and body weight 25 to 30 kg. The difference in shape and size of two sexes is discernible.

GOLDEN RETRIEVER

This breed of working gun dog with an excellent combination of brain and beauty was developed in Scotland. It is one of the most popular pet dog. Due to its docile and kind nature it has been found to be an excellent companion and guide specially to help persons with different kinds of physical disability like blindness and deafness, etc.

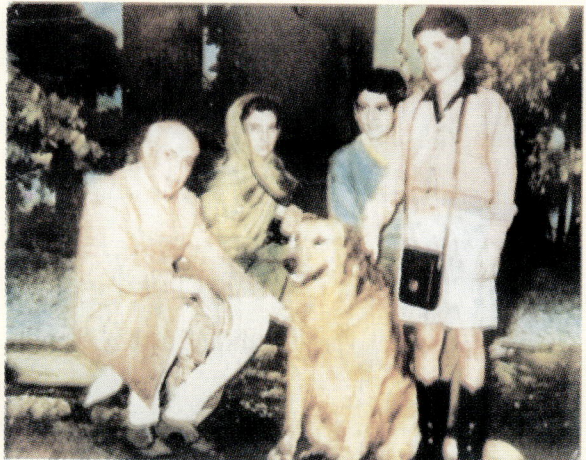

Fig. 42a Golden Retriever with Pt. Jawaharlal Nehru, Smt. Indira Gandhi, Rajiv and Sanjay

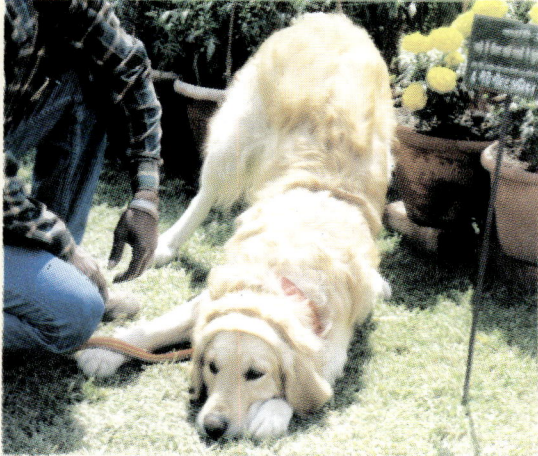

Fig. 42b Golden Retriever–Shaking Hand

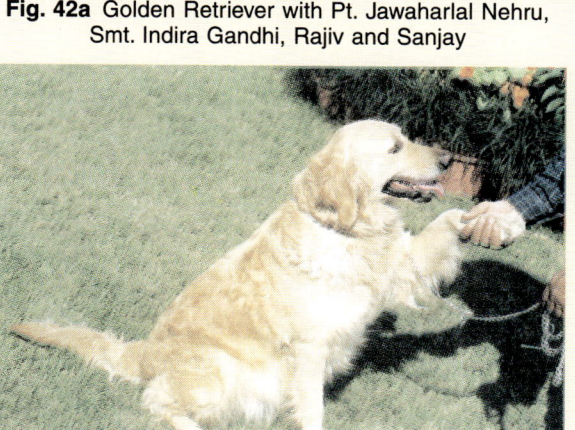

Fig. 42c Golden Retriever–Obeying Command

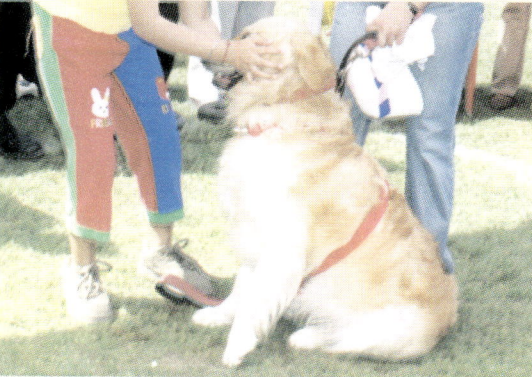

Fig. 42d Golden Retriever–At Show

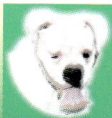

Head and Face: Head is large and convex with a clear stop. Nose bridge is long and straight. Muzzle is strong and nose is yellowish tan. Head and face are clean.

Mouth: The lips are flewed and teeth are arranged in scissors bite.

Ears: These are medium in length and flapped on either side of the skull.

Eyes: These are dark brown and set apart at the level of stop.

Neck: It is muscular, long, moderately arched and strong.

Body: Body is muscular with deep chest, well developed brisket, straight dorsal line and almost tuck up belly.

Tail: It is long, straight and well feathered.

Forequarters: Strong shoulders fuse well with the chest and moderately slope to shoulder joints. Upper arm is muscular. Limbs are boned and strong with straight forearms and supple pasterns.

Hindquarters: The thighs are muscular and limbs are thick boned and properly angulated.

Feet: These are round with close set and well arched prominent toes and padded soles fit for strong holdfast.

Coat: It is double coated animal covered with fine water resistant under coat and covered with flat or wavy long outer coat. The colour is different shades of golden yellow with glossy appearance.

Size and Weight: Height at withers is 55-60 cm for dogs and 50-57 cm for bitch with 30-35 kg and 27-32 kg body weight respectively.

GORDON SETTER/ENGLISH SETTER

This breed originated in Scotland and was refined by the Duke of Gordon during the first

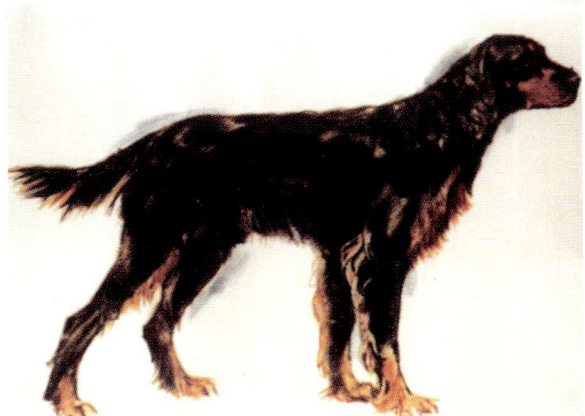

Fig. 43 Gordon Setter

quarter of the nineteenth century for hunting the game birds for which it became famous. It has further gained popularity as a gun dog in Britain and United States of America. The animals are a little larger than the other setters.

Head and Face: The head is moderate and face is medium size. Occiput is moderately convex which gradually slopes to blend with nasal bone at the stop. Nose is black and nostrils are wide.

Mouth: The lips are well developed and slightly flewed. Teeth embedded in black or flash marked black gums are arranged scissors bite.

Ears: These are set relatively high on the skull and are flat and triangular. Sometimes it may be carried erect in an alert dog.

Eyes: These are almond shaped, bright, brown, large and prominent and placed at the level of stop.

Neck: Medium size neck is muscled, somewhat rounded, slightly arched and strong. It blends well with the shoulders and brisket.

Body: It is slender and narrower than the other setters due to which it looks bigger. The dorsal line is straight and clearly slopes down the

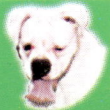

croup. The chest is deep and waist is relatively narrower than the other setter.

Tail: It is somewhat low set, straight and tapering from the root. The tail is reasonably flagged.

Forequarters: The height at withers is somewhat greater than that on the loin. Shoulders are strong and well developed muscles extend sloping upto elbow joint. Bones of fore limbs are thick and strong. Forearms are straight and moderate and pasterns are supple.

Hindquarters: These are compact with moderate slope over the croup and properly angled hind limbs with straight pastern. Legs are well feathered.

Feet: These are rounded. Toes are close set and arched, and sole is thickly cushioned and covered with cornified skin.

Coat: Body is covered with soft and fine hairs. Coat colour is black with tan markings generally on extremities, face, jowl and beneath the tail.

Size and Weight: The height at withers is 60-65 cm and body weight 25-33 kg. However, in certain conditions lighter animals have been also reported.

IRISH SETTER

This breed is also known as Irish red setter or only red setter due to rich mahogany solid colour body coat. It is a native of Ireland but it was refined in England. This sporting breed has been developed as a gun dog for assistance in hunting. It is very attractive, elegant and active dog.

Head and Face: The elongated head is lean, coarse and clean. The skull is oval and occiput is clearly defined. Stop is distinct and eyebrows are prominent. Square muzzle is less sloping anteriorly. Black nose is desirable.

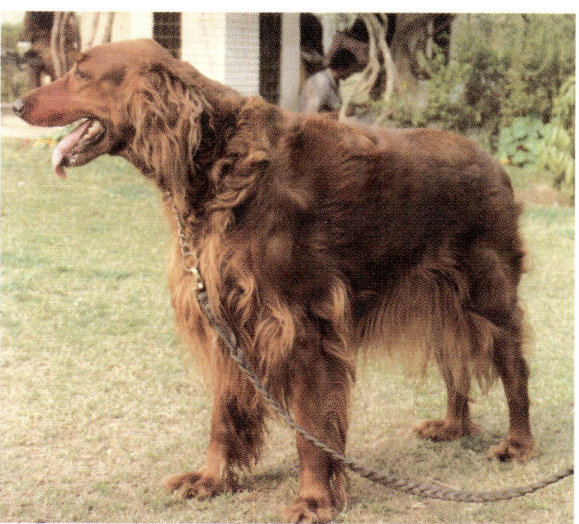

Fig. 44 Irish Setter

Mouth: The lips are smooth and level, and strong teeth are also level bite in most of the animals.

Ears: These are medium in size with fine texture. The ears are low set and reasonably posterior on the skull and hanging on the head.

Eyes: These are either dark brown or dark hazel.

Neck: It is moderately long, well muscled, coarse and reasonably arched and also free from prominence of throat.

Body: The dorsal line is sloping sharply from withers to root of the tail. The body is very broad anteriorly with deep chest and sharply sloping towards the loin. The muscular but reasonably tucked up loin is a little arched.

Tail: It is moderately long, low set, strong at root, tapering towards tip, carried straight and heavily flaged.

Forequarters: The well muscled powerful shoulders are close set with chest. The boned forelegs are straight, anteriorly smooth and positively feathered.

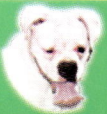

Hindquarters: Well muscled hips and thighs make hindquarters powerful. The hindlegs are long and muscular, and shannons are strong.

Feet: These are firm, close set, and strong with arched and feathered toes and padded sole.

Coat: The head, legs and ears are well feathered. The body is covered with silky, long, flat and straight hairs. The colour is rich chest nut or mahogany solid. However, white markings on chest, throat, toes or fore head or even blaze is permissible.

Size and Weight: The height at withers is 60 to 65 cm and body weight 27 to 29.5 kg. As in most of the cases bitches are lighter than the dogs.

IRISH WATER SPANIEL

This breed is largest of the all spaniel varieties and it is also quite different in general appearance and its tail is also long. There appears to be some close relationship of Irish Water Spaniel with Poodles. The ancestors of the Irish Water Spaniel appear to be present in the middle east much before the start of Christian era. It is a good gun dog but not much popular.

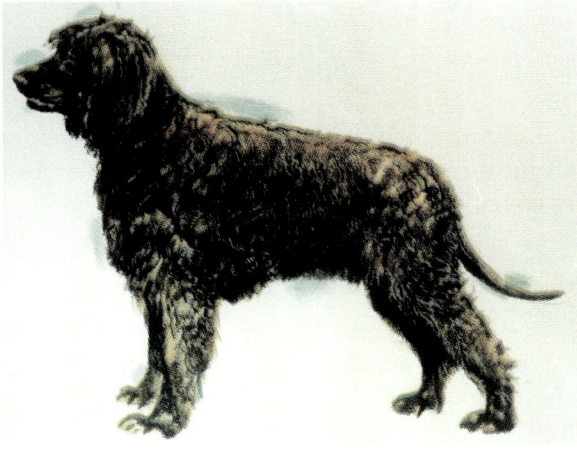

Fig. 45 Irish Water Spaniel

Head and Face: Moderately large head is well domed. Long muzzle is somewhat square and powerful. Smooth face is covered with curl coat. Nose is large and liver coloured.

Mouth: The lips are sharp and smooth, and teeth are strong. A well formed beard is present on chin.

Ears: Low set ears have long dropping leather covered with curled coat and reaching close to cheek.

Eyes: These are small, bright, active and brown.

Neck: It is moderately arched, powerful and covered with curls as on other parts of body.

Body: The muscular body is compact with short, broad and straight back. The chest is deep and ribs cage is capacious. The loins are wide and not tucked up.

Tail: It is short and straight with broader root and tapering tip. Low set tail is carried down to hocks. Initial part in continuation with croup is covered with curls and larger part is smooth upto tip.

Forequarters: The well muscled shoulders are powerful and sloping and strongly boned forelegs are straight.

Hindquarters: Muscular hips and thighs are powerful with angled stifles and low set hocks.

Feet: These are semicircular, large and spreading with toes and inter toes space is covered with hairs.

Coat: It is dense, curly and oily. The limbs are covered with ringlets upto feet. The anterior of hindlegs below hocks is smooth but posterior is reasonably feathered. Coat colour is dark liver.

Size and Weight: The height of dogs at withers is 52 to 60 cm and that of bitches 50 to 57 cm. The body weight ranges from 25 to 30 kg and 20 to 26 kg for the dogs and bitches respectively.

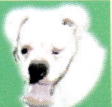

LABRADOR RETRIEVER

The dogs were present in New Found Land in early eighteenth century. This is a renounced intelligent breed of obedient dogs. These are sympathetic, gregarious and non-aggressive in nature. They are an excellent companion and also very good for guard and search work. Initially they were bred for hunting and water retrieving in all weather.

Head and Face: The head is broad and smooth with moderately convex occiput, pronounced stop, straight nasal bone, strong muzzle and broad nose.

Mouth: It is large with fine lips and strong scissors bite teeth arranged in strong gums.

Ears: These are reasonably large with blunt pointed tip which hang close to the head on either side.

Eyes: These are sharp and set at the level of stop.

Neck: It is well muscled, medium size and powerful.

Body: The body is muscular, broad and round with deep chest and sloping croup. Waist is broad but narrower than the chest.

Tail: It is thick at the base and gradually tapering to a blunt end. Its size is medium and carried straight while in action.

Forequarters: The shoulders are very strong, close to chest and moderately sloping forward. Limb bones are very strong and forelegs are straight. Pasterns are also straight and reasonably flexible.

Hindquarters: These are well built, slopy and strong. Bones are thick and strong and joints of limbs are properly angled to facilitate fast tracking.

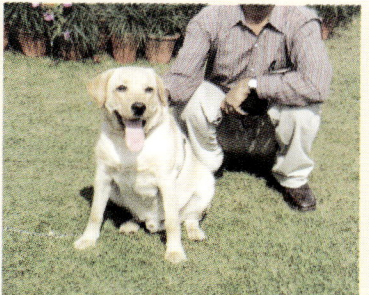

Fig. 46a Labrador–Whole Colour Brown

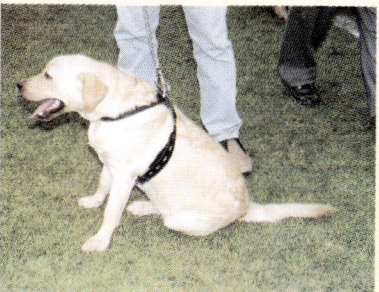

Fig. 46b Labrador–Whole Colour Brown

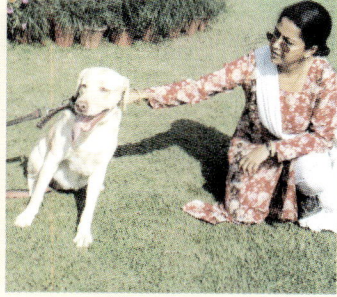

Fig. 46c Labrador–Whole Colour Brown with Flesh Nose

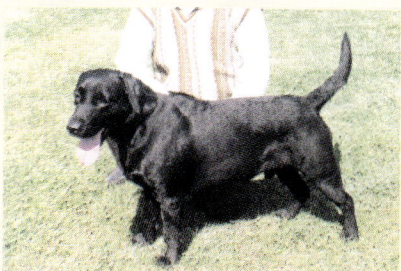

Fig. 46d Labrador–Whole Colour Black Standing

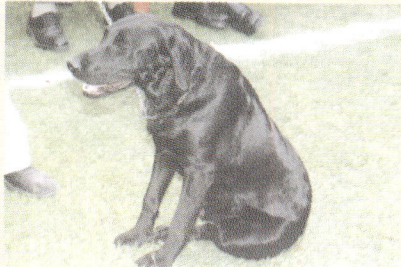

Fig. 46e Labrador–Whole Colour Black Sitting

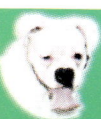

Feet: These are round with close set and arched toes. Soles are thickly padded.

Coat: Body coat is short, dense, smooth and glossy, and beneath this there is a fine under coat for protecting skin from cold and water. Colour of the body is single without any markings or shade. It is mostly chestnut but may be yellow, brown, chocolate and black uniformly.

Size and Weight: The males are a little larger than the females. Height of dogs at withers is 55-60 cm and that of bitches is 50-58 cm. Body weight mostly ranges between 25 to 35 kg.

POINTER

It is believed that Pointers were developed in Spain through cross breeding between Spanish Pointer and Foxhound. It is an excellent fast tracking gun dog. This breed is very obedient and eager sporting dog. Pointers have been found to be very efficient for birds hunting as these do not live the place after scenting them. Due to its affectionate nature and medium size, it has been found to be a good house dog.

Head and Face: Width of head is medium and forehead is shallow furrowed. The muzzle is strong and large nose is black but often there may be flesh marking. Stop is pronounced.

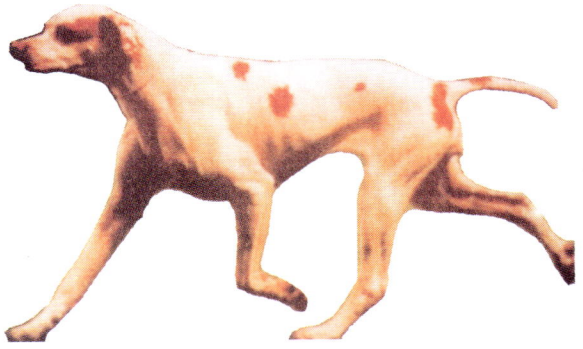

Fig. 47b Pointer in Gallop

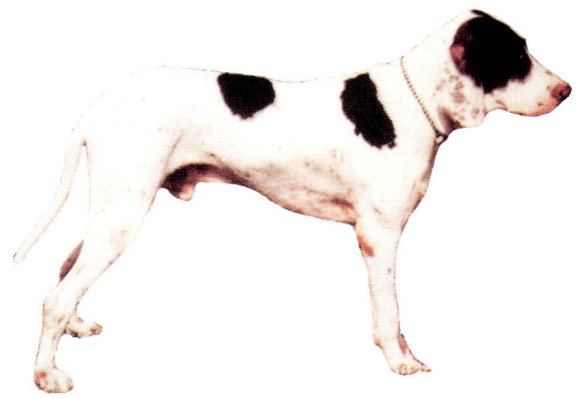

Fig. 47c Pointer in Standing

Mouth: It is moderate with levelled lips and strong teeth arranged in a scissors bite fashion.

Neck: Medium size neck is muscular, well blended with shoulders and slightly tapering upwards to merge with the jaws.

Body: It is muscular, compact, smooth and round. Withers are set higher than the straight back and slightly sloping croup. Chest is deep with well sprung ribs and somewhat projected brisket.

Tail: Medium length tail is slightly broad at the root and tapering distally to pointed tip. It is

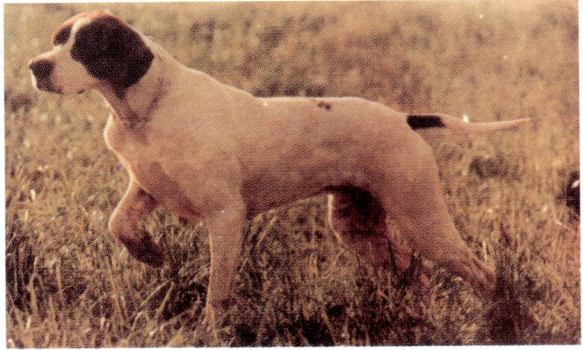

Fig. 47a Pointer in Action

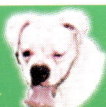

carried straight and slightly curved upwards in dog in action.

Forequarters: These are well muscled, smooth, fine and slightly sloping forward obliquely. Upper arm is sloping upto knee joint. Limbs are boned, strong and legs are straight. Pasterns are straight and flexible.

Hindquarters: Hindlimbs are well muscled from hips down the hock joints and straight downwards.

Feet: These are round with padded sole. The toes are moderately arched and properly set.

Coat: The body coat is short, fine, smooth and uniform, and its colour may be liver, black, orange, lemon with white patches. There may be sometimes self coloured or tri-coloured specimens. Another strain wire haired pointer is quite popular in Germany.

Size and Weight: Height at withers ranges from 60-65 cm and body weight 25-30 kg.

POODLE STANDARD

Standard Poodle was developed as a gun dog and its earlier development is considered to be in France, Germany and Russia where white, brown and black coated dogs were evolved respectively. Now other whole colour Poodles are also found. The Poodles are rarely presented original and commonly presented hair dressed. This is a gentle breed of good nature, active, elegant and intelligent. The coat of Poodles is cut in different styles like Lion trim, continental clip, Dutch clip and English saddle clip. Pups below one year of age are dressed as puppy clip. For this breed of dog regular grooming is very essential and it can not be taken in a casual manner.

Head and Face: The head is long, fine and somewhat rectangular with slight peak at the

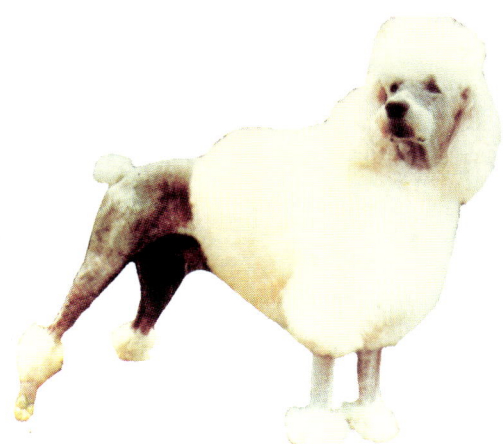

Fig. 48 Poodle

back part. Moderately broad skull joins bridge of nose at the stop. Strong face is well chiselled.

Mouth: The cheeks are flat and strong while teeth are embedded in black gums. Lips are levelled and smooth.

Ears: Long and wide ears covered with dense coat are low set and hang along the cheeks.

Eyes: The eyes may be either almond shaped or oval. The colour is black in black coloured variety and usually brown in white and light coloured varieties.

Neck: The moderately long neck is carried elegantly high and abundantly frilled.

Body: The body is short with moderately arched back, moderately wide; and deep chest with well sprung ribs provide attractive appearance to the animal.

Tail: The tail is set somewhat high and docked to almost half length.

Forequarters: Well muscled strong shoulders slope well and fore limbs are straight. Pasterns are straight.

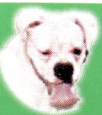

Hindquarters: The thighs are compact with developed muscles and properly angled stifle joint. The hocks are well down. Pasterns are moderately flexible.

Feet: Feet are small and oval with close set and arched toes.

Coat: Profusely grown dense coat is somewhat coarse and kept clipped in different styles by specialist hair dresser. Only whole colour or single colour coat is acceptable which may be white, black, cream, yellow, tan and many of other colours. Hairs are not shed in this breed.

Size and Weight: Average height at withers of adult dog is about 38 cm. However, values for body weight are highly variable and ranges from 9 to 14 kg.

RHODESIAN RIDGEBACK

Although the breed is called Rhodesian Ridgeback, it is a native of South Africa refined in Rhodesia and it is decorated with a ridge on the back. This breed was famous for driving away lions from the camp area. The distinct feature of this breed is the ridge on back formed of hairs growing in opposite direction. The dogs are amiable, loyal, dependable, robust and easy to train. Its grooming is easy and dog is agile.

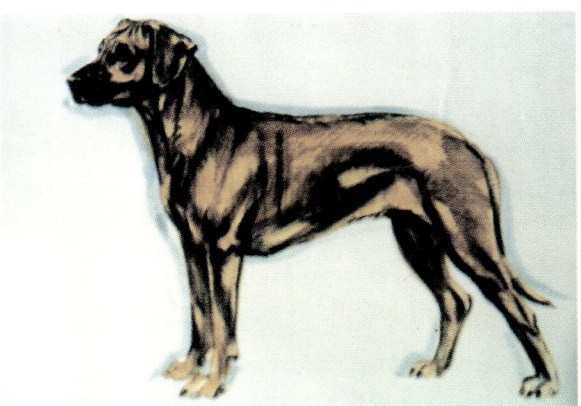

Fig. 49 Rhodesian Ridgeback

Head and Face: The head is fairly large, skull is flat and muzzle is broad. The stop is prominent and there is one or two vertical folds on the forehead, extending upto stop. The muzzle is long and strong.

Mouth: Upper lip is massive flewed and teeth are strong.

Ears: Long, drooping and fine ears are set apart on either end of occiput. The base is broad and leather with blunt pointed tip extends upto the level of cheek.

Eyes: These are round and bright, and set reasonably apart at the level of stop.

Neck: Well muscled strong and massive neck is closely blended with shoulders and moderately sloping upwards. It is moderately arched, fine, smooth and round.

Body: The body is compact and massive with deep chest, well sprung ribs, strong loins which is moderately arched and possesses distinct ridge.

Tail: It is broad at the base and tapering towards the tip extending to the level of hocks.

Forequarters: Muscular shoulders are sloping and powerful. The strong and boned forelegs are straight while pasterns are supple.

Hindquarters: The hind legs are well muscled, properly angled and strong.

Feet: These are compact with close set and well arched toes and padded sole.

Coat: Short body coat is dense, sleek and glossy. The colour is light to dark brown and there may be small white marks on brisket or toes.

Size and Weight: The height of dogs at withers is 62 to 68 cm and that of bitches 60 to 65 cm, and body weights 34 to 37 kg and 30 to 32 kg respectively.

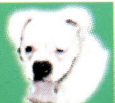

SUSSEX SPANIEL

This medium size attractive and elegant breed was evolved by cross breeding a few spaniel breeds resulting in the formation of a rich golden liver colour animal in Sussex county. In the life history of this breed, a stage arose and almost entire lot failed to litter puppies due to inbreeding. However, during later half of the twentieth century a pair from a litter helped in revival but still its extinction chances have not been overcome.

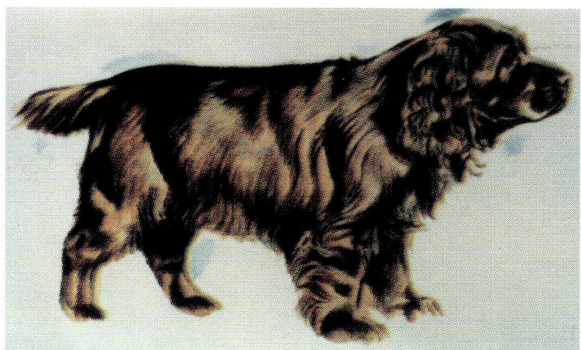

Fig. 50 Sussex Spaniel

Head and Face: The skull is round and wide, stop is prominent and muzzles are short and wide. The nose is liver colour.

Mouth: The mouth is strong with level lips and teeth.

Ears: Moderately low set drooping ears are thick, large and fringed.

Eyes: These are prominent, fairly large and light reddish brown.

Neck: It is muscular, sloping upwards, strong and slightly arched.

Body: The body is compact and strong with level dorsal line. The chest is deep, capacious and loin region is less tuckup.

Tail: Low set tail is docked living behind a longer stump of 15 to 18 cm, which is carried low.

Forequarters: The shoulders are muscular, sloping and powerful. The forelegs are boned, thickly feathered and straight.

Hindquarters: The hips and thighs are muscular, and legs are short, strong and well feathered.

Feet: These are circular, moderately arched, well padded with furred toes.

Coat: Profuse dense coat is flat. Its colour is rich golden liver with gold shaded tips.

Size and Weight: The height at withers is 38 to 41 cm, and body weight of dogs is about 20 kg and that of bitches is about 18 kg.

TIBETAN SPANIEL

Despite its name the breed has been evolved from the ancient dog found in Himalayan region of Tibet and India and the dogs were patronized by Buddhist monks and reared as companions and watch dogs. The dog is highly intelligent but somewhat scared of strangers. Affectionate with family members, sensitive and good companion, it is an alert and balanced animal.

Head and Face: The head is smaller in relation to body size and skull is slightly rounded. The muzzle is short and blunt. Stop is well marked.

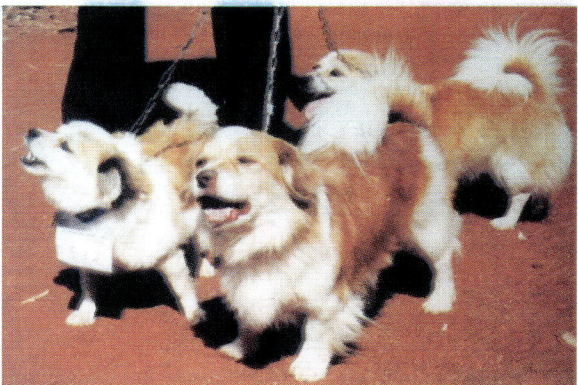

Fig. 51a Tibetan Spaniel

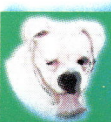

Mouth: It is slightly under shot but teeth are not exposed.

Ears: Large pendant ears are heavily feathered and are placed slightly lifted away from the side of the head.

Eyes: Less prominent eyes are dark brown and set reasonably wide apart almost horizontal at the level of stop.

Neck: Neck is short and heavily covered with long mane.

Body: It is longer than the height with straight dorsal line and moderately sloping croup. Chest is broad and brisket is prominent. Loin region is somewhat narrower than the chest but not tucked up.

Tail: The high set tail is plumed and carried over the back.

Forequarters: Broad and sloping close set shoulders are longer than the small legs down the elbow joint. The legs are bony and small, and pasterns are supple.

Hindquarters: Well muscled hips and thighs continue with almost straight pasterns.

Feet: The animals are hare footed with loose and long toes. Soles are padded.

Coat: The animal is double coated with dense and woolly under coat covered with long, silky and straight outer coat. The neck is covered with fluffy mane and frilled shoulders and brisket. The legs are well feathered. Coat colour is quite variable and may be golden, cream, fawn, brown, biscuit, white, shaded sable, red sable, black, parti-coloured or tri-colour.

Size and Weight: Height of dogs at withers is 26-28 cm and that of bitches 23-25 cm, and body weights of two sexes are 4.5 to 7.5 kg and 4 to 7 kg respectively.

WELSH SPRING SPANIEL

This is low set long dog of medium size. These dogs possess clean legs below the knees and hocks. This is an English breed of hard working and loyal dog, cheerful and independent. The animal is muscular, compact, active and very hardy.

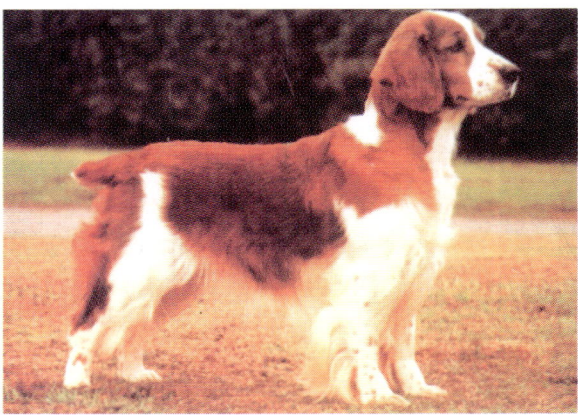

Fig. 51b Welsh Spring Spaniel

Head and Face: The domed skull is of medium length with clean stop. Moderately long muzzle is straight and somewhat square.

Mouth: The jaws are level and powerful with moderate flew. The teeth are strong.

Ears: These are slightly low set, comparatively small and pendulous hanging up to the cheek.

Eyes: Almond shaped eyes are a little oblique set and dark hazel.

Neck: It is muscular, long and clean with moderate arching.

Body: The body is muscular and compact with deep brisket. The chest is deep with well sprung ribs and less sloping towards the loin. The top line is sloping from withers to croup.

Tail: Slightly low set tail is always carried at level or low with the dorsal line and it is active.

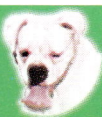

Forequarters: The muscular shoulders are powerful and medium size forelegs are boned and straight. The pasterns are short and supple. Entire forequarters are moderately feathered.

Hindquarters: The well muscled hindquarters are wide and strong with well angulated stifle and hock joints.

Feet: Thickly padded feet are semi circular, firm and cat like in appearance.

Coat: The shining silky coat is either straight or flat but never wavy. Its colour is bright red with white ventral part. White markings may be present on any part of body.

Size and Weight: The height of dogs at withers is 40.5 to 48 cm and that of bitches is 38 to 46 cm. Body weights ranges between 16 and 20.5 kg.

IV. Hound group

1. Afghan Hound
2. Basenji
3. Basset Hound
4. Beagle
5. Blood Hound
6. Borzoi/Russian Wolfhound
7. Dachshunds
8. Deer Hound (Scottish)
9. Grey Hound
10. Irish Wolf Hound
11. Norwegian Elk Hound
12. Otter Hound
13. Saluki
14. Whippet

AFGHAN HOUND

It is a large, hairy, extra ordinary beautiful and aristocratic dog of varied colour and moderate

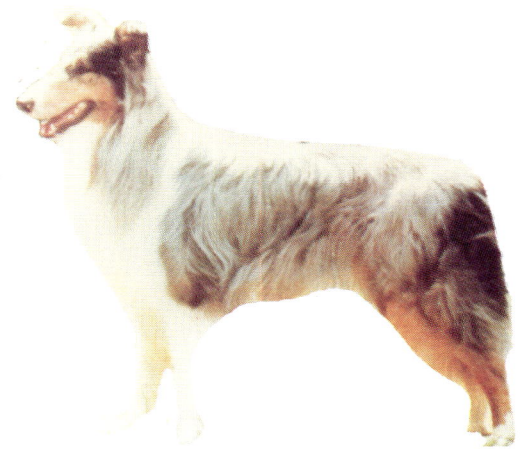

Fig. 52a Afghan Hound–Light Colour

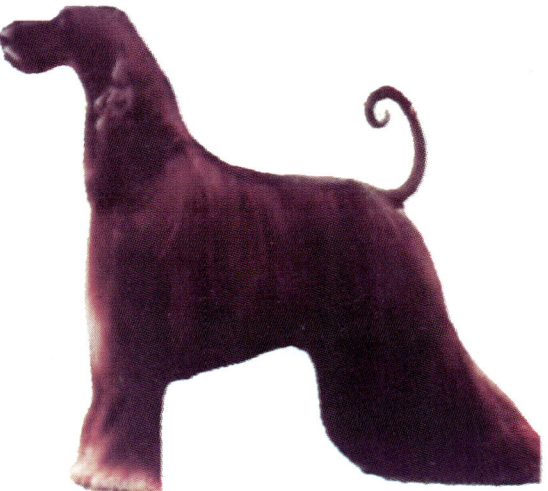

Fig. 52b Afghan Hound–Black

size. This breed originated in hills of Afghanistan and perhaps in Egypt simultaneously.

Head and Face: The head is moderately convex above the stop and straight downwards with prominent nasal bone. The jaws are fine and powerful and do not display abnormal flews. Nose is generally black but may be liver colour also. A tuft of long hair is found on the top of the head.

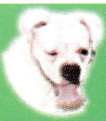

Mouth: The muzzle is long and fine. Strong teeth are embedded in black gums and, as usual, arranged in scissor bite.

Ears: The flat ears are drooping on either side of the head and covered with long silky hairs.

Eyes: Triangular and obliquely placed eyes with inner canthus in line with the stop are dark or golden and attractive.

Neck: Neck is narrow, long, powerful and moderately arched. It is profusely covered with very long silky hairs.

Body: The body is long, narrow and covered with fringed long silky hairs which are shorter on back. Chest is deep with well sprung ribs and loin is narrower.

Tail: Long hairy tail loops into a circle.

Forequarters: Sharp shoulders and long limbs are carried straight down the knee joint.

Hindquarters: Strong hindquarters slope slightly at croup. Feathering is quite prominent on the thighs.

Feet: These are long and flexible. Toes are moderately arched and covered under the coat. Nails are black or greyish black with pointed tips.

Coat: Outer coat is long except on the back region. It is silky and bright of almost all colour encountered in dogs.

Size and Weight: The height of dogs at withers is 67-74 cm and that of bitches is 61-69 cm, and body weights of both sexes ranges between 23-29 kg. Females of same litter are generally lighter than the males.

BASENJI

Among the spitz variety Basenji is the only breed covered with a smooth coat. This breed

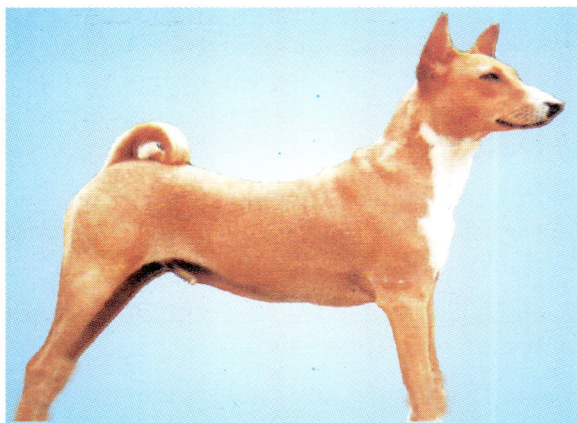

Fig. 53 Basenji

does not bark which is an unusual character and differentiate it from all the breeds. The anatomy of vocal organ (larynx) of Basenji is different than the all other breeds. This indicates the possibility of evolution of this breed for silent hunting. Basenji emits a different kind of mixed voice of loudness unusual for a dog. The animals are famous for cleanliness and do not emit doggy odour. The slender and strong Basenji is an independent, courageous, loyal, alert, intelligent and swift dog. This is a cheerful dog with drive for playing with children. It is an aristocratic animal of light frame and relatively long and almost vertical limbs. Balanced body with broad brisket and narrow loin appears like small variety of antelope.

Head and Face: The head of dog is flat and medium in width joining the face with a slight stop. The part above stop is somewhat greater than the lower part. The face is narrow towards nose. The side lines also taper to continue with jaws. Few fine longitudinal wrinkles are present on the forehead which are more prominent in pups. Nose is mostly black.

Mouth: The animals normally keep the mouth closed and tongue is usually not protruded. The muzzle is cone shaped and jaws are smaller.

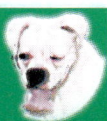

Teeth are embedded in strong black gums in a scissors bite arrangement and slightly overlapped by upper teeth.

Ears: Pricked ears of fine texture are moderately hooded and set forward on either side of skull sparing greater length of occiput. Erect ears bring the tips nearer to the centre of the skull.

Eyes: Obliquely placed almond shaped eyes are dark in colour, sharp and bright with unpredictable expression.

Neck: The fine neck is longer, moderately arched and strong. It is broader at brisket end and gradually tapers moderately towards jowl end. Gracefully held up neck exhibits alert disposition of an active dog.

Body: The body is smooth, compact and short with leveled back. The chest is deep with well sprung ribs which moderately slopes towards the waist. Sloping is less in females than the males. Two rows of well-formed teats are quite apparent on the ventral aspect of body arranged in pairs from pectoral to inguinal region in bitches. Sheath is tight in males.

Tail: Smooth tail is tightly curled set high over the croup with buttocks pulled beyond the root of the tail.

Forequarters: The forequarters are covered with compact muscles forming reasonable slope from withers to elbows. The elbows are placed close to the brisket in line with the ribs. The forelimbs are placed straight. The bones are fine and forearms are longer and straight. The pasterns are also quite long, straight and flexible.

Hindquarters: The strong hindquarters are covered with well developed and compact muscles providing great strength to the hind-limbs. The hocks are properly let down and in line with the long second thigh, slightly pushed back stifle and straight hindlegs.

Feet: Feet are thin, small and narrow with well arched toes and developed pad covered with coarse cornified skin. The nails are sharp pointed and short and forepaws are stronger than the hind paws.

Coat: The body is covered with close set short and fine single coat. Coat colour may be bright red, brown red, tan black and tan or pure black with feet, chest and tip of the tail white. There may be one or more of the blaze, collar and legs white.

Size and Weight: Average height of dogs is about 43 cm and bitches 40 cm, and body weight of corresponding sex is about 11 and 10 kg.

BASSET HOUND

These are tiny short legged dogs evolved in France about 400 years back and first exhibited in a show at Paris. It has drive for hunting and strong will power. These dogs like to live in large courtyard and natural environment. It is friendly and make a good companion.

Head and Face: Long head is provided with moderate wrinkles on the fore head. Broad muzzle is heavily flewed overlapping the lower

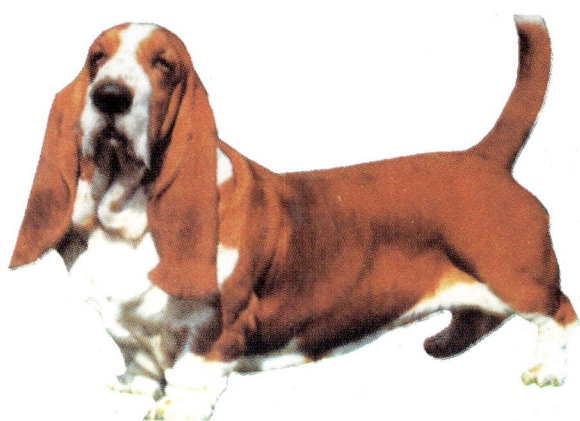

Fig. 54a Basset Hound

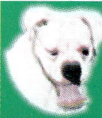

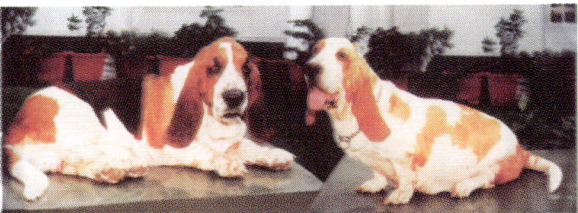

Fig. 54b Basset Hound–Pair

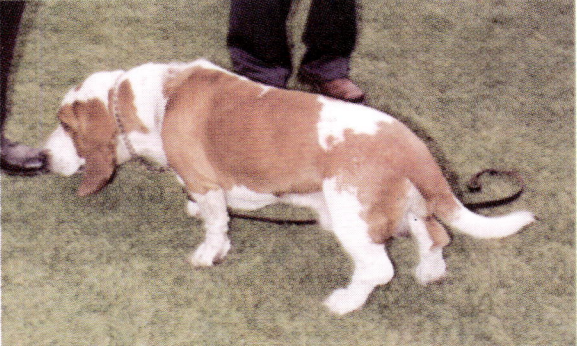

Fig. 54c Basset Hound–At Show

jaw. Nose is normally black in dark coated animals. Face is often decorated with natural markings. Occiput is convex.

Mouth: The mouth is broad and blunt. Strong scissors bite teeth embedded in black gums are not visible due to overlapping flew.

Ears: Very long drooping ears hang like pendulum and reach to the level of throat or even below.

Eyes: Obliquely placed almond shaped prominent eyes are sagacious brown or hazel or dark. There may be characteristic semicircular symmetrical markings over the inner canthus of both eyes.

Neck: The neck is usually short and heavy with loose skin.

Body: The body is longer than the height and frame is made of strong bones. The back is straight and deep chest is broader whereas tapering towards the waist is rather less.

Tail: Beautiful tail is slightly curved at the distal end. It is long, strong and tapering.

Forequarters: Shoulders are well muscled and strong. Forelegs are short, strong and bones of limbs are thick and heavy. Pasterns are short but reasonably flexible.

Hindquarters: It is almost in level with the dorsal line. Limbs are strong and lower legs are straight below moderately bent stifle.

Feet: Large feet are broad and semicircular. Toes are slightly arched and each one is visibly distinct. Sharp nails are short and pointed. Pad is thick and formed of cornified skin.

Coat: Body coat is short and smooth, which is mostly tri-colour and may be also lemon colour, tan and white and many other colour encountered in hound breeds. Different kinds of markings on head, face, legs and body are common features.

Size and Weight: There appears to be no specific distinction in shape and size available in the records. The height of adults at withers may be 33-39 cm and weight 15-23 kg.

BEAGLE

Actual origin of Beagle is not known but it is one of the earliest dog breeds of Britain which was used preferably for the hunting of hare in olden days. The friendly dog is alert and capable to cope even with odd situations and can adjust in all kinds of diversified situations. This is one of the most wanted companion.

Head and Face: The head is fairly large and occiput is somewhat domed. Head and face are distinguished by the distinct stop. Muzzle is wide and flews are flappy overlapping the lower jaw. Nose is black and blunt.

Mouth: It is well developed and wide. Strong scissors bite arranged teeth are embedded in

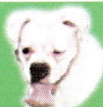

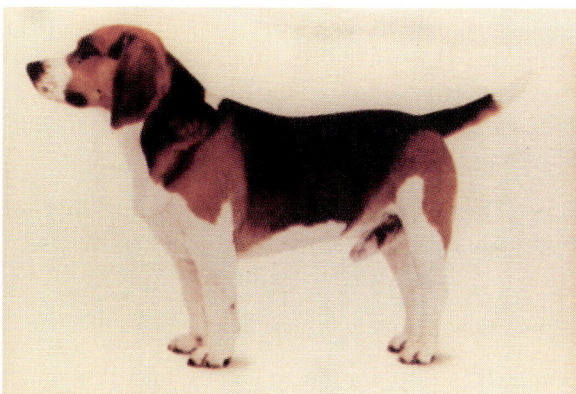

Fig. 55a Beagle

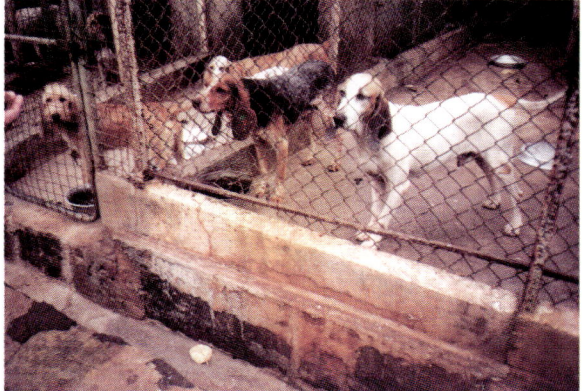

Fig. 55b Beagle Group in Enclosure

black gums. Teeth are generally not visible as dogs keep the mouth shut by nature.

Ears: Ears are drooping, flappy, smooth, broad at the base and hanging low from either side of the head. Tips are rounded and length reached to the level of larynx or sometimes even a little longer.

Eyes: Obliquely set almond shaped eyes at the level of stop are clean and dark brown in colour.

Neck: It is medium, fine, smooth, strong and slightly arched.

Body: The body is muscular, smooth and powerful. Withers are placed at a higher level than the croup. Back is straight, and sloping beyond croup is non-significant. Chest is broad, deep and muscular. Brisket is rather heavy due to prominent muscular development. As usual, waist is narrower.

Tail: Thick tail of medium length is held high.

Forequarters: The level of muscular and smooth forequarters is higher than the hindquarter dorsally. Legs are strong and straight. Pasterns are medium, straight and flexible.

Hindquarters: Hindquarters are strongly muscular and smooth with little slope over croup. Legs below stifle are straight and bones are reasonably thick.

Feet: Feet are round, and moderately arched toes are close set.

Coat: Body coat is short, dense, smooth and weather proof. It is mostly tricoloured with a mixture of black, tan and white. Legs are generally white. Other colours are also acceptable.

Size and Weight: Height at withers ranges from 32 to 40 cm and weight from 9 to 18 kg. This great variation in size and weight is probably due to difference in breeding stock of different regions.

BLOOD HOUND

It is a very old breed and has descended from the Celtic hound of Middle East. It is a docile, lovely and gentle dog with magnificent olfactory sense, calm nature and good for guarding and companionship. The dog is clean but excessive drooling of saliva is an unwanted trait. This is a large size breed.

Head and Face: The head is large with somewhat oval occiput, prominent forehead, distinct stop and black nose. The skin is loose and wrinkled on head and face. Muzzle is almost equal to skull.

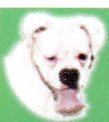

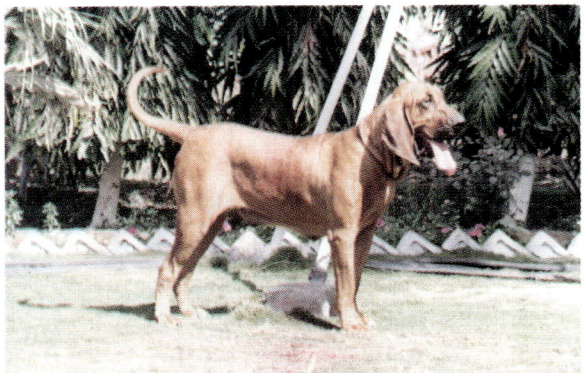

Fig. 56a Blood Hound–Whole Colour Brown

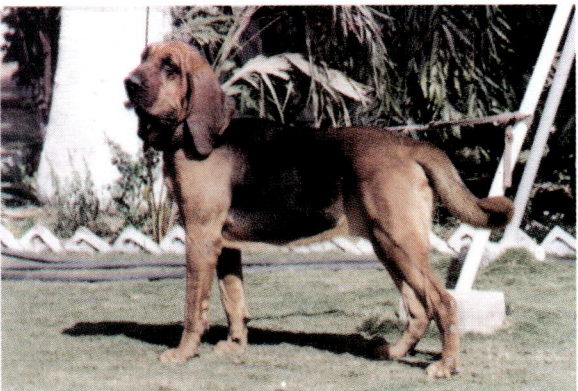

Fig. 56b Blood Hound–Black Shaded Coat

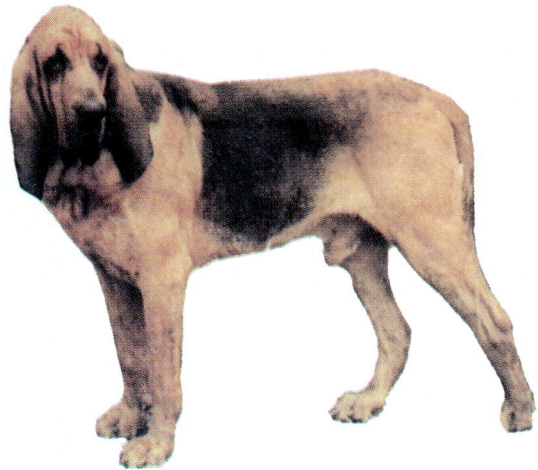

Fig. 56c Blood Hound–Black shaded coat

Mouth: Mouth is short and upper lip is pendant. Tips of the tongue remain protruded drooling saliva most of the time. Teeth arranged in close scissors bite are not visible until mouth is opened.

Ears: These are very long, hanging and low set on the skull. The structure of ears helps in tracking scent during trailing.

Eyes: These may be dark, hazel brown.

Neck: It is fine, long and strong and can reach to ground easily. It is carried high.

Body: Muscular, compact, smooth and strong with deep chest and broad brisket. Dorsal line slopes sharply to continue straight over the back and loin which mildly slopes down the croup. Waist is relatively less narrow than the rib cage.

Tail: It is thick, fine and extends upto stifle joint. The tail is carried high over the back when animal moves.

Forequarters: Shoulders are fine, strong and slope obliquely to join with upper arm. Forelegs are boned, strong and straight.

Hindquarters: These are formed of well developed muscles smoothly sloping to stifle joint. Hindlimbs are strong with usual bent at hock joint and forming moderate angle downwards.

Feet: These are rounded and toes are close set and slightly arched. Pads are thick and cornified. Nails are black and sharp pointed.

Coat: The coat is formed of short and coarse hairs. Coat colour may be black with head and quarters tan or liver and tan or reddish brown or roan.

Size and Weight: Height at withers of dogs is 63-69 cm and that of bitches 58-63 cm with body weight 25 to 45 kg.

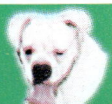

BORZOI/RUSSIAN WOLF HOUND

The ancestors of Borjoi were introduced in Russia from Arabia and crossed with a local Russian Collie type dog with thick, heavy and wiry coat. The crossbreeds were refined through breeding to modern Borjoi with stable traits.

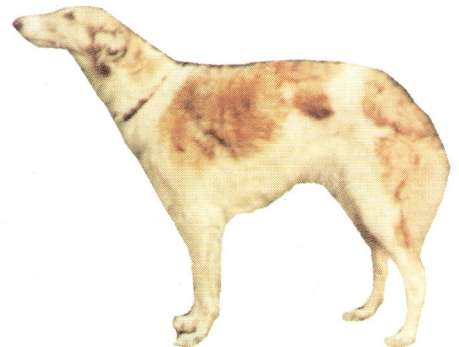

Fig. 57 Borzoi

The breed is docile, quiet, beautiful, elegant, large, fast and ferocious. It is famous for style.

Head and Face: The head is fine, long, thin and narrow with domed skull and shallow stop and narrow muzzle. Inner canthus of eyes is almost half way between the top of occiput and tip of the nose. Nose bridge is elongated and somewhat rounded. The nose is black and cheeks are fine.

Mouth: It is long and narrow exhibiting almost all teeth when open. Lips are level and teeth are prominent and strong.

Ears: The small, fine and responsive ears are laid back on the neck.

Eyes: The obliquely set almond shaped eyes are dark in colour.

Neck: It is moderately long, narrow above and wider at shoulders, strong and slightly arched.

Body: It is long and arched with deep chest and tucked up loin. Croup slopes sharply down the lumbar region.

Tail: The feathered long tail is carried low.

Forequarters: The shoulders are long, strong and blended with the chest. Brisket is strong. Fore limbs are bony, straight, long and strong with short pasterns.

Hindquarters: The hips are drooping and thighs are well muscled. The angulation of hind legs appear pulled due to arching of back.

Feet: These are rounded with moderately arched toes and padded sole.

Coat: The body is covered with long, silky and wavy hairs. The mane is long, tail is feathered but coat is short at head, face, ears and lower part of limbs. The neck, chest, body and hindquarters are properly frilled. The coat colour may be white, various shades of golden, tan shaded with black, uni colour or with white markings.

Size and Weight: Height of dogs at withers is 73-74 cm and that of bitches 68-69 cm. Body weights of both sexes range between 34 and 46 kg.

DACHSHUND

Dachshund are German breeds developed during the sixteenth century for hunting and different names like badger creeper, badger digger, burrow dogs and dachsel have been used in olden days. These dogs gained popularity as pets and companions and now these are spread to different countries including India.

These are intelligent, sprited, cheerful and affectionate animals with drive to play with the children. The shape and size of dogs are very characteristics and easy to recognize.

These dogs are identified as two main type: normal dachshund and miniature dachshund

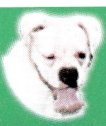

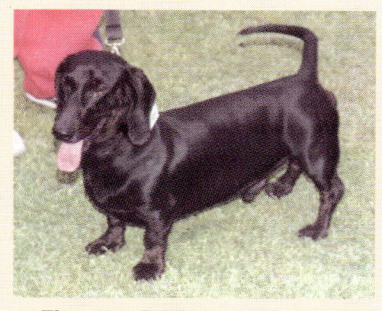

Fig. 58a Dachshund–Smooth
Haired Black

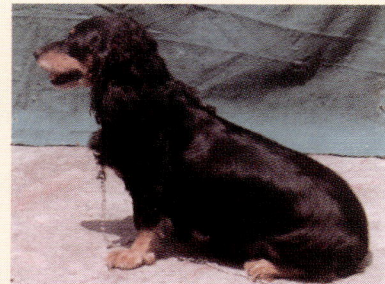

Fig. 58b Dachshund–Wire Haired
Black

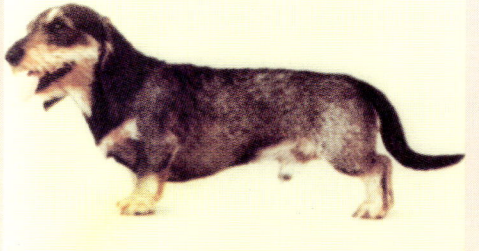

Fig. 58c Dachshund–Wire Haired Bridle

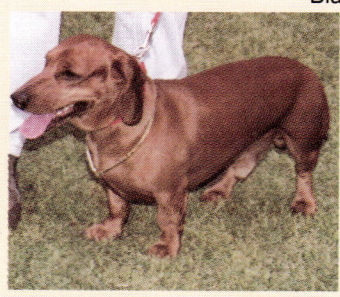

Fig. 58d Dachshund–Smooth
Haired Miniature Brown

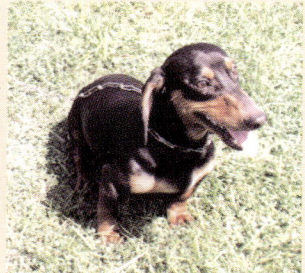

Fig. 58e Dachshund–Smooth
Haired Miniature with Tan Face

and each type is further distinguished into long haired, wire haired and smooth varieties on the basis of body coat.

Head and Face: The head is slightly convex and face is long and tapering. There is no stop. Head and face are smooth and often a shallow vertical furrow is present on the forehead down to start of the bridge of the nose. Nose is black.

Mouth: These dogs mostly keep their mouth closed. Upper jaws are slightly flewed and both jaws are strong. The number of teeth is almost 42 and arranged in scissors bite.

Ears: These are long and set drooping like flaps on either end of the occiput. The base of ear is broad and tip is rounded. These are smooth in smooth variety and fringed in hairy variety.

Eyes: These are oval, prominent and either dark red or black.

Neck: It is long and projected forward and upward. It is smooth in smooth variety and fringed in hairy variety.

Body: The body is very long, compact and powerful with moderately deep chest and relatively less sloping towards the waist. Dorsal line is almost straight up to end of loin with slightly sloping croup. Brisket is protruding.

Tail: It is thick at the root and tapering at the end, and carried straight. The tail is flagged in hairy breeds.

Forequarters: Shoulders are muscled and strong and limbs are boned, very short and supple.

Hindquarters: These are well muscled and powerful with properly angled limbs.

Feet: These are rounded with arched toes and padded soles.

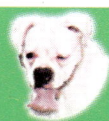

Coat: (*a*) Hairy type–Coat is made of shiny either straight or wavy long hairs covering all over the body except the skull and face.

(*b*) Smooth type–Coat is short, dense, smooth and free from curling.

Colour of the coat may be dark red, tan red, dark brown with tan shades , brindle black and tan, but not white.

Size and Weight: (*a*) Large type–Height at withers may ranges from 20-25 cm and weight 8-12 kg. (*b*) Miniature type–Height at withers may be 12-20 cm and weight 3-5 kg.

DEER HOUND (SCOTTISH)

This breed has been also named as Scotch Grey Hound and Highland Grey Hound. These dogs were probably first brought to Great Britain and later on refined in Scotland with heavier and weather tolerant coat. This breed is known for its aristocratic and romantic behaviour but now it is found rare.

Head and Face: The head and face together are

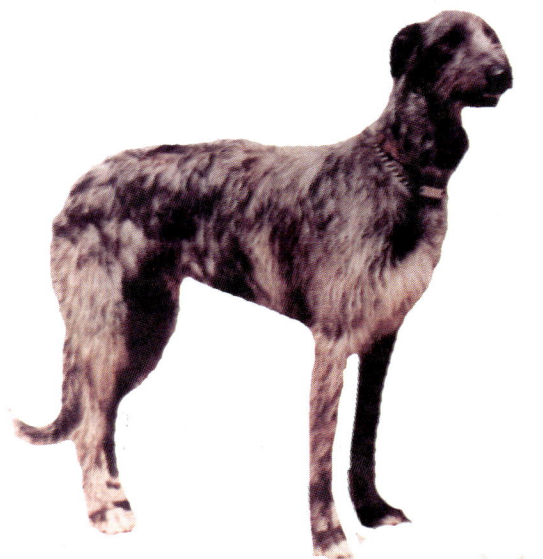

Fig. 59 Deer Hound (Scottish)

conical with broad occiput, tapering muzzle and shallow stop. The nose is usually black but blue in blue and fawn coloured dogs. There are long and coarse hairs all over and also moustache of silky hair.

Mouth: The mouth is long with level and fine lips. Upper jaw is a little over shot. The teeth are prominent.

Ears: High set ears are folded and feathered. The ears are raised erect in aggressive dogs.

Eyes: These are deep set in sockets, moderately full and may be brown, dark or hazel in colour. The eye brows are fully developed.

Neck: The long neck is covered with rarely spread mane of harsh hairs.

Body: It is more or less similar to Grey Hound. The chest is deep and flat with tucked up waist. Arched loin is sloping posteriorly upto root of the tail. The back should be arched and straight one is unwanted.

Tail: Feathered tail is thick at the base and gradually tapering towards the tip and normally reaches upto the ground.

Forequarters: The shoulders are compact and sloping well forward to join strong arms. Long and boned forelegs are perpendicular. The pasterns are short and almost straight.

Hindquarters: The hips are set apart and legs are properly angled for fast propulsion.

Feet: These are well padded and compact with close set and arched toes.

Coat: The body is covered with harsh and wiry hairs of medium length. There is moderate mane and fringe on all the limbs. Soft and woolly coat is not liked. Preferred body coat colour is dark blue-grey. However, there may be wide range of greys, brindles, reddish fawn,

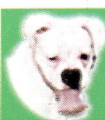

sandy red or yellow. White marks on chest and toes are acceptable.

Size and Weight: The body weight of dogs is 38.5 to 47.75 kg and that of bitches is 29.5 to 36.5 kg, but higher limits of 50 kg and 43 kg for the corresponding sexes have been accepted in America.

GREY HOUND

The origin of Grey Hound is Egypt where it was patronized in ancient time for hunting large animals like deer and wild hogs and also for racing. The sporting dogs are slim with exposed ribs and other bones, and tucked up loin. In standing position it is vigorous, robust and most graceful. Daily extensive exercise is necessary for keeping the dogs fit for games and show. The dog has extremely stable temperament and relaxed poised attitude and great stamina and speed.

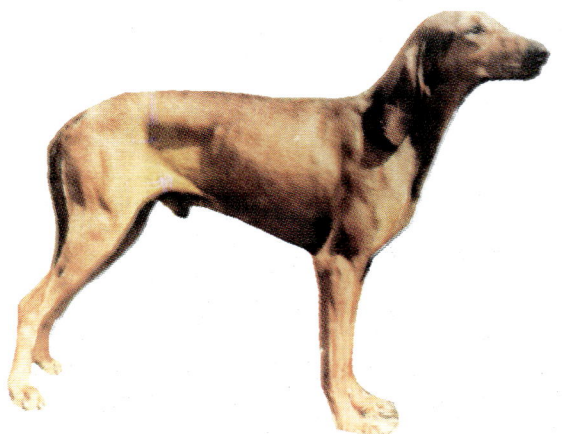

Fig. 60b Grey Hound (Italian)

Mouth: Narrow and sharply leveled lips are normally kept closed. Teeth are strong.

Ears: Small ears are thin and rose shaped exposing the inner surface.

Eyes: Almond shaped dark eyes are set oblique with inner canthus at the level of stop.

Neck: It is long, fine and sloping upwards with prominent hollow of the neck in racing dogs and full in show dogs.

Body: It is long with straight, broad and somewhat arched back. Belly is tucked up. Chest is deep with well sprung ribs and ribs are visible in hunting and racing dogs but smooth in show specimens. Brisket is well muscled and powerful. Sloping down the croup is prominent.

Tail: Long tapering fine tail is shallow curudal and hanging.

Forequarters: Well muscled shoulders are sharp and smooth. Long and strong fore limbs are straight. Pasterns are also straight but flexible.

Hindquarters: The thighs are kept pushed back in standing dogs and pasterns are long and

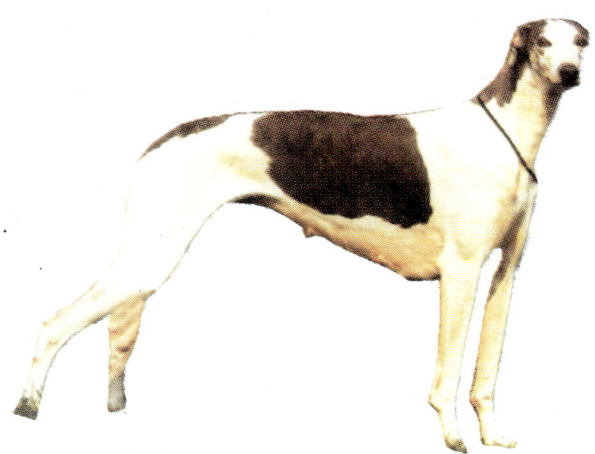

Fig. 60a Grey Hound

Head and Face: Head is long with chiseled and long sharp muzzle. Nose is pointed and black. Fore head is slightly convex, shallow stop and straight bony nose bridge. Muzzles is long and sharp.

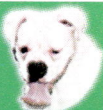

straight. Bones and tendons of limbs down the stifle joints are clearly visible.

Feet: These are irregularly rounded with thick padded and coarse sole. The toes are well arched and knotty in appearance. Nails are strong and pointed.

Coat: It is fine, short and smooth. Its colour may be red, brown, black, fawn cream, brindle, pied and white. Both whole colour and mixed colour animals are found.

Size and Weight: Height at withers of the dogs is 70-80 cm and that of bitches is 65-70 cm; and body weight ranges from 25 to 35 kg.

IRISH WOLF HOUND

This is considered to be one of the oldest and tallest breed of the world which has descended to present form. This had been a legendary hound of Ireland. These well-built strong dogs are very gentle but due to their large size and large food requirements the owners of this breed are now limited as hunting has almost become an activity of past.

Head and Face: The skull is long with flat fore head and shallow stop. The muzzle is long and moderately tapering to end in a blunt oral end. The nose is black.

Mouth: The upper lip is flewed and teeth are strong.

Ears: Small ears are low set and hang folded back towards the neck.

Eyes: These are big and dark, and set diagonally with inner canthus at the level of stop.

Neck: It is muscular, long, strong and moderately arched. It is heavily covered with coarse ruff. The long hairs over the crest form mane.

Body: Muscular and compact body is

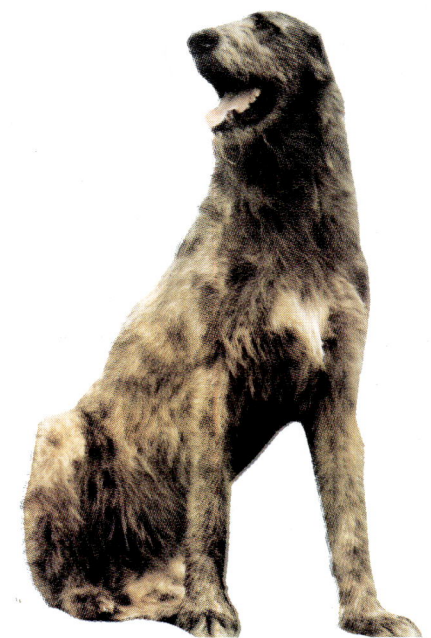

Fig. 61 Irish Wolf Hound

moderately arched. The chest is deep with long rib cage and sloping loin. The croup is sloping.

Tail: It is low set, long, slightly curved, moderately thick at the base and gradually tapering distally. It is covered with harsh hairs.

Forequarters: Muscular shoulders are very strong, moderately sloping and boned forelegs are straight. The pasterns are short and supple.

Hindquarters: Muscular thighs are strong with well let down hock joints.

Feet: These are moderately large and round with close set and arched toes and padded sole.

Coat: The hairs are rough and hard on body, head, face, legs and jaws. The colour may be grey, red, black, fawn, brindle, white or other such shades.

Size and Weight: The minimum height of dogs at withers is 77.5 cm and that of bitches is 71

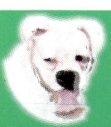

cm. Similarly minimum body weights of corresponding sexes are about 54 and 41 kg respectively.

NORWEGIAN ELK HOUND

Originally it is a working dog of arctic area and a member of spitz variety. Elkhounds are very tactical breed and used for hunting elks. The dog is very strong, active, alert, hard and imaginative. It is highly docile and loyal and famous for devotion towards the family members of owner. Over-feeding spoils the physique and performance of dogs which is highly undesirable. Thus, the dog should be kept active and well maintained for efficient performance.

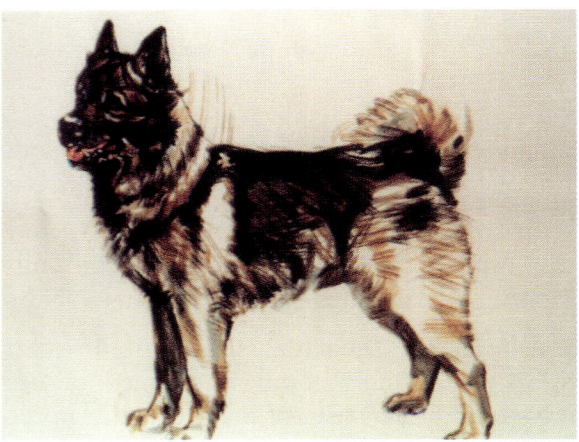

Fig. 62 Norwegian Elk Hound

Head and Face: The skull is broad and a vertical furrow is visible on the forehead. The muzzle is broad at the level of distinct stop and tapers to blunt oral end. The nose is black.

Mouth: Lips are smooth and fine, and strong teeth are arranged scissors bite.

Ears: Triangular pricked medium size ears set high on skull face forward. The tips are pointed.

Eyes: Almond shaped and moderately big eyes are obliquely set at the level of stop. These are dark brown.

Neck: The neck of medium length is firm, muscular and blended with shoulders and brisket. It is strong and carried raised in alert manner.

Body: The body is short, muscular and compact with wide and straight back, deep and capacious chest and less sloping waist region.

Tail: Bushy tail curl slightly over the back.

Forequarters: The shoulders are muscular and powerful which slope moderately forward to join the upper arm. Boned legs are straight and a little shorter than the upper part above the elbow joint. The pasterns are moderately angled and supple.

Hindquarters: The hindquarters are sloping with moderately angled hindlimbs suitable for quick propulsion.

Feet: These are oval and compact with close set and arched toes. The soles are thickly padded and covered with thick keratinized skin.

Coat: The body is covered with water resistant dense coat abundant on neck, body and tail and short on head, face, ears and lower part of limbs. The hairs are longer on ventral aspect of neck and on brisket, belly, under side of tail and posterior aspect of hips. The thighs and hind legs are feathered. Colour is various shades of grey with black tip of hairs.

Size and Weight: The height at withers is 45 to 51 cm and body weight is about 20 to 25 kg. and heavier animals are unwanted.

OTTER HOUND

Packs of this dog were used for hunting otters and that is the genesis of the name Otter

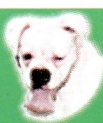

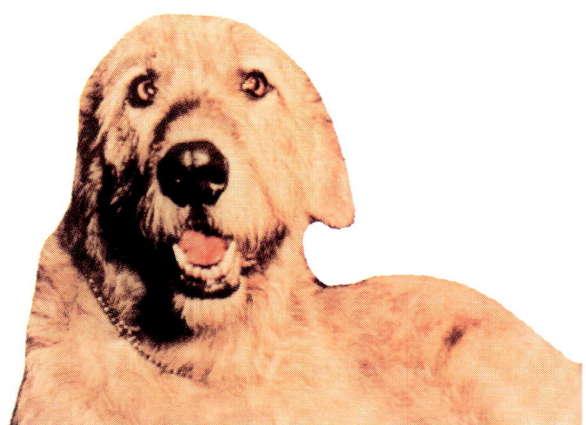

Fig. 63 Otter Hound–Face

Hound. This breed has been evolved from the genetic amulgamation of active breeds like Airedale, Blood Hound and Spaniels. This is a working breed and possesses very sensitive nose and can follow otter moving submerged in water. Otter Hounds may swim for few hours for hunting otters. This shows the strength and stamina of the dog. Now-a-days this breed is diminishing at a fast rate as otters are now not hunted.

Head and Face: The head is broad, muzzle is wide, stop is shallow and nose is generally black.

Mouth: Flewed upper lip over shot the lower lip. The teeth are strong.

Ears: These are long, feathered and hanging. The leather may reach upto the level of throat.

Eyes: Small Eyes are placed in line with the stop.

Neck: Although medium in size the neck appears small due to heavy feathering of rough coat.

Body: The body is longer than the height. The dorsal line is straight. There is no sway during walk in compact body. The chest is moderately deep.

Tail: Feathered medium size tail is carried high above the back.

Forequarters: The shoulders are muscled but less oblique. The boned forelegs are straight. Pasterns are small and less flexible.

Hindquarters: The thighs are thickly muscled and powerful. The legs are well angulated for efficient propulsion during swimming.

Feet: Round feet are large and padded.

Coat: The under coat is dense and fine while outer coat is harsh, and both layers are oily. These results in emitence of strong doggy odour and require occasional washings. Coat colour is gizzle or sandy with well defined black or tan colour.

Size and Weight: The height at withers ranges between 61 to 69 cm and body weight between 30 to 35 kg.

SALUKI

It is a breed of Grey Hound group of dogs and Saluki is perhaps one of the earliest breed of this family. The dog is probably evolved in an ancient Arabian town 'Saluk' from where it spread to Europe, Indian sub-continent and other countries. Another theory of its origin is a crossbred of Indian and Egyption Grey Hounds.

The Saluki is an elegant, graceful, intelligent, agile and affectionate dog with slender body and graceful disposition. At present two varieties, i.e. smooth and feathered are found.

Head and Face: The head is clean with slightly domed occiput and long, narrow and thin face with slightly arched muzzle. Nose is black or flesh marked and blunt pointed. Stop is moderately formed.

Mouth: The jaws are long and narrow with somewhat projected upper jaw. The teeth

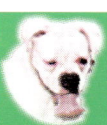

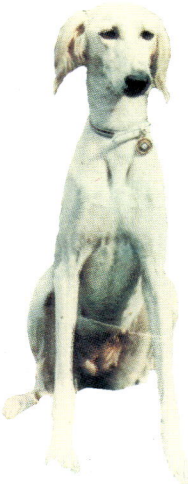

Fig. 64 Saluki

arrangement is either level or scissors bite. Flew is rudimentary and lips are smooth.

Ears: The hanging long ears may extend upto the cheeks and these are covered with long and hanging silky hairs in feathered animals and smooth in others.

Eyes: The large eyes are obliquely set with lower level of inner canthus at the level of stop. Colour of eyes may be light to dark brown.

Neck: It is long, smooth and fine with moderate arch, and carried gracefully high.

Body: The body is elongated, smooth with wide back and prominently arched loins. The chest is deep and narrow which extends to sloping and tucked up belly.

Tail: The low set tail is naturally curved at the distal part. It is well feathered on the under side in feathered variety.

Forequarters: The shoulders are muscular, compact and sloping. Forelegs are boned, long and vertical down the elbow joint. Pasterns are moderately formed.

Hindquarters: The strong hip bones are set apart and covered with well developed compact muscles sloping down to hock joint. The hindlimbs are well angled and hocks are low. Pasterns are almost straight.

Feet: The length of feet is moderate and the toes are well arched and feathered. The sole is cushioned and covered with cornified skin.

Coat: The coat is short, smooth and glossy in smooth haired, and moderately long, wavy and silky in feathered variety. Almost all colours, viz., white, fawn, tan, brown, cream, golden and black whole colour or with patches and tricolour are found. Beautiful feathering of ears and tail adds to the elegance of the dog.

Size and Weight: The height at withers ranges between 58 and 72 cm, and body weight 13 to 30 kg. As usual, females of same litter are usually shorter and lighter than the males.

WHIPPET

Whippet may be described as a miniature form of Grey Hound for persons who have not yet seen the animal. However, this breed of dog is smaller than the Grey Hound, more refined, symmetrical, gentle and lovely. The animal is affectionate, docile, more disease resistant and easy going. It has long life and makes a very good companion.

Head and Face: The head and face together are cone shaped with occiput forming the base. The skull is broad and proportionate to type, while muzzle is tapering. Stop is shallow.

Mouth: It is long and narrow with level lips. Well developed teeth are embedded in strong gums.

Ears: These are small and rose shaped, fine and smooth.

Eyes: Dark eyes are prominent, bright and alert but small in size.

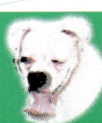

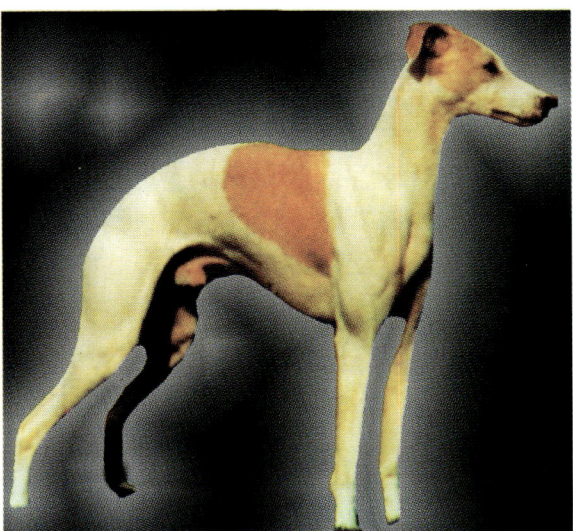

Fig. 65a Whippet—Red and White

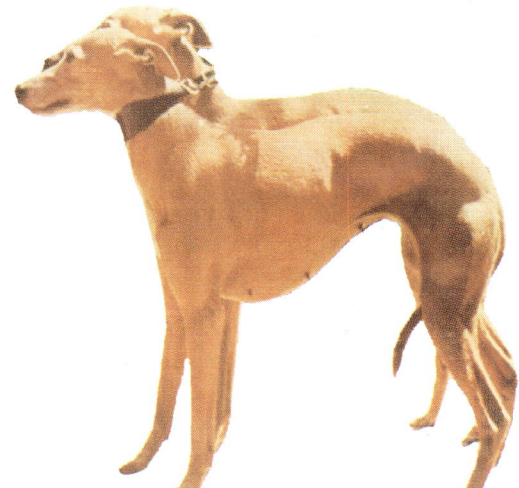

Fig. 65b Whippet Pair—Whole Colour Red

Neck: Long and muscular neck is elegantly arched and carried high in alert dogs.

Body: The body is long, fine and smooth with moderately arched back. Chest is deep and narrow with well defined brisket while loin is tucked up and tapering behind the xiphoid. The croup slopes down to merge with the hip.

Tail: Long and tapering tail hangs between the legs in standing dogs but carried upward delicately curved in dogs on run.

Forequarters: The blades of oblique shoulders extend upto the spine and closely set together at the withers. The upper arm is well muscled and sloping to merge with the bony legs. The pasterns are supple.

Hindquarters: These are very strong with well muscled broad thighs. The dog usually stands with hindlegs ready to spring on the ground and showing great driving power.

Feet: These are neet with loose set and well arched toes. The thick and strong pads are very rough.

Coat: Fine and short coat closely covers the body which makes grooming and cleaning very easy. All colours are acceptable but any solid colour is preferred.

Size and Weight: The height of dogs at withers is 46 to 55 cm and that of bitches is 44 to 53 cm. Body weights of dogs are 8 to 13 kg and that of bitches 5.5 to 10 kg.

V. Terrier breeds

1. Airedale Terrier
2. Australian Terrier
3. Bedlington Terrier
4. Border Terrier
5. Boston Terrier
6. Bull Terrier
7. Bull Terrier Miniature
8. Cairn Terrier
9. Dandie Dinmont Terrier
10. Fox Terrier (Smooth haired)
11. Fox Terrier (Wire haired)
12. Irish Terrier
13. Kerry Blue Terrier

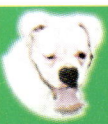

14. Manchester Terrier
15. Norfolk Terrier
16. Norwich Terrier
17. Scotish Terrier
18. Sealyham Terrier
19. Skye Terrier
20. Tibetan Terrier
21. Welsh Terrier
22. Yorkshire Terrier

AIREDALE TERRIER

Its origin is Airedale and it possesses high terrier characteristics. The breed was recognized at a show in England during the last quarter of nineteenth century and since then gained more popularity, and also spread to other countries. The dog is smart, active, gay and sporting. Later on its popularity recorded some decline due to its large size and it is also time consuming to keep it clean.

Head and Face: The head is made of a long and almost flat skull of moderate width. The broad and long muzzle is strong and stop is almost rudimentary. The nose is black.

Mouth: The level lips are tight and teeth are strong.

Eyes: These are small, V-shaped with rounded tip hanging upto the level of the outer canthus of eyes.

Ears: Small eyes are set oblique with inner canthus at the level of rudimentary stop.

Neck: The neck of moderate length is clean, smooth, muscular and blended with shoulders and brisket.

Body: Strong and compact muscular body is short and level. The chest is deep with moderately sprung ribs.

Tail: The straight tail is set high and carried almost perpendicular.

Forequarters: Long and muscular shoulders are close set with chest. The boned forelegs are straight and pasterns are short and less supple.

Hindquarters: These are compact and long with well laid down hocks.

Feet: Small, round and compact feet are well padded, and toes are close set.

Coat: It is coarse, dense and wiry. Colour of body is black or Zizzle with tan markings on ears, head, sides of skull and legs.

Size and Weight: Average height of dogs is about 59 cm and that of bitches is 57 cm and body weight 20 kg approximately.

AUSTRALIAN TERRIER

The ancestors of this breed were introduced from British Isles but due to specific changes in phenotypic look the evolved breed became Australian Terrier. This is a dwarf variety with small limbs, long body, long coat and alert disposition.

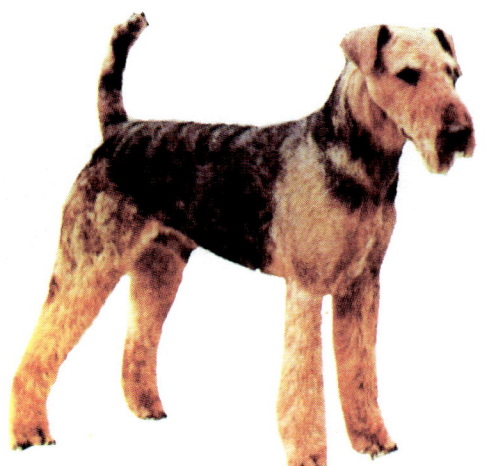

Fig. 66 Airedale Terrier

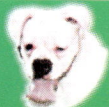

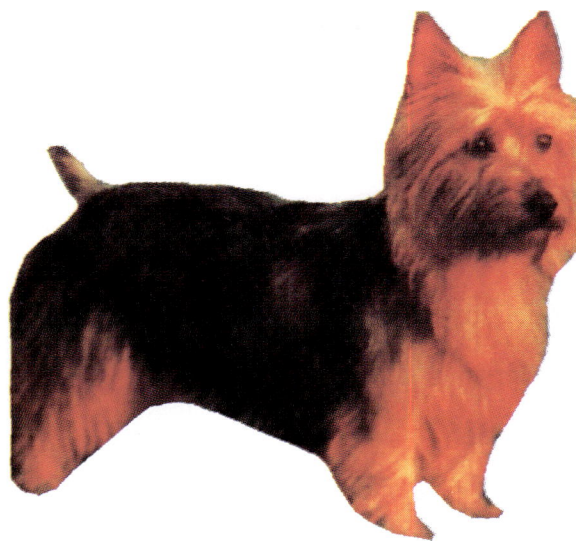

Fig. 67 Australian Terrier

Head and Face: The head is long, skull is flat and stop is shallow. The muzzle is long and powerful with flat nasal bone and black nose.

Mouth: The jaws are level and conical and teeth are arranged level bite.

Ears: Small and pricked ears are set high on the skull. The parietal surface is smooth and frontal surface is covered with fine and soft hairs.

Eyes: Almond shaped small eyes are set almost in line with the shallow stop. These are dark in colour.

Neck: It is long and broad and covered with dense mane.

Body: The body is long with straight back and deep chest with well sprung ribs. Loin region is relatively less sloping.

Tail: Stump of docked tail is carried high.

Forequarters: Well blend muscular shoulders are strong and blend with small, boned and straight fore legs. The pasterns are supple.

Hindquarters: These are muscular and strong with slightly bent hock joints.

Feet: These are round, small, clean and padded with moderately arched toes and black nails.

Coat: The body is covered with long hairs all-over except the muzzle, part of ears and lower of limbs. The colour of body coat may be blue, red, sandy or silver grey. There may be tan markings on legs and face with some of the coat colours.

Size and Weight: Body weight of animals may range from 4.5 to 6.2 kg.

BEDLINGTON TERRIER

This breed shows the mingled characteristics of Terrier and Hound. It is an animal of moderate size and pleasing personality as desired in a good companion. The dog is kept well trimmed of rough hair.

Head and Face: The head is pear shaped with round nose bridge without any stop and black or brown nose.

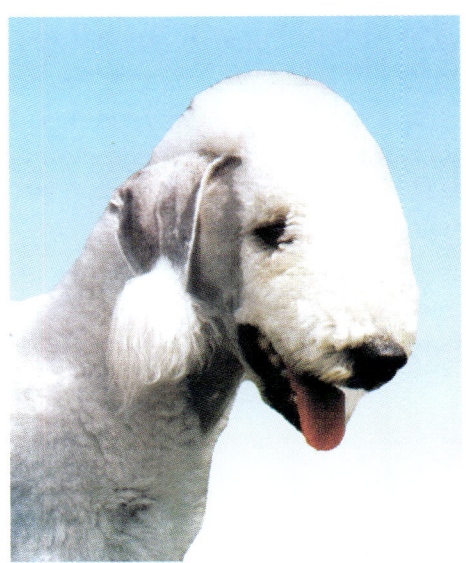

Fig. 68 Bedlington Terrier

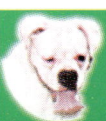

Mouth: The jaws are level or pincer like with strong teeth.

Ears: Long filbert shaped and low set drooping flat ears are placed across the cheek.

Eyes: These are small and bright with dark or lighter colour depending on the coat colour.

Neck: It is long and tapering without defined throat.

Body: Muscular body is flat and flexible with deep chest, rounded back, arched loin, and prominent brisket and sloping croup.

Tail: Low set, tapering with thick base and gracefully lifted diagonally.

Forequarters: The shoulders are close set, compact, well muscled upto arms and boned legs are vertically placed. Pasterns are short and supple.

Hindquarters: Muscular hind quarter is strong and hind legs appear longer than the forelegs due to arching of loin.

Feet: These are long with arched toes and thickly padded sole.

Coat: The coat is thick and crimbled. It has tendency to twist. Clipping is common for this breed. The colours are blue, blue and tan, liver or sandy.

Size and Weight: Height of dogs at withers is 41.5 cm and that of bitches is 39.5 cm, and body weight for both sexes ranges between 8 and 10.5 kg.

BORDER TERRIER

It is fearless, bold, agile and accommodative besides being friendly with children. Origin of this little dog is the hills at the border of England and Scotland. Border Terriers do not like fighting with other dogs. The dog is clean,

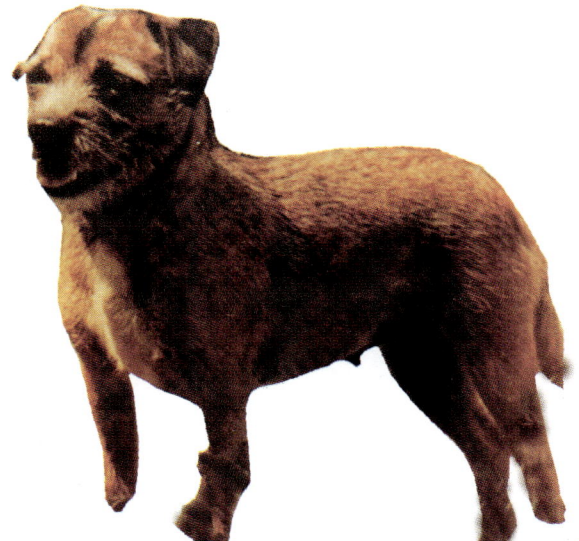

Fig. 69 Border Terrier

small, handy, loyal and gentle due to which it has greater popularity.

Head and Face: The prominent head resembles with the head of otter due to wide skull and small but broad and strong muzzle. Nose should be preferably black. Stop is shallow.

Mouth: Upper lip is flewed with shaded and smooth margin. The teeth are mostly scissors bite but may be level bite also.

Ears: Small V-shaped drooping ears are set apart on either side of the skull. These drop forward along the cheek.

Eyes: These are almond shaped, dark and almost in line with the stop.

Neck: It is short, muscular, fine and smooth.

Body: The barrel shaped body is compact and rounded with little sloping from chest to waist. Brisket is clean and there is almost no sloping at croup.

Tail: It is thick, medium and almost straight. It is never docked.

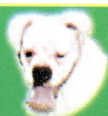

Forequarters: The shoulders are close set to chest and smooth with moderate forward slope and joining the muscular arm which extends down as straight forelegs. Pasterns are supple.

Hindquarters: The hips and thighs are well muscled and powerful. The limbs are moderately angulated.

Feet: These are small and padded with arched and close set toes. The nails are black.

Coat: Under coat is very short and dense whereas outer coat is harsh and dense. Coat colour may be red, brown, fawn, gizzle and tan. Sometimes blue and tan animals are also found.

Size and Weight: Average height at withers is 25 cm. The body weight of males is 6 to 7 kg and that of bitches is 5 to 6 kg.

BOSTON TERRIER

This breed was evolved in United States of America through inter-crossing between English Bulldogs and White English Terriers. The breeding was managed to retain almost

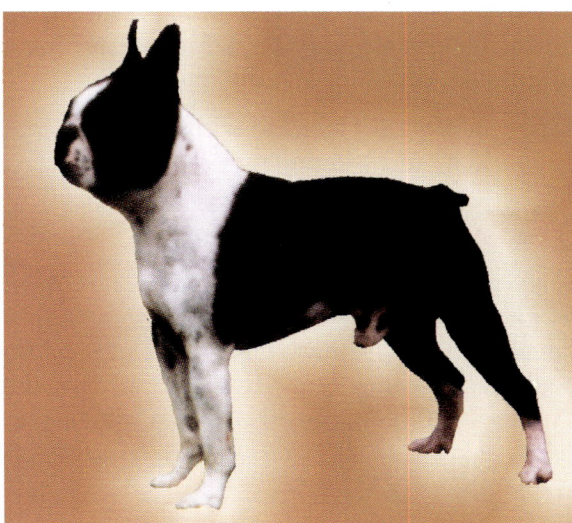

Fig. 70 Boston Terrier

Bulldog like face. It is a compact dog of medium size, active, alert, intelligent, patient and well mannered. It makes a good companion dog.

Head and Face: The square head is short with moderately convex forehead and broad blunt face like that of Bulldog. Nose is short, pulled back and black. Stop is clear and length between stop and nose tip is shorter than the part above the stop.

Mouth: Muzzle is broad and strong with flappy flew of upper lip. Lower lip long but not overshot. Generally mouth is kept close. Strong teeth are embedded in black gums.

Ears: Ears are large, triangular with broad base and pointed tip. These face side-wards and distance between bases of ears is wide.

Neck: It is short, fine, strong and well set on the shoulders.

Body: Compact and muscular body is short with straight dorsal line and slopping croup. Chest is deep with well-sprung ribs and posterior portion moderately tapers up to waist region.

Tail: It is short, twisted and carried low and turned to side.

Forequarters: Shoulders are broad, strong and obliquely set. Arms are boned, strong and straight. Pastern is long, almost straight and flexible.

Hindquarters: Hindquarters are well muscled and strong with moderately pushed back hock and straight downwards.

Feet: These are rounded with slightly arched and close set toes and curved pointed nails. Pads are well developed and coarse due to cornification.

Coat: Body coat is short, smooth and fine. The colour is brindle with white blaze, flew, brisket and pasterns or toes and some part of tail.

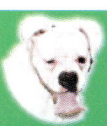

Size and Weight: Height of adults at withrs is 38 to 43 cm and body weight 11 to 12 kg.

BULL TERRIER

This breed has been evolved from the cross-breeding between Bulldog and Terriers to evolve a lighter and agile breed during first half of nineteenth century. These are friendly with amicable temperament, obedient and loyal but not ferocious. These medium sized animals are excellent guards and good companion.

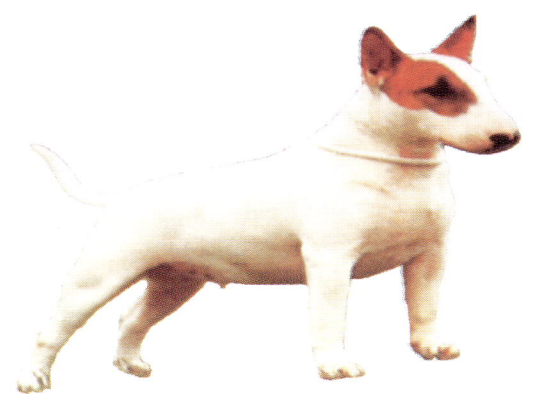

Fig. 71 Bull Terrier

Head and Face: Long head is ovoid and face is elongated. Front is straight without stop. Nose is black and sometimes may leave flesh marks.

Mouth: It is long and lips are sharp and smooth. Flew is almost unnoticed. Sharp and strong scissors bite teeth are present embedded in dark gums.

Ears: These are long, erect, triangular, pointed, set reasonably backwards and tips are apart than the base. Inner surface is almost devoid of hairs.

Eyes: Almond shaped obliquely set small eyes are dark and narrow with sharp glint.

Neck: Muscular, fine, smooth and long neck is moderately arched.

Body: Body is rounded, robust and strong with broad and deep chest, well sprung ribs and strong and wide brisket. Back is somewhat convex beyond the saddle and moderately slopping in the croup region. Waist is a little narrower than the chest.

Tail: It is thick at the base and gradually taper to blunt tip, and slightly upwards curved is carried horizontal.

Forequarters: Shoulders are strong and muscular, and fore limbs are bony, short and straight, while pasterns are short, straight, slightly forward and flexible.

Hindquarters: Muscular hips and thigh are powerful which slopes down to slightly angular hocks and a little forward carried lower limbs.

Feet: These are semi circular with clean arched and knotty toes. Soles are well padded and coarse.

Coat: Smooth coat is made of short and hard hairs. Its colour may be white with black, brindle and black or brindle markings.

Size and Weight: Height at withers ranges from 50 to 54 cm and weight from 23 to 28 kg.

BULL TERRIER MINIATURE

It is a miniature strain of Bull Terrier evolved in Great Britain. This breed was probably developed from a native breed of nineteenth century. Another contributor to add in the development of this breed is old toy bull terrier. This is an active tiny breed of playful companion dogs.

All the physical features of this miniature breed are similar to Standard Bull Terrier except the

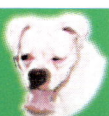

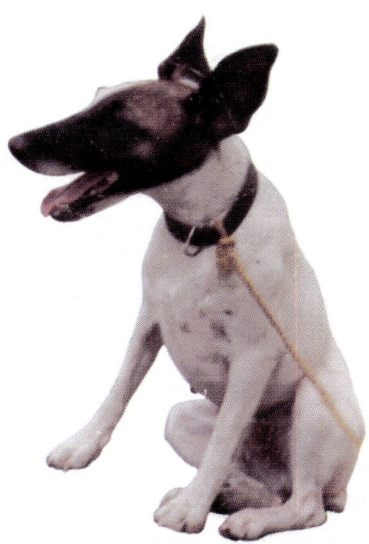

Fig. 72 Bull Terrier–Miniature

maximum height restricted to 35.5 cm and maximum body weight not more than 9 kg.

CAIRN TERRIER

It is a small hairy breed of Scotland. A sturdy dog is useful game and working breed. It is affectionate and good companion in small houses.

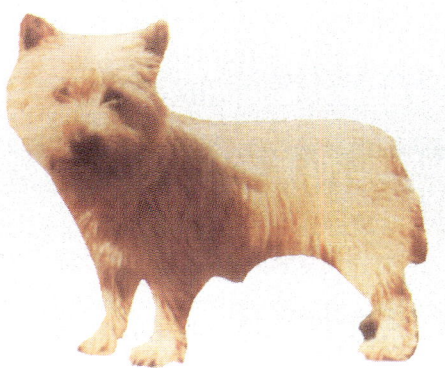

Fig. 73 Cairn Terrier

Head and Face: Proportionate to body and covered with long hairs; display clear shallow stop differentiating the fore head and muzzle. Nose is black.

Mouth: Mouth is usually kept open but tongue dose not protrude in general. Canines are prominent and teeth are arranged in scissors bite manner. Lips are black.

Ears: These are short, triangular, placed well apart living wide occiput, pricked and face forward. Inner side is clean.

Eyes: These are deep set in line with the stop and dark hazel in colour.

Neck: It is proportionate to body, highly frilled and moderately arched.

Body: Body is long and hairy with straight dorsal line.

Tail: It is bushy.

Forequarters: Shoulders are strong and straight limbs are short.

Hindquarters: Well muscled strong hindquarters are reasonably angled at stifles and hocks but straight downward.

Feet: These are semicircular and covered with hairs. Soles are well padded and rough.

Coat: It is double coated animal. Under coat is short, dense and fine, while outer coat is long, fringed and coarse may be red, sandy, grey, brindle or brindle and black.

Size and Weight: Height at withers is about 25 cm and weight is 5-6 kg.

DANDIE DINMONT TERRIER

This small size dog of long body and short legs was evolved from interbreeding between Terriers at the border of England and Scotland. The fur on head appears like a wig.

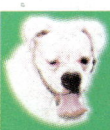

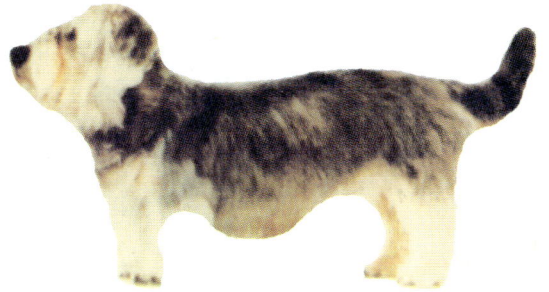

Fig. 74 Dandie Dinmont Terrier

Head and Face: Large dome shaped convex head is broad at the level of ears. The muzzle is short and cone shaped, and nose is black.

Mouth: It is short with slightly overshot and smooth upper lip. The upper teeth are level and slightly overlapping.

Ears: These are low set, long, hanging and heavily feathered. These reach upto the cheeks.

Eyes: These are large, round, prominent, alert and dark in colour.

Neck: It is moderate and carried almost straight over the shoulders and brisket. It is covered with soft ruff.

Body: It is long and flexible with somewhat depressed shoulders, straight back, moderately arched loin and sloping croup upto the root of the tail. The chest is deep but body appears like a barrel due to low sloping towards the waist.

Tail: It is long, fully feathered and curved like a shallow sickle or single edged sword. The length of tail may be 20 to 25 cm.

Forequarters: The shoulders are little depressed and forelegs are small and straight.

Hindquarters: The hips are dropped, thighs are strong and smallhind legs are properly angled.

Feet: These are round, feathered and padded with moderately arched toes.

Coat: The body coat is a mixture of soft and coarse hairs of light to dark grey colour which is described as pepper or mustard colour. The furred head is very attractive and entire body is well feathered.

Size and Weight: The height at withers may range from 20 to 28 cm, and body weight from 8 to 11 kg.

FOX TERRIER (Smooth Haired)

It is evaluated as one of the best Terrier and lively pet. It is active, obedient and courageous dog, and makes a very good companion. This breed is very popular in United States, Canada, India and Australia. The name evolved from its use for fox baiting in ancient time.

Head and Face: The head is flat and long face is made of powerful tapering muzzle and black nose. Bridge of nose is continuous with the skull without any defined stop.

Mouth: Mouth is long and lips are without any flew. Strong teeth are arranged scissors bite.

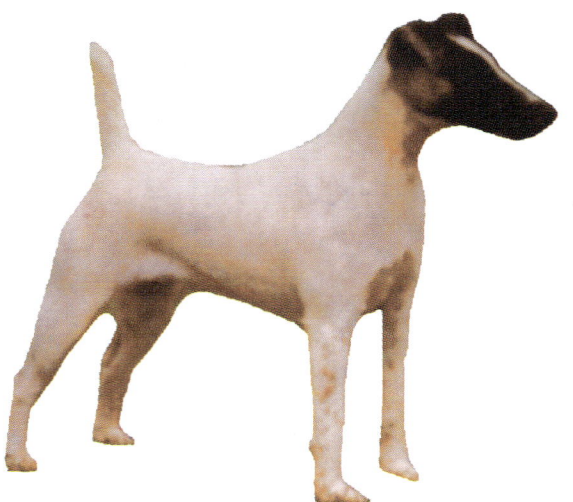

Fig. 75 Fox Terrier–Smooth Haired

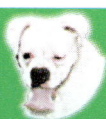

Ears: These are small, high set and drop forward.

Eyes: Almond shaped dark eyes are set oblique.

Neck: It is long, stout, compact, fine, slightly arched and normally kept proudfully high.

Body: Body is moderate, well muscled, compact and straight dorsally. The chest is moderately deep and backward slope is small.

Tail: It is smooth and docked living behind a stump of about 10-15 cm.

Forequarters: Strong, muscular and smooth shoulders join strong upper arms and continue with bony and straight fore arms and supple pasterns.

Hindquarters: Well muscled and powerful hindquarters slope down proportionately to thigh and boned lower limbs. Pasterns are supple.

Feet: These are rounded with close set and arched toes.

Coat: It is short, dense and smooth and white colour has black, tan or dark brown markings of different size generally patches.

Size and Weight: Height at withers is 35 to 40 cm and body weight 7 to 8 kg. Bitches are generally lighter than the dogs.

FOX TERRIER (Wire Haired)

Probably it is an English breed, which is active, attractive and playful. It is a good barker. This is highly wanted house dog. This breed is perhaps a mutant of smooth haired fox terrier and it was developed much later than its ancestors.

Head and Face: Head is flat and face is elongated oval. Muzzle is long, stop is absent and nose is thinner.

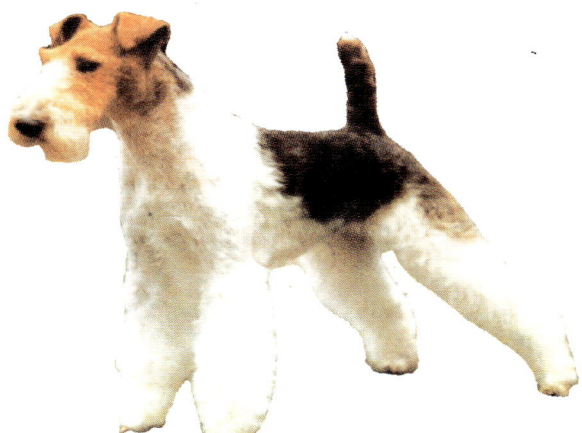

Fig. 76 Fox Terrier—Wire haired

Mouth: It is long with levelled lips. Teeth are scissors bite and canine teeth are long.

Ears: These are small and set high on the skull. Pinnae are V-shaped with round tip and half fold forward to lie over the cheeks.

Eyes: Almond shaped with almost half curved upper lid and dark eyes are characteristic for the breed.

Neck: Neck is moderately long, muscular, slightly arched and held high.

Body: It is muscular, compact and straight dorsally with deep chest, broad brisket and slightly sloping waist. Body is shorter than the limbs.

Tail: It is docked living behind a stump of 8-10 cm

Forequarters: These are clean and muscular with boned straight limbs.

Hindquarters: These are powerful and less angular.

Coat: It is longer, dense and moderately curled to produce characteristic appearance of the breed. Colour is white with brown or black patches.

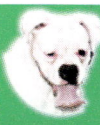

Size and Weight: Height at withers measures 35-40 cm and weight is 7 to maximum 8 kg.

IRISH TERRIER

This breed was perhaps first time recognised during the last quarter of the nineteenth century. It is a native of Ireland and it was evolved as a gun dog with retrieving ability. These are tough, courageous, active and easily trainable dogs of non-agitative temperament. It is a kind, lovable and dignified animal displaying a well developed beard.

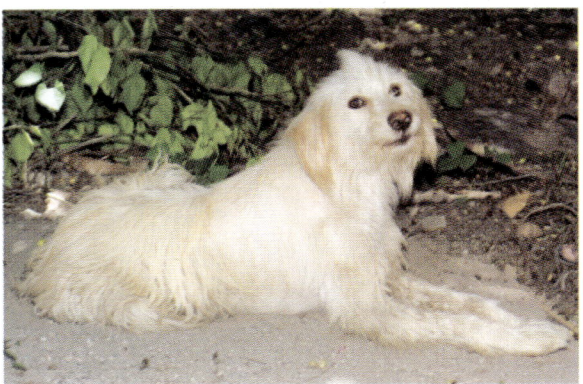

Fig. 77 Irish Fox Terrier–Smooth Haired

Head and Face: Long head is narrow between the ears which extends upto the level of well defined stop. The sockets of eyes are prominent. The muzzle is long, narrow and bonny with straight nose bridge.

Mouth: The upper jaw is a little over shot and slightly flewed. Teeth are strong and even bite.

Ears: Forward dropping medium size ears are set a little back on the skull. The leathers hang upto the level of throat.

Eyes: These are dark, bright, active, a little sunken and small, and placed almost in line with the stop.

Neck: It is moderately long with broad shoulders and gradually sloping upwards.

Body: It is muscular with straight top line, sloping croup and deep but somewhat flat chest. Muscular loin is slightly arched.

Tail: It is docked to live behind a long stump of about three fourth of its length. The smooth tail stump is set high and carried gaily.

Forequarters: The compact shoulders are fine, well muscled and less sloped. Boned forelegs are straight. The pasterns are short and straight.

Hindquarters: The hips and thighs are muscular and strong. Powerful hindlegs are moved straight. The shannons are short and straight.

Feet: These are round, small and strong with arched toes and padded sole.

Coat: It is short, coarse, wiry and broken. It is more dense and crisp on legs but without any feathering. Whole colour red, brownish red or yellow red coats are typical for the breed.

Size and Weight: The height at withers is about 45 cm, and desired body weights of dogs and bitches are about 12.5 and 11 kg respectively.

KERRY BLUE TERRIER

There are many stories about the genesis of this breed, which was probably refined in Kerry county of Ireland. The blue coat colour was established through selective breeding. This breed was known as Irish Blue Terrier also for several years. It is a medium breed slightly taller than Bedlington and shorter than Airedale Terrier. The puppies born black gradually change to characteristic blue coat following puberty. The breed has spread to many countries but mostly in limited number.

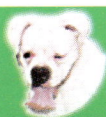

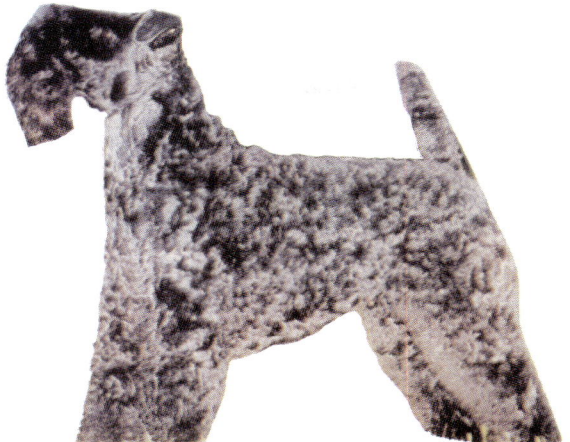

Fig. 78a Kerry Blue Terrier

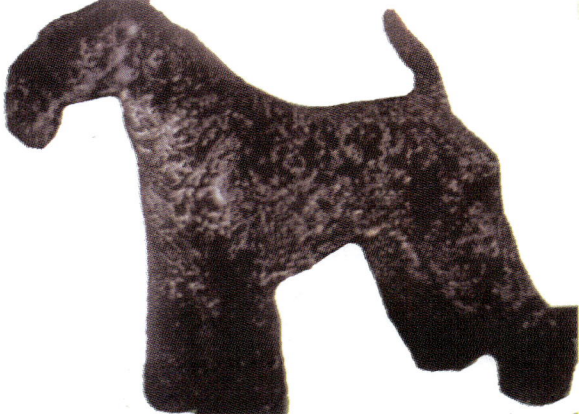

Fig. 78b Kerry Blue Terrier

Body: It is short and compact with deep and capacious chest, less sloping loin and straight dorsal line.

Tail: Docked tail with moderate stump is set high and displayed erect.

Forequarters: Flat shoulders are close to chest upto elbow joints. The straight forelegs are moderately boned and powerful. Pasterns are also straight.

Hindquarters: Proportionately muscled large and developed hindquarters are carried on moderately angulated strong limbs.

Feet: These are round, small, close set and well padded with black nails.

Coat: Body is covered with profusely growing wavy, soft and silky coat of various blue shades. There may be small white patches on chest.

Size and Weight: The height of dogs at withers is 45 to 48 cm and body weight 15 to 17 kg. The bitches of same litter are mostly lighters.

MANCHESTER TERRIER

It is an English breed of Manchester, which has been refined through selective breeding to modern standard. At one stage the breed was

Head and Face: Elongated head with almost flat skull and rudimentary stop is well balanced. The face is long, strong and deep with little tapering towards oral end. The nose is black.

Mouth: It is long and strong with level lips and strong level bite teeth embedded in dark gums.

Ears: These may be small to medium in size, V-shaped, bent downwards and placed forward at the level of forehead. These are fine and smooth.

Eyes: Small and dark Eyes are placed oblique.

Neck: The neck is broad at shoulders and sloping upwards with somewhat hollow jawl.

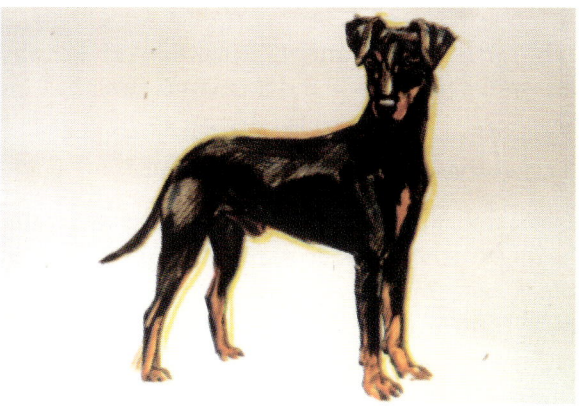

Fig. 79 Manchester Terrier

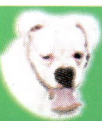

threatened but later on it was revived and its popularity increased. The animal is smooth and fine.

Head and Face: The wedge shaped head with broad occiput and tapering muzzle is characteristic for the breed.

Mouth: The teeth are level set.

Ears: Medium size ears are set high, face forward and carried half bent.

Eyes: Dark eyes are small, bright and set moderately oblong with inner canthus at the level of shallow stop.

Neck: It is fine, smooth, broad at the base and slightly sloping upwards, a little arched, muscular, strong and elegant.

Body: The body is well muscled, compact and round dorsally. Back is straight and croup is moderately drooping. Broad and deep chest with well sprung ribs reaches upto elbow joint. The belly is slopy and tuckedup to certain extent.

Tail: It is smooth, tapering and carried almost straight at the level of back.

Forequarters: The strong shoulders are smooth and close set with chest, moderately sloping. Boned forelegs are straight and pasterns are reasonably flexible.

Hindquarters: Hip and thigh are powerful, limbs are well angled and hind Sannan is straight.

Feet: These are round, thickly padded and arched toes are close set.

Coat: Short and smooth coat is made of glossy hairs which make grooming easy. Colour is black with tan markings on different parts of face like muzzle, dorsal point of eyes and cheeks, and side of chest, knees and vent etc. A thumb mark like impression above the feet and light penciling of toes are specific features.

Size and Weight: The height of adult dogs at withers is an average 40 cm and that of bitches is 37.5 cm. Body weight of both sexes should not exceed 10 kg.

NORFOLK TERRIER

Probably nothing specific is known about the evolution of this breed and it has been perhaps developed from some short legged terriers. The breed was standardized during the early years of twentieth century in England. In early years two varieties, one with erect ears and another with drooping ears existed but during third quarter of the twentieth century only drop eared variety continued as Norfolk Terrier and that with erect ears were separated as a new breed Norwich Terrier in Britain.

Norfolk Terrier is a small, low set dog with coarse body coat. It is a good working variety.

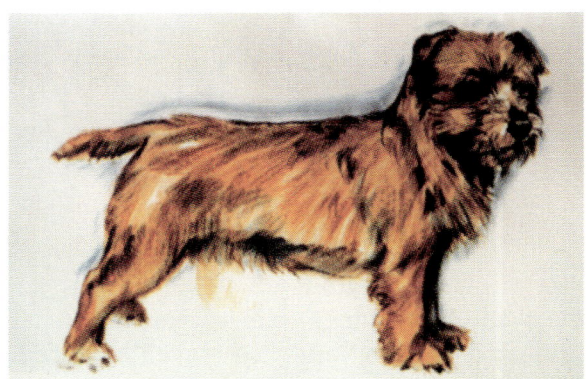

Fig. 80 Norfolk Terrier

Head and Face: The skull is moderately round and muzzle is foxy. The strong muzzle is shorter than the skull. The stop is prominent and nose may be liver colour.

Mouth: The teeth are scissors bite and strong, and jaws are smooth and clean.

Ears: Medium length ears are dropped and placed close to cheeks. The tips are rounded.

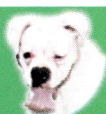

Eyes: These are moderate in size, bright, dark and active.

Neck: It is medium in length and covered with frilled mane.

Body: Elongated muscular and compact body appears somewhat cylindrical with much less narrowing of the loin region. The withers are little higher and posteriorly back is straight upto croup. The chest is deep reaching upto elbow.

Tail: It is medium docked.

Forequarters: These are muscular and powerful. The arms are strong and forelegs are boned and short.

Hindquarters: Well muscled and powerfully strong hindquarters with proper angulation of limbs for propulsion are the characteristics.

Feet: These are round with arched and close set toes. The soles are padded.

Coat: The outer coat is made of coarse, wiry and straight longer hairs on the body, neck and upper part of limbs. However, hairs on ears, muzzle and skull are short. Coat colour may be all shades of red, black, tan and wheaten. White markings are usually not liked but do not disqualify for show.

Size and Weight: Average height of dogs at withers is about 25 cm.

NORWICH TERRIER

This breed was separated from the Norfolk Terrier in Great Britain during the year 1965 and it included the variety with pricked ear. It is not only the ears but otherwise also its morphology is much different than the Norfolk Terrier. It is a small breed of longer body carried on small feathery limbs.

Head and Face: The skull is broad and a little rounded with almost flat forehead and distinct

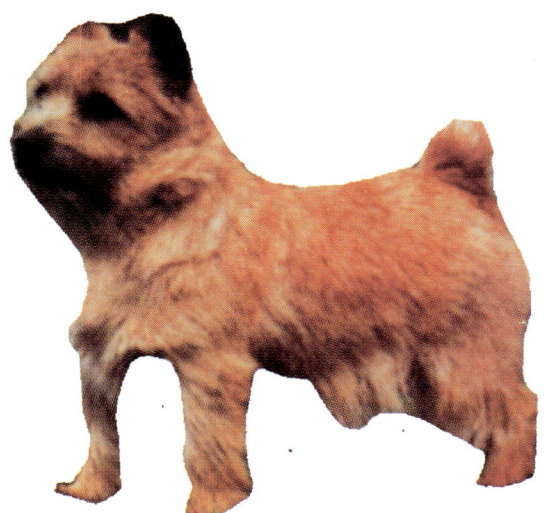

Fig. 81 Norwich Terrier

stop. The muzzle is longer than the distance between centre of the occiput to upper end of stop. Nose bone is straight and nose is black with upward extended shade.

Mouth: The lips are smooth and teeth are scissor bite with very prominent canines.

Ears: Medium size erect ears face forward. The tips are blunt pointed and base is set apart on the skull.

Eyes: Almond shaped eyes are somewhat obliquely set on either side of nose bone at the level of stop. These are dark shaded and bright.

Neck: It is moderately long and carried high. The neck is heavily frilled with long and straight hairs.

Body: It is short, compact and rounded dorsally. The chest is deep with well sprung ribs and sloping towards waist is moderate.

Tail: As per breed requirement it is medium docked.

Forequarters: Well muscled powerful shoulders are laid back properly into short and

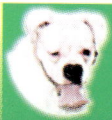

boned straight forelegs. The pasterns are small and flexible.

Hindquarters: These are powerful with good propulsion ability due to angulation of hind-limbs.

Feet: These are round with arched toes and well padded.

Coat: The hairs on neck and shoulders are more coarser and longer than the rest of the body. Entire body is covered with moderately long straight and also wiry hairs, which are softer on brisket and abdomen but short on head, muzzle and ears. Coat colour may be all shades of red, brown, black and tan. White markings are unwanted.

Size and Weight: Average height at withers is about 25 cm.

SCOTTISH TERRIER

It is a small, compact and sturdy dog. Earlier this was known as Abardeen terrier, which was registered with the name of Scottish Terrier during the last phase of the nineteenth century.

Head and Face: The head is long and narrow

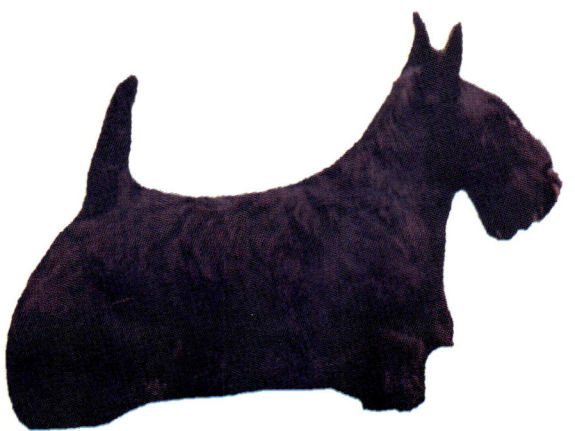

Fig. 82a Scottish Terrier

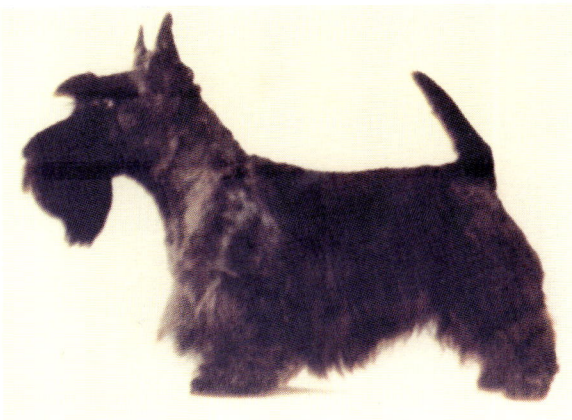

Fig. 82b Scottish Terrier

with a distinct stop. The nose is large and muzzle is broad.

Mouth: The lips are level and teeth are large and strong.

Ears: These are clean, smooth and pricked. The ears are set high on the skull and face forward.

Eyes: The almond shaped eyes at the level of stop are dark brown and alert.

Neck: Moderately long neck is muscular and blended with the sloping shoulders.

Body: The body is short and muscular with straight dorsal line. The chest is deep and broad.

Tail: It is thick at the base and tapering to end in a blunt pointed tip. It is carried up right.

Forequarters: The shoulders are sloping and shortforelegs are straight.

Hindquarters: The hips and thighs are muscular and very powerful. The legs are moderately angled and short.

Feet: Circular feet are well padded with arched toes.

Coat: It is a double coated breed with short, dense and very soft under coat. The outer coat

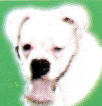

is rough, dense and wiry. The coat colour may be black, brindle or wheaten. However, sandy, iron grey and gizzled animals are also found in USA.

Size and Weight: The height of this breed at wither is about 25 to 28 cm. The body weights of dogs may range from 8.5 to 10.5 kg and that of bitches from 8 to 9.5 kg.

SEALYHAM TERRIER

This breed was evolved in middle of the nineteenth century in a town of Wales. This is one of the aristocratic, beautiful, charming, active and free moving dog. It is a good natured and affectionate companion of small size.

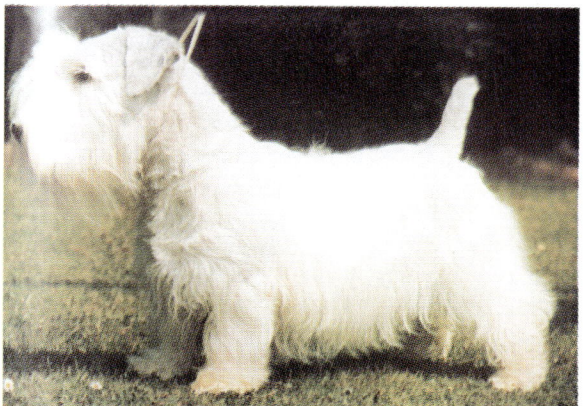

Fig. 83 Sealyham Terrier

Head and Face: A little domed head is broad between the ears and without a defined stop. The bridge of nose is somewhat arched. The muzzle is large and more or less rectangular. It possesses a beautiful beard. The nose is black.

Mouth: The flew is developed and covered with long hairs.

Ears: These are medium in length with rounded tip and reaching upto the cheeks. The ears are dropping, V-shaped and clean.

Eyes: The medium size and round eyes are dark in colour.

Neck: It is reasonably long and muscular with broad base and gradually sloping towards the jawl. The neck is moderately arched.

Body: The length of body is medium and back is level. The chest is broad and deep with well sprung ribs.

Tail: Dock of tail is carried straight.

Forequarters: Muscular shoulders are close set on chest and sloping. The forelegs are boned and straight.

Hindquarters: Well muscled hips and thighs are powerful and properly angled at the stifle joint.

Feet: Rounded feet with loose toes are cat like.

Coat: The coat is long, coarse and wiry and its colour is generally whole white or white with shades of lemon, brown or badger pied markings on head and ears.

Size and Weight: Maximum height of these dogs is about 30 cm at withers, and body weights are about 9 kg and 8 kg for dogs and bitches respectively.

SKYE TERRIER

This breed was evolved by cross-breeding between local Terriers and Maltese about three hundred years ago. It is a furious and intolerant dog which does not allow handling by strangers. A very loyal, cute, active and very long dog moves in a pleasing flaring style. The loyalty of one of the skye named Greyfriare Body has become immortal in the form of a memorial as he could not part away even after the death of his master and remained along his grave for about ten long years.

Head and Face: The head is long, flat and strong. The jaws are short, wide and powerful.

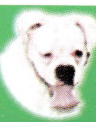

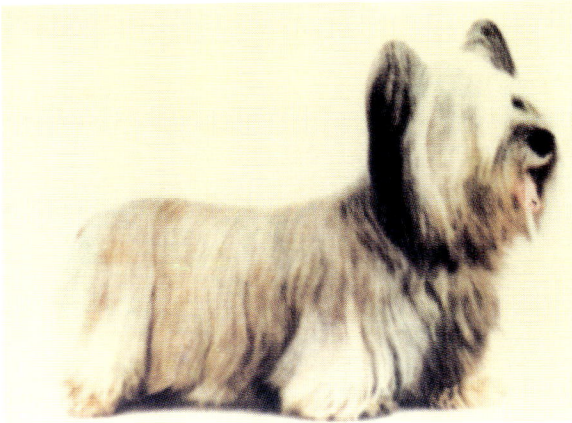

Fig. 84 Sky Terrier

Mouth: It is profusely covered with long hairs. The lips are level and teeth are arranged scissors bite.

Ears: These may be either erect or dropped. Prick ears are shorter than the drop ears. These are heavily feathered and black.

Eyes: Medium size eyes are dark brown.

Neck: Slightly crested neck is long and strong.

Body: The body is long and low set with straight top line, slightly raised loin and deep chest.

Tail: It is heavily feathered with pendulous upper part and somewhat curved lower part which is carried as a continuation of sacral vertebrae.

Forequarters: The shoulders are broad and strong and boned forelegs are very short.

Hindquarters: The hips and thighs are muscular and hindlegs are angulated and short.

Feet: These are long and projected forward.

Coat: It is a double coated small animal. The under coat is short, soft, dense and woolly. The outer coat is very long, coarse and straight which envelopes entire body upto ground. Long hairs along dorsal line appear parted. Any coat colour with black nose and ears are accepted.

Size and Weight: The height at withers is about 25 cm and body length is about 50 cm but from tip of the nose to tip of the tail, these dogs may measure upto 100 cm. Body weight of dogs is about 11.5 kg and that of bitches is about 10 kg.

TIBETAN TERRIER

Despite its name Tibetan Terrier, it is not included in the Terrier group in Britain and clubbed with utility group. This breed closely resembles with the Lhasa Apso but due to longer legs it is like Spitz. It is an old breed patronized in monasteries of Tibet for centuries. They were given as presents to nomadic tribes for lucky achievements. The dogs are used for guard, watch and retrieve lost objects. The long hairs clipped in summer are used for weaving after mixing with yak hair.

Head and Face: Medium size skull slightly narrows from ears to eyes and stop is quite prominent. The muzzle is short and nose is black.

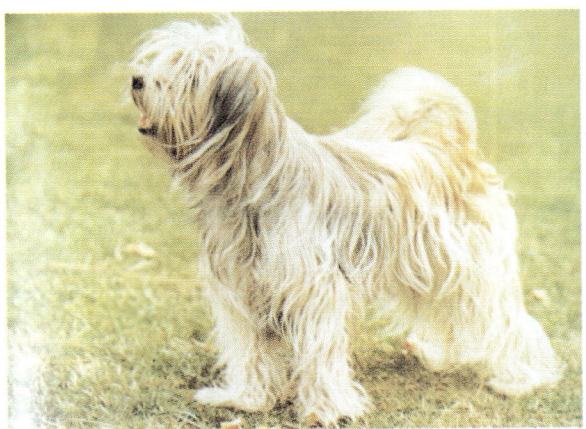

Fig. 85 Tibetan Terrier

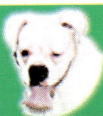

Mouth: Jaws are level but a little under mouth is acceptable.

Ears: These are V-shaped, drooping and heavily feathered.

Eyes: These are placed wide apart, large size and dark with dark eyelids.

Neck: It is short and covered with heavy mane.

Body: The body is squar. Dorsal line is straight, rounded and compact. Chest is moderately deep and loin is less sloping. Croup is sloping.

Tail: Tail of medium length is set gaily high, heavily feathered and carried over the back.

Forequarters: Strong shoulders slope obliquely and bony forelegs are heavily furnished.

Hindquarters: Well muscled hindquarters are heavily furnished and strong pasterns are straight.

Feet: These are large, round, heavily furnished and well padded.

Coat: Double coat with fine, soft and woolly under coat covered with long and straight feathering all over the body may be white, cream, golden, grey, black, parti-coloured or tricolour.

Size and Weight: The height of adult dogs may be 35 to 40 cm and bitches are little smaller and lighter.

WELSH TERRIER

It is considered to be an ancient breed of tiny dog appears like a Miniature Airedale. The dog has been probably descended from the English Black Terrier with characteristic wired hairy terrier. The breed gained popularity during the last quarter of the nineteenth century. It is affectionate, agile, active and obedient dog, which can be trained easily.

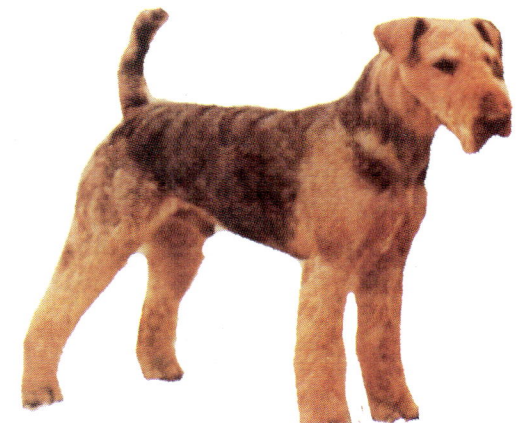

Fig. 86 Welsh Terrier

Head and Face: The skull is clean, flat and wide between the ears. The muzzle is deep and powerful, and stop is shallow. The nasal bone is straight. The head is more masculine and nose is black.

Mouth: The lips are level. The jaws are powerful and level teeth are very strong and embedded in thick gums.

Ears: The V-shaped half turned small ears are set moderately high on the lateral aspects of skull. These are turned forward at the level of the cheek.

Eyes: Bright small almond shaped eyes are set prominently. These are dark.

Neck: It is moderately long, thick and a little arched.

Body: Muscular body is compact with wide rib cage, almost straight dorsal line, deep chest and less tuck up loin.

Tail: Docked tail is carried high.

Forequarters: The shoulders are long, sloping and close set with chest. The muscular legs are straight and strong.

Hindquarters: These are powerful with

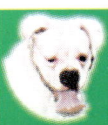

muscular thighs and well let down hocks. The hindlegs are well boned.

Feet: These are small and elongated round like a cat.

Coat: Short coat is close set, dense, coarse and wiry. The coat colour is preferably black and tan but may be black gizzle and tan but tan black below hocks and penciling of toes are disqualification.

Size and Weight: Maximum height of this breed at withers should not be more than 39.5 cm and body weight may range from 9 to 9.5 kg.

YORKSHIRE TERRIER (YORKY)

This is a hairy toy breed developed and refined from the Yorkshire small working dog. There is also a view that the quality and appearance have been produced through the blending of genes from English Terriers and Maltese by several breeding manipulations. This glamorous breed is equally liked by men and women. This breed was listed during later part of the nineteenth century in England and United States of America. Now it is one of the few most popular breeds of dog throughout the world.

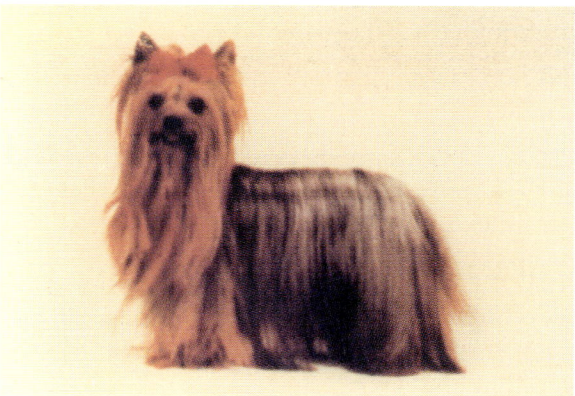

Fig. 87a Yorkshire Terrier–Hair Dressed

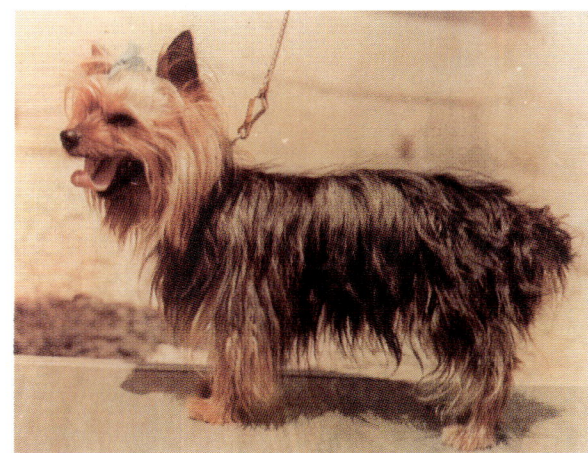

Fig. 87b Yorkshire Terrier

Head and Face: The head is small and flat. The muzzle is moderate and strong, and stop is defined. Frontal part of head and nose bone is fine and smooth, and nose is black.

Mouth: The lips are even and teeth are strong.

Ears: These are small V-shaped and mostly pricked but may be half bent. These are covered with short hairs.

Eyes: These are oblong, medium, dark and bright. Area above upper eyebrow is usually dark shaded.

Neck: It is proportionate to body, carried high and covered with dense, long straight hairs.

Body: It is compact, dorsally straight and heavily feathered.

Tail: Medium length frilled tail is carried a little higher than the level of the back.

Forequarters: The shoulders and tiny straight legs are densely covered with long hairs.

Hindquarters: Similar to forequarters these are also covered with dense long hairs.

Feet: These are round with moderately arched toes and strong black nails.

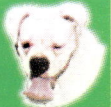

Coat: It is made of long, straight, fine, silky and glossy hairs. Coat colour may be dark steel blue which is darker on dorsal surface. The chest and legs may be bright tan. Coat may be golden tan also.

Size and Weight: The height at withers is about 23 cm and body weight is about 3 kg.

VI.   Toy Breeds

1. Affen Pinscher
2. Chihuahua
3. Maltese
4. Pekingese
5. Pomeranian
6. Poodle Toy
7. Poodle Miniature
8. Pug
9. Shih Tzu
10. Silky Terrier

AFFEN PINSCHER

This is a very small breed of pleasing and playful dog. It is a native of Germany. These dogs are like a small monkey in appearance. Some of these dogs are decorated with a chin tuft and a few others possess moustache.

Head and Face: The head is round and forehead is dome shaped. The muzzles are short and pointed. Entire face is feathered. Nose is black.

Mouth: It is short and level. The lower jaw is a little longer than the upper one. The teeth on two jaws mesh.

Ears: These are prick, triangular and set high on the skull. At some places ears are also clipped.

Eyes: These are big, round, shining and black.

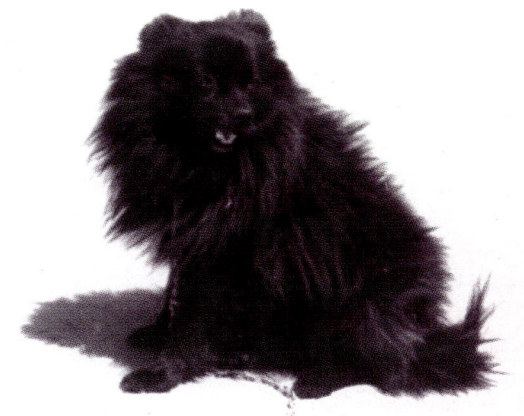

Fig. 88 Affen Pinscher

Neck: The neck is moderately arched, medium in length and profusely feathered.

Body: The body is almost square. The top line slopes a little upto loin. The chest is deep and loin is slightly narrower than the rib cage.

Tail: High set tail is docked to live behind a short stump.

Forequarters: The shoulders are muscular and sloping forward. The forelegs are boned and straight, and pasterns are short.

Hindquarters: The hips are sloping. The hind-legs are almost straight due to very little angulations at stifles and hocks.

Feet: These are round, small, close set, compact and furred.

Coat: The long coat is wiry. The hairs on face, chin and legs are long and shaggy. The head and neck are covered with profusely growing hairs. Coat colour is mostly black but may be black with tan markings, grey, red or other combinations.

Size and Weight: The height at withers is about 26 cm and body weight 3.5 kg but smaller specimens are desired.

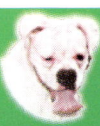

CHIHUAHUA

It is one of the small breeds developed in Mexico but now-a-days most popular in United State of America followed by Europe. It may be also seen in Indian metropolitan cities. Another group claims it a Chinese breed brought to Mexico by Spanish traders. A third suggestion of its development is by Aztec Indians. Due to its tiny size this breed is very popular amongst the families living in the limited space of apartments and also companion for the elderly persons.

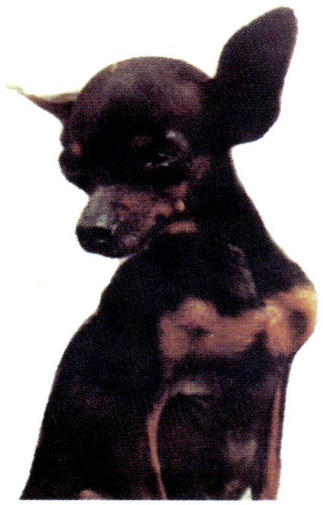

Fig. 89 Chihuahua

Head and Face: Apple shape fine head is convex in a shape of dome at the occiput. Muzzle is sharp. Stop is prominent. Nose is black but may be partly flesh colour in light colour animals.

Mouth: Mouth remains mostly close. Lips are sharp and fine.

Ears: These are long, erect, triangular, blunt pointed, smooth and set apart on the sides of domed occiput.

Eyes: These are round, very black, prominent and in line with the stop.

Neck: It is long, fine, strong and reasonably arched.

Body: It is compact, smooth and longer than its height.

Tail: Curved tail may be carried either over the croup or on the sides.

Forequarters: Smooth and continue with boned short and straight limbs.

Hindquarters: Slightly drooping at the croup and downward continue with moderate angles at joint.

Feet: These are flat with low arched toes and padded sole.

Coat: Coat may be short or long. The former is smooth, close fitted and shiny with feathering tail while later are long coated, fringed ear and bushy tail. Coat colour may be cream, golden, light brown or mixture of these colours.

Size and Weight: Height at withers is 12-15 cm and weight 1 to 2.5 kg. Smallest specimen of 24oz only has been recorded.

MALTESE

It is a lap dog or toy breed originated in Malta and refined in Italy. This small and beautiful creature is completely covered in luxuriant and long silky hair. Its gay disposition, smartness, volatile spirits and good behaviour attract many friends Specially it is liked by ladies and young children. The dog is very intelligent, sensitive, lively and alert. To keep it tidy regular grooming is essential.

Head and Face: The head is balanced and face below stop is about one third. The nose is quite prominent and black.

Mouth: It is small with level lips and covered with silky coat. Teeth are arranged scissors bite.

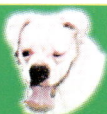

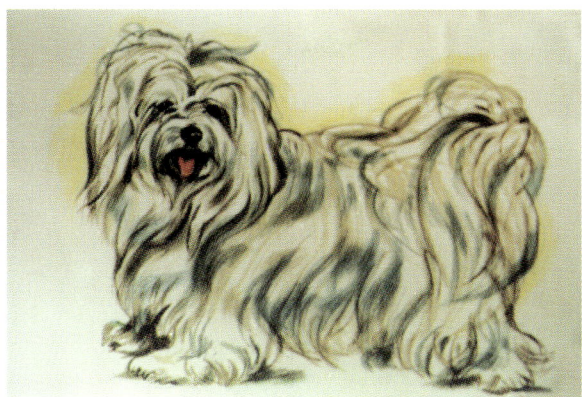

Fig. 90 Maltese

PEKINGESE

It is a Chinese breed of Spaniel group popularly famous as a lap dog. The dog is tiny, balanced and beautiful toy, which is playful and makes a good companion particularly of children because it is never aggressive but fearless and barking. Now these have spread to many countries. It is also popular among the ladies in most of the advanced sophisticated families.

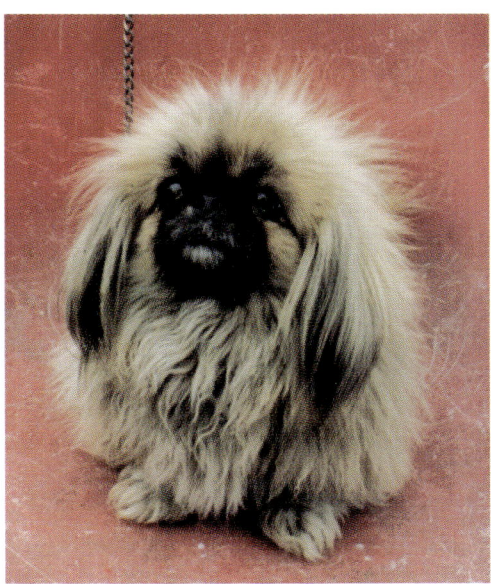

Fig. 91 Pekingese

Ears: These are long, fully feathered and hanging closely on either side of head.

Eyes: These are dark brown with black ring and set somewhat apart at the level of stop.

Neck: Medium size and strong neck is set on the sloping shoulders.

Body: It is short and cobby with straight back. Well sprung ribs provide large space for lungs and heart.

Tail: It is fully feathered and well arched over the back.

Forequarters: The balanced shoulders are compact and short legs are straight.

Hindquarters: Properly angulated hindlegs are short.

Feet: These are rounded with close set and moderately arched toes.

Coat: Coat is formed of straight and long luxuriant silky hairs of 20-25 cm length and without curling or mat formation. Colour is pure white. Rarely light lemon colour is accepted.

Size and Weight: Height of dogs at withers is 20-27 cm and that of bitches is 20-23 cm. Body weights of both sexes ranges between 3 to 4 kg.

Head and Face: The head is wide and sunken in bush of long hairs. Short muzzle is wrinkled on the face. Stop is defined and nose bridge is short. Black nose is broad and face is clean.

Mouth: It is small and long incisors and canines are often visible on the lower jaw. Lips are black.

Ears: The ears are set level with skull and frame the face. These are hidden beneath the dense coat of long hairs.

Eyes: These are big, round, dark and set wide apart at the level of deep stop.

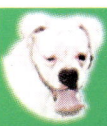

Neck: It is short, thick, highly frilled and hidden in long mane.

Body: It is compact and pear shaped, and longer than the limbs. Entire body is covered under a cover of dense and long outer coat.

Tail: Heavily feathered tail is set high and carried moderately curled over the croup and may also cover some part of loin.

Forequarters: The forelegs are short, heavy boned and bowed.

Hindquarters: The hind limbs are proportionately angled, short and thick.

Feet: These are somewhat flat and slightly turned outwards.

Coat: It is double coated animal covered with a fine, dense and woolly under coat, and a long, straight and thick outer coat. Its colour has wide range viz., red, brown, cream, fawn, black, white, golden and brindle etc.

Size and Weight: Height at withers of dog is 15-20 cm and body weight 3-5 kg.

POMERANIAN

Originally Pomeranian were larger than the modern one and evolved from the dogs of arctic region bred in Prussian state of the ancient Pomerania. There appears to be some relationship with Samoyed and Finnish Spitz breeds. Pomeranians became very popular by first decade of the twentieth century because it got the patronage of Queen Victoria during the last years of nineteenth century. Original Pomeranians were perhaps the hybrids of phenotypically similar breeds and earlier breeders observed that few very small pups in litters discarded as runts grow well without any deformity in the dogs of smaller body size. At present mostly people prefer tiny Pomeranians of pure white fluffy coat appearing like a

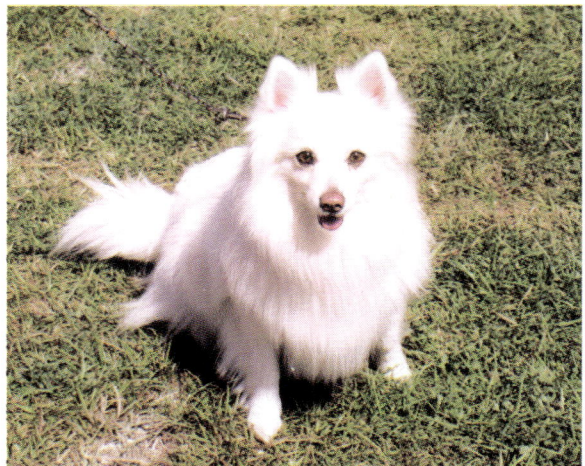
Fig. 92a Pomeranian–White

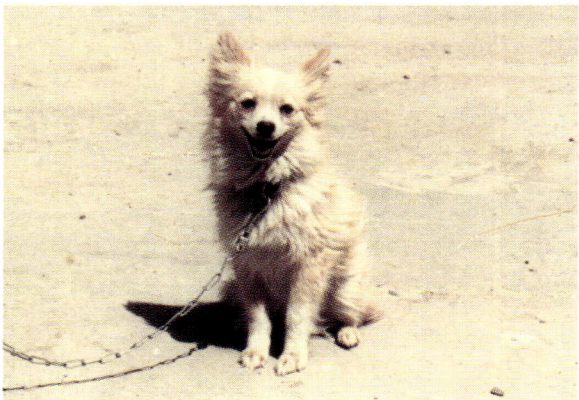
Fig. 92b Pomeranian–Brown

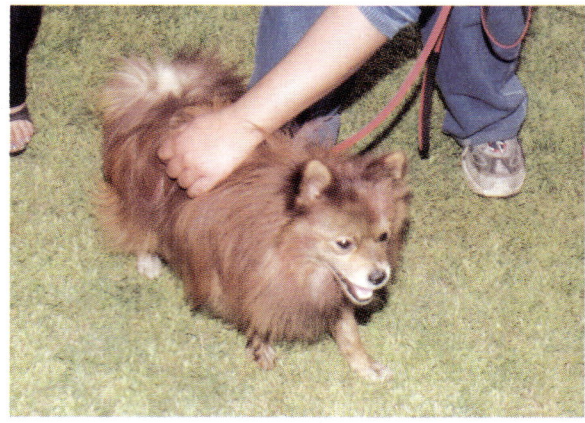
Fig. 92c Pomeranian–Golden

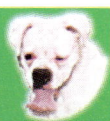

puffball. This is a very intelligent animal which can be trained easily to a very high level of performance.

Head and Face: The face of Pomeranian is fox like i.e. wedge shaped. The skull is flat and larger than the muzzle. The head above stop is covered with long hairs but face is mostly cleaner. The stop is quite prominent and anterior part extends upto nose. Nose is black in most of the animals. In some coloured strains the nose may be self coloured but it is never white. Head and face are smooth, sharp and the face is covered with sharp coat. Short pricked ears are placed apart and occiput is wide.

Mouth: The jaws are well aligned and do not possess unusual flews. Teeth are levelled. Hog mouth (Undershot) and parrot mouth (Overshot) are undesired and disqualification.

Ears: The ears are short, erect and close set on the skull reducing the length of occiput. The ears are covered with long hairs growing around and on the dorsal aspect of the ears.

Eyes: Somewhat oval shaped eyes are medium sized, bright and dark coloured. The eyes display good intelligence. A black rim around the eyes in white, cream and orange (bright brown) is commonly present.

Neck: The neck is short and well set on shoulders. It is frilled by covering of soft hair coats.

Body: The body is compact, chest is deep and back is short and straight. The body is covered with puffy coat.

Tail: The plumed tail is carried turned over the back. The tail is normally carried flat and straight. The hairs on tail are long, coarse and feathery.

Forequarters: The shoulders are clean and legs are medium in length and straight. These are well feathered.

Hindquarters: Entire hindlimbs upto hocks are fully feathered and made of fine bones.

Feet: Small feet are compact, moderately arched and covered with long hairs hiding the nails.

Coat: It is double coat animal covered with an undercoat of fluffy and woolly fibres and outer coat of long, straight and coarse hairs covering the entire body. The coat grows abundantly in the region of neck, chest and shoulder. Similarly hindquarter is covered with long hairs feathering from top of the croup to hocks. Coat length is also reasonably long and dense on the back and belly.

All whole colours free from any admixture are acceptable. The colours available are white, black, brown, pale, orange, cream and blue. Parti coloured specimen are allowed to compete with mixed Pomeranians.

Size and Weight: Height of dogs may be 30-32 cm and that of bitches 29-31 cm; and average weight may be 1.5 to 2.5 kg for both sexes.

POODLE TOY

Poodle Toy is a smallest replica of the Poodle Standard and has become more popular due to

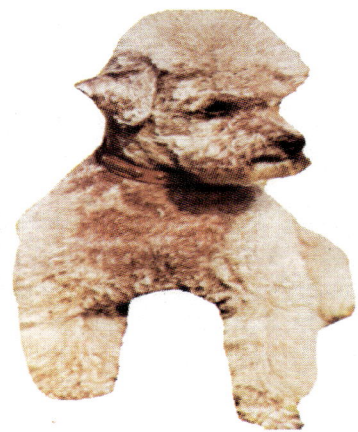

Fig. 93 Poodle Toy

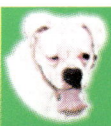

its good nature. It is an excellent companion. Poodle Toy is clipped in same fashion to its taller cousin. The differences are only height and weight. Height of Poodle Toy should be less than 28 cm at withers.

POODLE MINIATURE

In all respect of physical appearance and also in behaviour its a middle level replica of Poodle Standard. Its height at withers ranges between 27.5 and 37.5 cm. The dogs below 27.5 cm are toys and taller than 37.5 cm are standard Poodles.

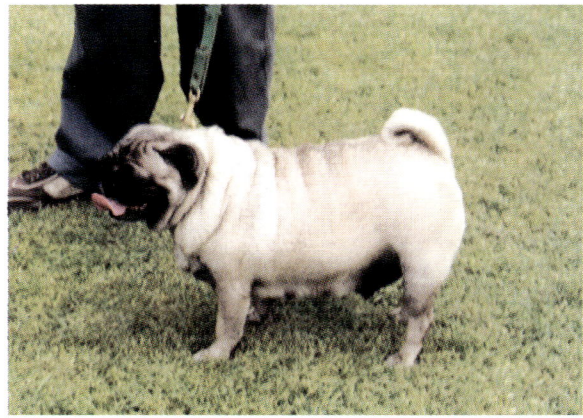

Fig. 95a Pug–Light Colour

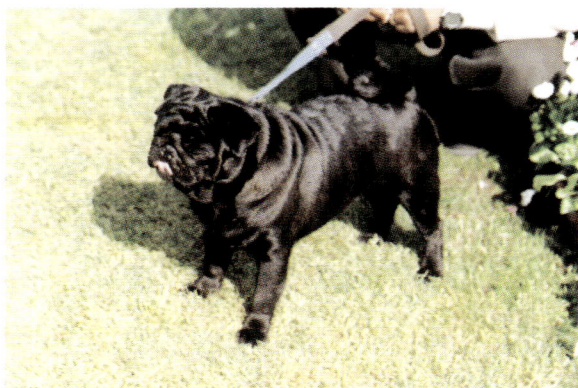

Fig. 95b Pug–Dark Colour

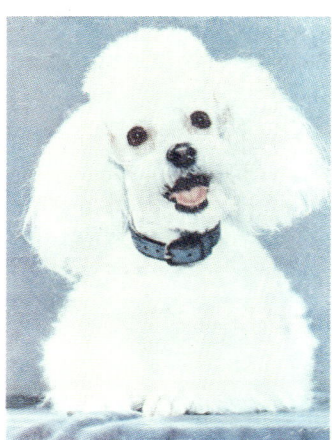

Fig. 94 Poodle Miniature

PUG

This small and affectionate breed was brought to Holland from China during the terminal years of the sixteenth century and refined to present form in Britain. Initially it was named Pu or Poo and Dutch Pug which finally remained only Pug. This is a sturdy member of toy breeds. The Pugs are affectionate and loyal companion of very good nature. They are generally quite, docile and vivacious. These animals can be adapted in wide range of living conditions but very hot weather in some

tropical countries is highly uncomfortable for the pugs. The shape of animal is square and cobby.

Head and Face: Massive and large club shaped head is very strong and covered with prominent wrinkles on the fore head. The face is pulled and nose bridge is short. Stop is shallow. Muzzle is short, blunt and wrinkled.

Mouth: The muzzle is short and black, and lips are flewed. Nares are short and nose is black with flesh mark. Oral opening is marked with inverted V-shaped flesh mark.

Ears: Soft, thin and small ears are present

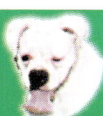

drooping on either side of skull along the line of occiput.

Eyes: These are large, bright and almost round with dark colour rim.

Neck: It is short and massive, and covered with wrinkled skin.

Body: The compact body is moderately heavy with well knit muscles. Straight dorsal line moderately slopes down the croup. Brisket is broad and prominent. A few prominent skin folds are seen in sitting dogs.

Tail: A characteristic smooth tail is tightly curled over the haunches.

Forequarters: Well muscled shoulders are heavy and blend with withers upwards and upper arm below. Thick boned fore arms are straight. Pasterns are short, thick and supple.

Hindquarters: Well muscled heavy and strong hindquarters are carried by thick and strong bones. The stifle and hock joints are moderately bent. The pasterns are proportionate, broad and flexible.

Feet: These are somewhat elongated semicircular with slightly arched toes covered with smooth coat partly overlapping the base of the toes. The soles are thickly padded and covered with coarse and cornified skin.

Coat: Glossy, short and fine coat is uniformly smooth all over the body. The colour of muzzle, eyes and ears are clearly darker than rest of the body. Coat colour may be apricot yellow of light brown.

Size and Weight: Height of adults at withers ranges from 25 to 28 cm and body weight 6.5 to 8.5 kg.

SHIH TZU

It is toy breed of arrogant behaviour. Chinese meaning for Shih Tzu is a lion dog, which was adopted from the Indian word singh for lion. Originally from Tibet this breed spread rapidly to other parts of China and other neighbouring countries thousands of years before as there was a custom in Tibet during sixteenth century to gift a pair of this breed to dignified visitors. The dogs are heavily feathered and cover ground like a hovercraft.

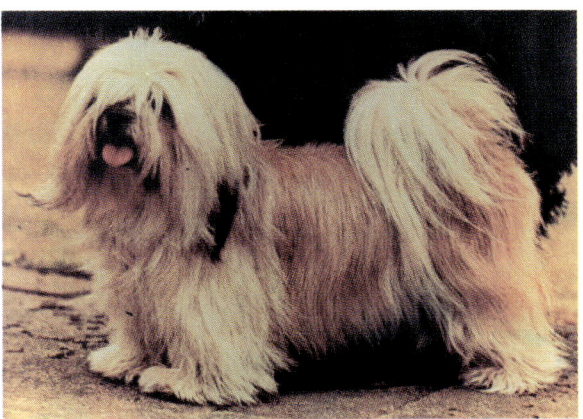

Fig. 96 Shih Tzu

Head and Face: The head is round and broad between the eyes, and covered with long hairs falling on the entire face except the nose. They possess fine long beard and whiskers. A bunch of well arranged flower like hairs are present behind the nose on bridge of the nose. Nose is black.

Mouth: It is short, wide and covered in long hairs. The mouth is level and a little under hung.

Ears: The drooping long leathered heavily coated ears are set below the crown of the skull.

Eyes: The eyes are large, dark and round.

Neck: Medium size heavily feathered and moderately arched neck is well blended with shoulders and brisket.

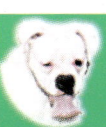

Body: The body is longer than the height. The back is level, and chest is deep and broad with well sprung ribs.

Tail: The high set tail is heavily plumed and carried gally curled over the back.

Forequarters: Heavily boned short legs are muscular, strong and straight.

Hindquarters: These are covered with very long hairs covering even the toes.

Feet: These are round, arched, well padded and covered in long feathering.

Coat: The under coat is fine, dense and woolly whereas outer coat is very long, straight and profuse. The colour may be any common colour with white blaze. A white tail tip is preferred.

Size and Weight: The height of this breed is about 27 cm and body weight preferably 4 to 6 kg but may be upto 8 kg.

SILKY TERRIER

This breed was evolved from cross-breeding between Australian Terrier and Yorkshire Terrier. It is also believed that at some stage of breeding programme blood of Norwich Terrier was introduced. Initially it appeared as Sydney Terrier during the early years of the twentieth century. After a few decades the name was changed to Australian Silky Terrier which is now popular as Silky Terrier.

Head and Face: A little longer skull than the muzzle provides wedge shaped appearance. The stop is shallow on the lower end of the flat fore head. The nose is black.

Mouth: The mouth is short, lips are smooth and teeth are arranged scissors bite.

Ears: Erect ears are set high on the skull.

Eyes: These are small and dark.

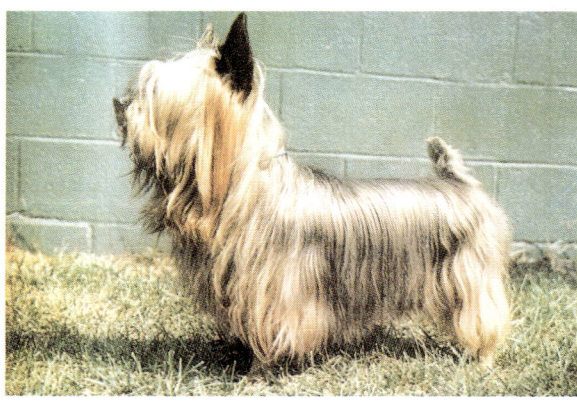

Fig. 97 Silky Terrier

Neck: It is medium, muscular, slightly arched and covered with ruff.

Body: It is longer than the height with almost straight top line and inconspicuous rounding at the loins. The brisket is prominent.

Tail: Docked tail is set high, carried erect and does not possess plume.

Forequarters: The shoulders are close set and moderately sloping. The forelegs are boned and small. Dewclaws are cut off in early life.

Hindquarters: The small hindlimbs are appropriately angulated at the joints.

Feet: These are in line with the frontal aspect of legs, strong, padded and arched.

Coat: The under coat is soft and woolly. The profuse outer coat is flat, fine and silky. The length of coat over the body from occiput to base of the tail may be 12 to 15 cm, and it appears parted along the dorsal line. Hairs on head and face are shorter and on lower part of legs much shorter. Coat colour is commonly blue or tan. Different shades of blue may be silver blue, slaty blue or pigeon blue but tan should be always deep.

Size and Weight: The height at withers should

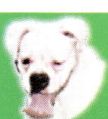

not be less than 20 cm and may reach upto 25 cm. The body weight is 3.5 to 4.5 kg approximately.

VII. Indian Breeds of Dog

1. Bhutia/Bhotia
2. Bhutia Bully
3. Bangra Tehri
4. Banjara/Sanehta/Tazi
5. Chippiparai
6. Combai
7. Himalayan Sheep Dog
8. Gaddi
9. Mudhol
10. Rajapalayam
11. Rampur Hound
12. Gangetic Hound

BHUTIA/BHOTIA

This is a Mastiff type large size and heavily feathered dog of Indo-Tibetan Himalayan region. This breed has been named due to its close affiliation with the Bhutia community where it has been developed for guarding, protection and companionship. This is an excellent breed of loyal, powerful and ferocious dogs, and capable of tolerating wide climatic variations.

Head and Face: The head is massive with square and prominent skull, broad muzzle, flat nose bridge and wide nostrils. Stop is distinct.

Mouth: The lips are fine and level, and strong teeth are arranged scissors bite.

Ears: Medium size, low set drooping ears are triangular with blunt pointed tip.

Eyes: These are moderately sunken and black or hazel. The arch of eye brow is prominent.

Neck: Well muscled, massive and medium size fluffy neck is carried almost at the level of shoulders.

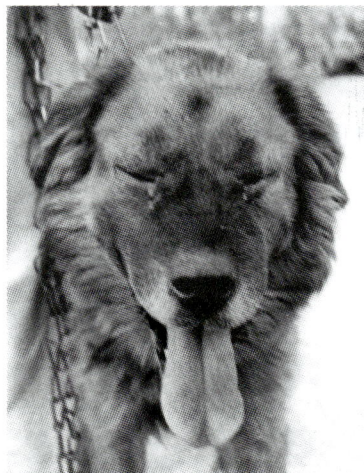

Fig. 98a Bhutia—Front View

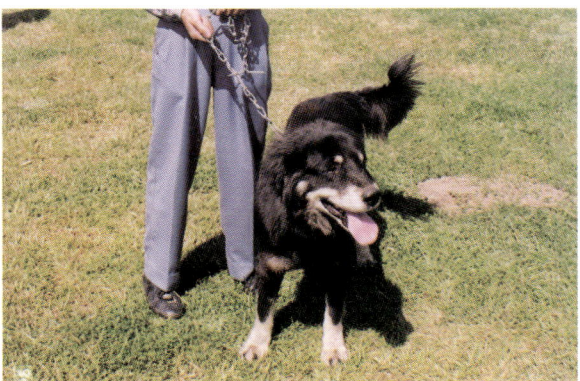

Fig. 98b Bhutia—Blackish Grey with Round Mark on Eyes

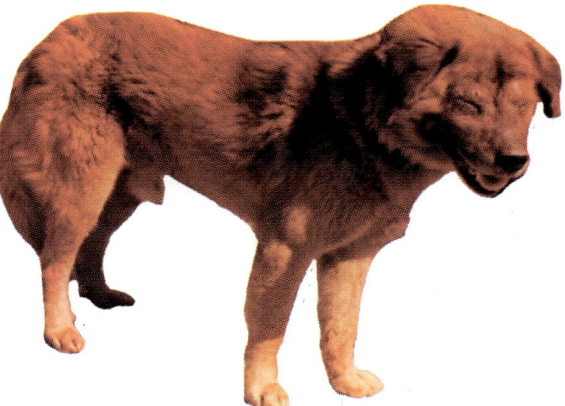

Fig. 98c Bhutia—Whole Colour Red

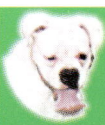

Body: It is muscular, compact and broad with straight dorsal line and sometimes moderately contoured loins and sloping croup. The chest is deep and broad with well sprung ribs and sloping towards waist region is less.

Tail: Fox like heavily feathered tail may reach upto hocks. It remains hanging in quite animals but often carried loose curled while working.

Forequarters: The shoulders are heavily mus-cled, powerful and less sloping. The upper arms are strong. The forelegs are medium size, boned and straight. The pasterns are flexible.

Hindquarters: The hips and thighs are powerful and legs are moderately angled.

Feet: These are wide, rounded and thickly padded with close set and arched toes.

Coat: The coat is dense, medium size and harsh. The colour is mostly black or brindle with tan shaded limbs. Different shades of brown, brownish tan and mixtures are also found.

Size and Weight: The height at withers is 40 to 50 cm and body weight 20-30 kg.

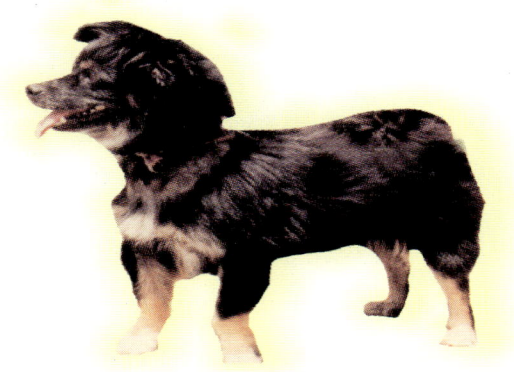

Fig. 99 Bhutia Bully

BHUTIA BULLY

These are miniature variety of Bhutia and preferred as companion. The dogs are cute, agile, playful and heavily covered with long coat. The size is much less than the standard. The height at withers is about 20 cm and body weight 3-10 kg.

BANGRA TEHRI

This breed often gives appearance of Rajapalayam in most of the physical characteristics. This appears a combination of Mastiff and Hound. Some believe it to be of Tibetan origin but actually it is wide-spread in east Tehri state of Himalayas. The dog is tall, amicable, active, loyal and good for guarding

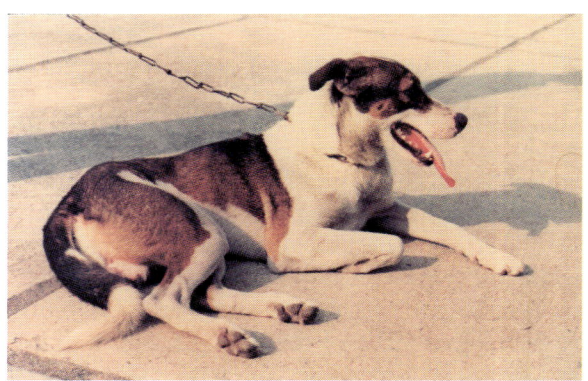

Fig. 100 Bangra Tehri

and also for protection of man and domestic animals from the wild animals.

Head and Face: The head is almost flat and square. The stop is shallow and muzzle is long and broad with broad oral opening.

Mouth: It is large with moderately flewed upper lip. The teeth are arranged scissors bite.

Ears: These are small and set high on the skull. The ear flaps are half bent.

Eyes: Almond shaped black eyes are set apart obliquely at the level of stop.

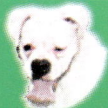

Neck: Medium size moderately arched neck is loose folded on the ventral aspect.

Body: It is long and moderately raised at the shoulders and arched on the loins. The croup is sloping. The chest is deep and moderately wide with less tucked up loin.

Tail: Low set tail is broad at the root and tapering towards the half curved distal third. It is covered with short hairs.

Forequarters: The well muscled compact shoulders are very powerful. The heavily boned forelegs are long and straight. The pasterns are short and less supple.

Hindquarters: The hips and thighs are very powerful and limbs are moderately angulated.

Feet: These are rounded and well padded. The toes are close set and prominently arched.

Coat: It is short, dense and coarse. Coat colour may be black with tan shaded extremities or various shades of orange to fawn.

Size and Weight: The height at withers may be 45 to 60 cm and body weight may range from 50 to 60 kg.

BANJARA/SANEHTA/TAZI

This slender tall breed of long and narrow body was evolved by the nomadic tribes of northern India. This multipurpose breed has been developed for hunting, guarding and companionship as these tribes live in mobile camps consisting of several families of the same group. This is one of the Indian hound class. The dogs are easily adaptable due to their close linkage and loyalty for the owner. They are famous for tracking the owner even after several months, if some how trapped by the another family.

Head and Face: The skull is square and coarse with almost flat occiput, vertical furrow on fore

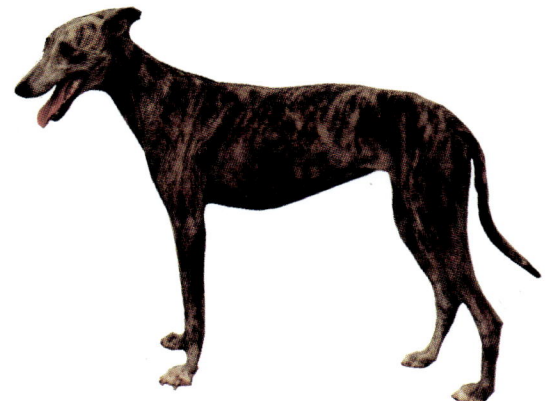

Fig. 101a Banjara/tazi-brindle

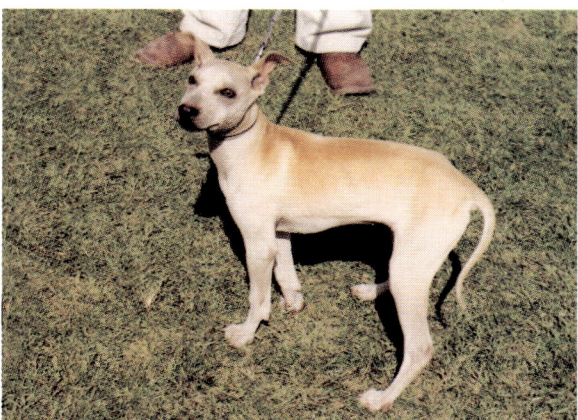

Fig. 101b Banjara/Tazi–Whole Colour Brown

head, well defined stop and deep eye sockets. Bridge of nose is narrow and straight and nose is black.

Mouth: Muzzle is long and narrow. The lips are fine and smooth and tongue remains wet and protruded most of the time.

Ears: These are small, half bent and set apart on either end of the skull.

Eyes: These are sunken and close set at the level of stop, and dark in colour.

Neck: Medium size compact neck appears fused with shoulders and brisket.

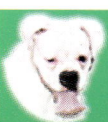

Body: It is long with raised shoulders and arched loin. The dorsal line is slightly convex or straight. The chest is moderately deep and narrow and waist is tucked up.

Tail: The low set whip like tail is broad at the base and tapering down to reach upto hocks or even longer in some animals.

Forequarters: The shoulders are compact, moderately sloping and slightly higher than the back. Boned forelegs are clean and straight. The pasterns are short and supple.

Hindquarters: These are sloping, compact and strong. The hind legs are well angulated for providing better propulsion.

Feet: These are circular with close set and well arched toes and thickly padded sole.

Coat: It is short, dense and coarse. The colour is mostly brindle, hyaena like, mottled with blue or grey and may be also black and striped tan or zebra marked.

Size and Weight: The height at weathers is 40-60 cm and body weight 20-30 kg. The females are lighter than the males.

CHIPPIPARAI

It is a member of Grey Hound variety evolved

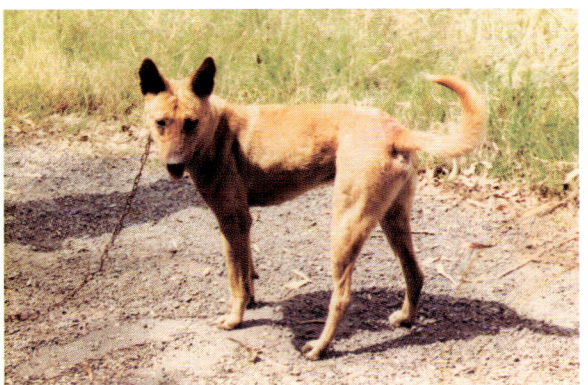

Fig. 102 Chippiparai

for hunting from the local dogs of ancient Tamil Nadu region. This is also known as Thambai dog. These are elegant, alert and active dogs popular for hunting and guarding.

Head and Face: The skull is flat and occiput is narrow due to high set ears. The forehead possesses central shallow groove. The stop is clear and strong muzzle is conical.

Mouth: The lips are fine and smooth, and the teeth are arranged scissors bite.

Ears: High set pricked ears are broad at the base and turned forward. These are fine and inner surface is devoid of hairs.

Eyes: Almond shaped obliquely set eyes are dark colour or black.

Neck: It is moderately muscular, fine and smooth with broad base fused with the shoulders and brisket may depict a vertical shallow furrow. It is slightly arched.

Body: The muscular body is compact with deep chest, well sprung ribs and narrower waist. The shoulders are slightly higher, dorsal line is straight loin is a little arched and the croup is sloping.

Tail: Low set medium size tail is moderately thick and carried in line with the croup but distal half is shallow curved.

Forequarters: The compact and powerful shoulders are almost straight but upper arm is well angled. The boned forelegs are long and straight. The pasterns are also long and moderately supple.

Hindquarters: The close set hip and thigh muscles are fine, smooth and tapering upto hock joints. The legs are well angulated to work like a spring while trailing.

Feet: These are smooth, circular and deeply padded with well arched toes.

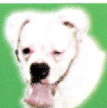

Coat: It is very short, dense, smooth and glossy. However, parts of ears, face, legs and under side of legs are covered with thin coat. Common coat colours are different shades of whole colour black or brown.

Size and Weight: The height at withers is mostly 50 to 60 cm and body weight range is 50 to 60 kg.

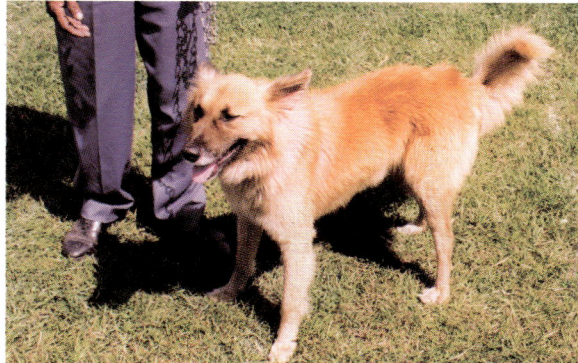

Fig. 103 Combai

COMBAI

This breed was also developed in the Combai Village area of Tamil Nadu for guarding and companionship. The body is almost square shape. The animal is docile, faithful and easy to manage.

Head and Face: The head and face together are conical from occiput to oral end. The skull is flat and square, stop is shallow and muzzle is long. The nose is liver colour in brown and black in others.

Mouth: The lips are smooth and level, and strong teeth are deeply embedded in thick gums.

Ears: These are medium size, high set and half bent.

Eyes: These are bright, oblique and brown to black.

Neck: It is muscular, compact, short and moderately arched.

Body: It is short, muscular and almost barrel shape due to less sloping from chest to waist. The chest is deep and ribs cage is capacious.

Tail: Medium size smooth and tapering tail is carried high and slightly turned forward.

Forequarters: Entire forequarters from shoulders to pasterns are heavily boned. The upper arms are loose set with the chest. Forelegs are long and straight and the pasterns are slightly narrower and supple.

Hindquarters: The hips and thighs are heavily muscled and powerful. The legs are well angulated and hocks are very prominent. The sannons slope a little forward.

Feet: These are ovoid with close set and moderately arched toes. The soles are well padded.

Coat: It is very short, smooth, fine and glossy. The coat colour is mostly black, different shades of brown or brindle.

Size and Weight: The height at withers may range from 55 to 60 cm, and body weight 30 to 35 kg.

HIMALAYAN SHEEP DOG

This is an ancient breed of medium to large size dogs which are well known for their intelligence, loyalty, sturdyness and capability for working in the harsh climatic conditions of Himalayan region. These dogs are capable of sorting out sheep of their flock from mixed flock on grazing land. It is a member of Mastiff group and found across the Himalaya.

Head and Face: The head is moderately large and almost square shape with prominent skull. The stop is shallow, muzzle is short and bridge of nose is straight. Nose is black.

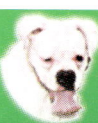

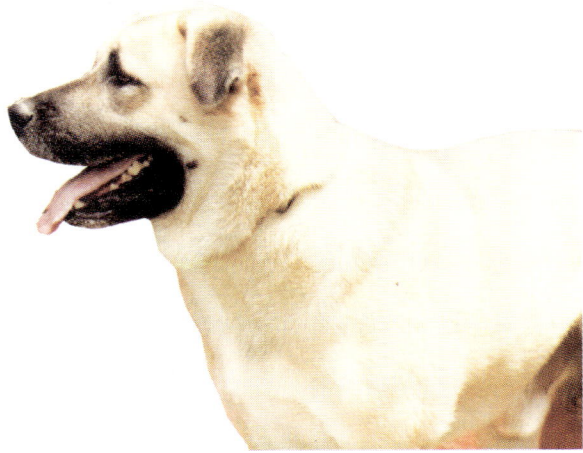

Fig. 104a Himalayan Sheep Dog

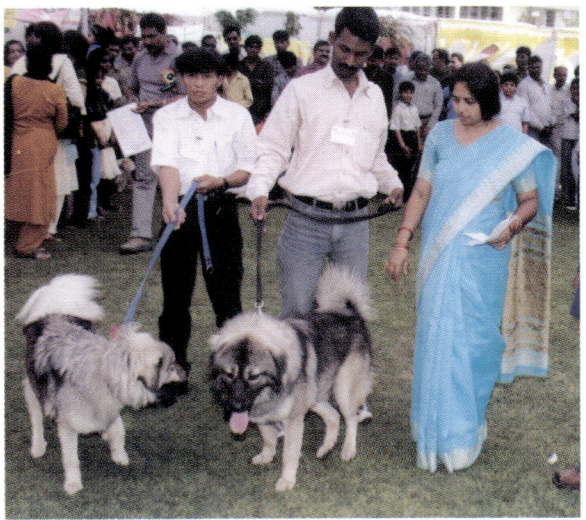

Fig. 104b Himalayan Sheep Dog at Show

Mouth: It is short and level with fine lips. The teeth are scissors bite and strong.

Ears: Low set and broad based ears drop like flap on either side of the head. The leathers are medium size and blunt pointed.

Eyes: Almond shaped eyes are small and set apart obliquely. These are black.

Neck: Medium size broad neck is moderately arched and fluffy.

Body: It is muscular, compact and dorsally rounded with straight dorsal line but slightly raised withers. The chest is deep and broad with well sprung ribs and moderately sloping loin. The brisket is prominent.

Tail: It is loose curled above the level of back and thickly flaged.

Forequarters: The shoulders are muscled, compact and moderately sloping. Boned forelegs are straight and fine. The pasterns are short and supple.

Hindquarters: The croup is sloping and hips and thighs are powerful. Boned hindlegs are properly angled for working in difficult terrain of hilly and mountainous region.

Feet: These are rounded with fine, close set and moderately arched toes and thickly padded sole.

Coat: The body is covered with uniform short, dense and smooth coat which grows longer during winter or in dogs at high altitude. The colour is mostly whole creamy white but other colours generally different shades of fawn are also found.

Size and Weight: The height at withers ranges from 50 to 70 cm, and body weight ranges from 30 to 40 kg. The bitches are distinctly lighter than the males.

GADDI

It is an Indian tropical breed evolved from dogs of Yamuna riverine of Meerut region thousands of years ago by the demon 'Mahidand' once famous for terror in the region. This is a heavy breed of Mastiff group. This is a courageous and powerful guard dog.

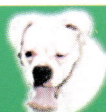

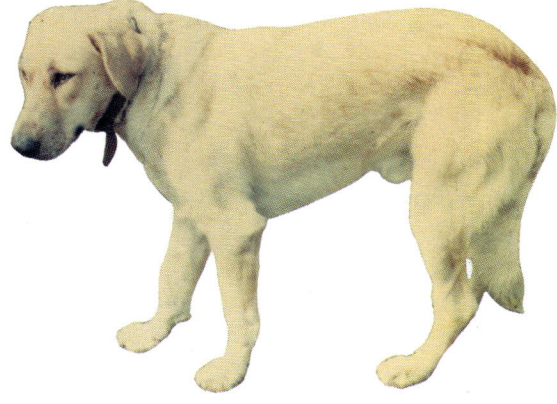

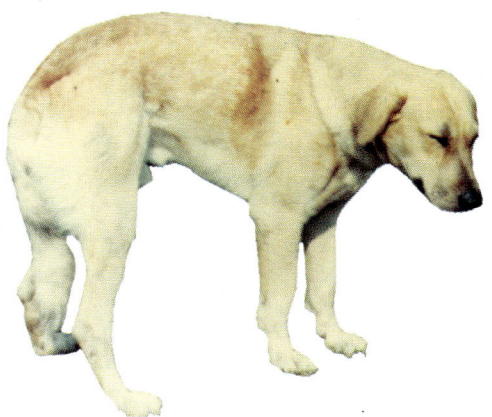

Figs 105 a and b Gaddi

Head and Face: The skull is broad, prominent, square and fine with shallow but defined stop. The nasal bone is longer than the length between top and stop. The muzzle is broad.

Mouth: The upper lip is flewed. The lips are level and strong teeth are arranged scissors bite.

Ears: Medium size drooping ears are low set, broad at the base and rounded tip. These are fine and smooth.

Eyes: Small eyes generally appear drowsy. These are small, dark and obliquely set.

Neck: Medium size muscular neck is smooth and moderately sloping from shoulders to base of the occiput. It is slightly arched.

Body: Muscular body is compact, fine and smooth with somewhat arched loins and a little higher set shoulders. The chest is deep and broad with well sprung ribs and less sloping towards the waist.

Tail: The tail is hairy, long and feathered.

Forequarters: The compact shoulders are less sloping and close set with the chest. The upper arm is muscular and elbow joint is prominent. Boned forelegs are straight and medium in length. The short pasterns are well supple.

Hindquarters: The croup, hips and thighs are well muscled and powerful. The hindlegs are moderately angled.

Feet: These are rounded and broad with close set and arched toes. The soles are thickly padded.

Coat: The body is covered with short, dense and smooth hairs but tail and posterior aspect of limbs are well feathered. Body coat often grows longer during the winter season. The colour is white or grey and belly region may be lighter. Some specimen may be lemon colour to light orange.

Size and Weight: The height at withers may be 50 to 70 cm and body weight 25 to 50 kg. The males are heavier than the females. Great variation in shape and size is due to indiscriminate breeding.

MUDHOL

It is a hound variety of Karnataka and adjoining region of Maharashtra. The dog is lean, moderately tall and bony. This breed has been developed for hunting and also protecting domesticated animals from the wild animals. The utility of this breed is now decreasing.

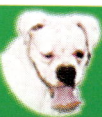

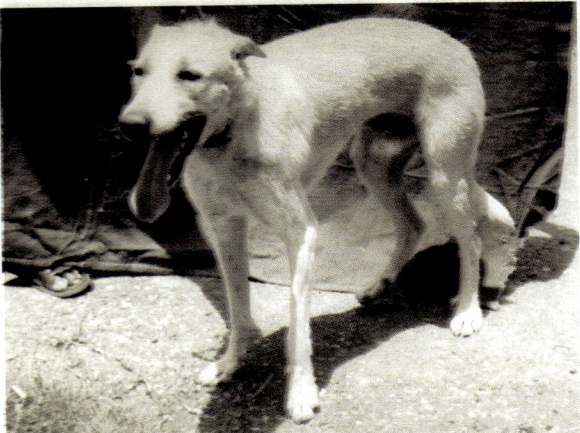

Fig. 106a Mudhol

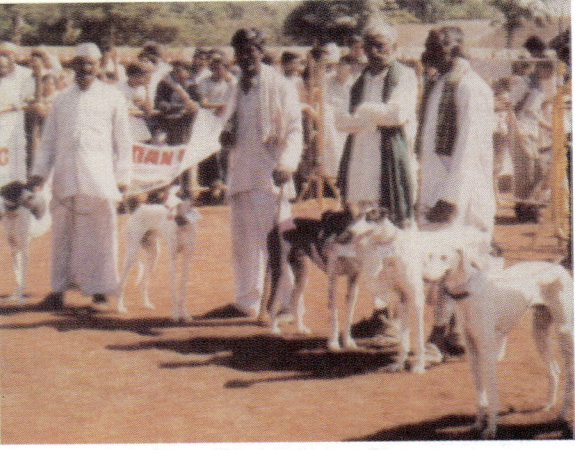

Fig. 106b Mudhol at Show

Eyes: These are large, oblique set and dark.

Neck: It is moderately long, compact and fused with the shoulders and prominent brisket. It is moderately arched.

Body: It is arched at shoulders, straight upto loins and then sloping down posteriorly. The chest is deep and broad but loin region is tucked up. The body is thin with reasonably exposed bones.

Tail: Whip like straight tail is broad at the base and tapering to the tip. It is fine and thin.

Forequarters: These are thin and boned from shoulders to toes. The shoulders are sloping, upper arms are little deflated and forelegs are long and straight. Similarly the pasterns are long and supple but a little narrower than the forelegs.

Hindquarters: The hips and thighs are lean and legs are well angled and put apart in standing dogs. The rear pasterns are put moderately forward in standing dogs.

Feet: These are elongated oval with moderately arched toes and padded sole.

Coat: It is very short, smooth and glossy. The colour is mostly black or tan but may be black and tan.

Size and Weight: The height at withers is about 55 to 60 cm and body weights are 25 to 30 kg.

Head and Face: The skull is smaller than the muzzle with slightly convex occiput and rudimentary stop. A central furrow on fore head extends down the stop. The nose bridge is long and flat. Entire head and face are thin and boned. The nose is broad and black.

Mouth: The lips are level and smooth, and teeth are arranged either scissors bite or level.

Ears: Medium size ears are set high on the skull and half bent. The bent part is placed at a higher level than the occiput. These are fine and smooth.

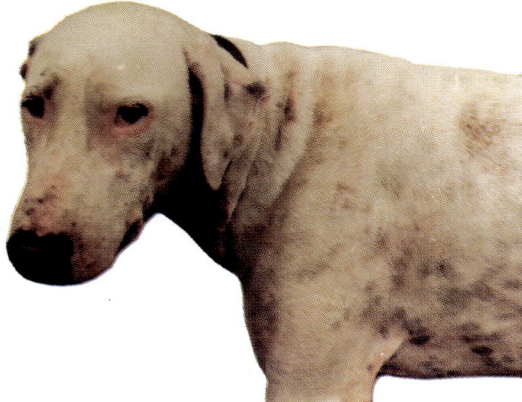

Fig. 107a Rajapalayam –Front View

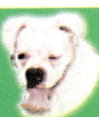

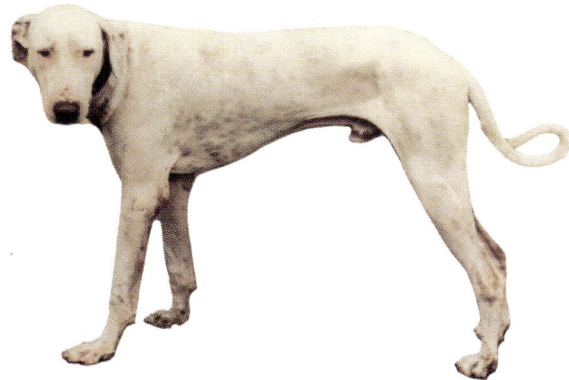

Fig. 107b Rajapalayam–Lateral View

RAJAPALAYAM

This is a famous hound breed developed in the Rajapalayam village of the Kerala State of India. This graceful, long, slender and fast trecking dog is famous for hunting and guarding.

Head and Face: The skull is short with domed occiput, prominent forehead, shallow stop and long muzzle. The bridge of nose is fine and straight. The nose is black or may be flesh marked.

Mouth: The lips are fine, smooth and level. The teeth are strong and arranged scissors bite.

Ears: Medium size triangular ears are fine, thin, smooth and dropped over the cheeks.

Eyes: Almond shaped eyes are sharp, bright and set apart at the level of stop.

Neck: Long, fine and smooth neck is moderately arched, sloping and fused with the shoulders and powerful brisket.

Body: It is muscular, compact and straight dorsally with a little arched shoulders and loins. The chest is deep but narrower and waist is tucked up.

Tail: Whip like tapering and smooth tail is long with upward curvature of the distal half. Hanging tail extends below the hock joint.

Forequarters: The compact and powerful shoulders are less sloping. The boned and straight forelegs are long with narrower and less supple pasterns.

Hindquarters: The hips and thighs are muscled, thin, boned and limbs are well angulated for effective trailing.

Feet: These are coarse with well arched toes and padded sole..

Coat: Short and smooth coat is glossy at head and coarse on the body. The colour is whole white. Grooming of the dog is very convenient.

Size and Weight: The height at withers is 45 to 65 cm and body weight 40-60 kg.

RAMPUR HOUND

This is also known as Eastern Hound. The animals are thin, slender, fine, bony and tall. The dogs are elegant, amicable, loyal and easy to be trained. This is a hunting breed used for capturing and trailing small hares to large size deer and antelopes. This breed was developed by the Nawab of Rampur in India.

Head and Face: The skull is narrow with prominent forehead, shallow stop and tapering narrow muzzle. The nose is black.

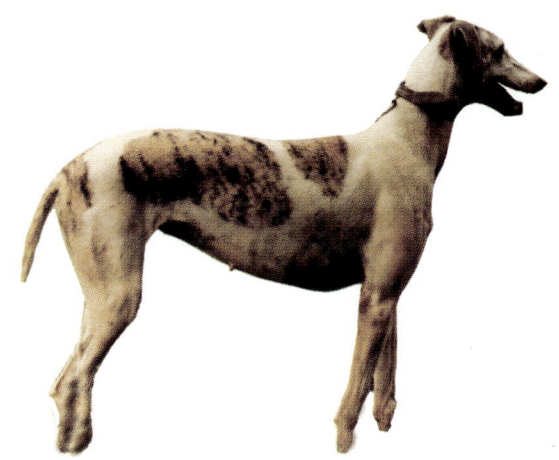

Fig. 108a Rampur Hound

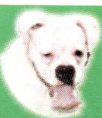

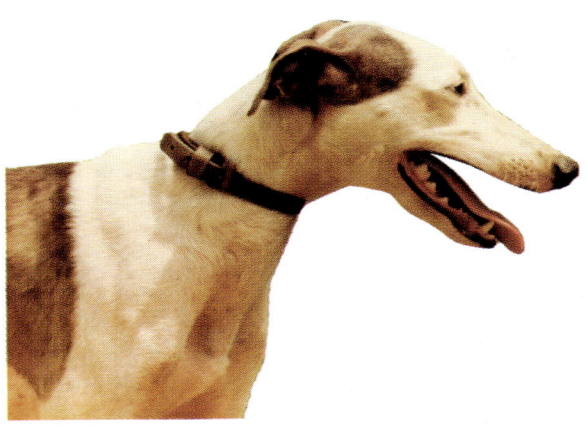

Fig. 108b Rampur Hound–Anterior Part

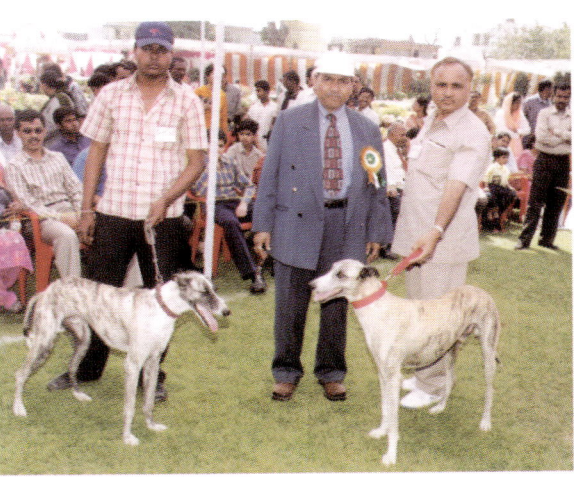

Fig. 108c Rampur Hound

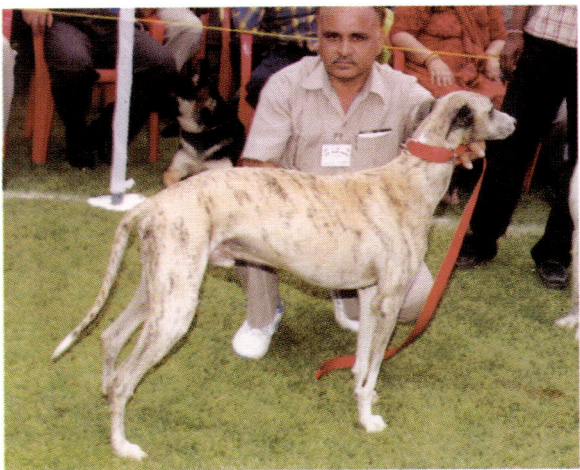

Fig. 108d Rampur Hound

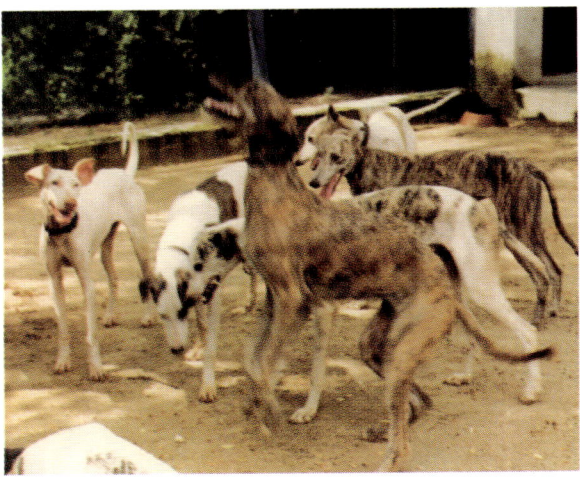

Fig. 108e Rampur Hound–Group

Mouth: The lips are fine and smooth, upper lip slightly overlaps lower lip. The teeth are very strong.

Ears: These are small, set apart and half bent with moderately exposed inner surface.

Eyes: Almond shaped black eyes are set obliquely at the level of stop.

Neck: It is moderately long, smooth, fine, compact, moderately arched and fused with the shoulders and brisket.

Body: It is long, narrow, moderate arched and shoulders are placed a little higher than the loin. The croup is sloping. The chest is deep but narrow and loin is deeply tucked up.

Tail: Whiplike slender, tapering and fine tail may reach down the hocks. It is low set but carried in line with the back while running.

Forequarters: The shoulders are compact, moderately sloping and powerful. The boned

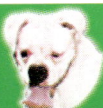

forelegs are long, perpendicular and strong. The pasterns are short, almost straight and less flexible.

Hindquarters: The hips are slopy, thighs are compact muscled and limbs are well angled for effective propulsion.

Feet: These are circular, thin and close set with well arched toes and padded sole.

Coat: It is short, dense, fine and smooth. The colour is brindle, tan stripped and various shades of fawn, grey and many other colours.

Size and Weight: The height at withers ranges from 50 to 70 cm and body weights ranges from 25 to 35 kg.

GANGETIC HOUND

This is one of the tall breeds of Indian dog found distributed in the rural areas. The dog is preferred by farmers specially those living away at farms for guarding the standing crops and also in the orchards of mango, guava and plumb during the crops. This breed is famous for loyalty. It is also kept for assistance in hunting.

Head and Face: The head is moderately domed with slightly convex forehead and shallow stops. Face is chiselled.

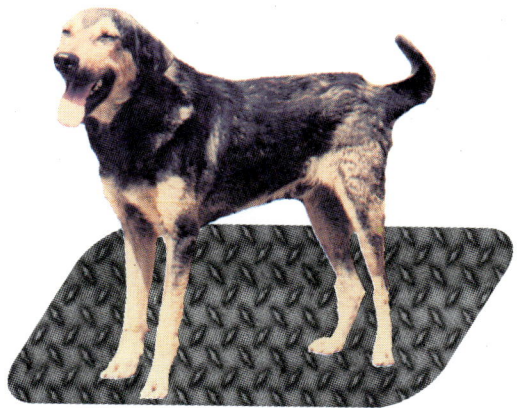

Fig. 109 Gangetic Hound

Mouth: The muzzle is moderately broad and upper jaw is slightly flewed. The teeth are arranged scissors bite and embedded in massive and black gum. Bridge of nose is straight and smooth.

Ears: Medium size blunt pointed ears are present drooping on either end of occiput.

Eyes: These are relatively small and set oblique with inner canthus at the level of stop.

Neck: It is massive, compact and fused with the shoulders. The arching is moderate.

Body: Massive body, moderately slopy from chest to waist. The body is compact with broad chest, tight brisket and well-sprung ribs. The dorsal line is straight upto posterior end of back and crop is drooping.

Tail: It is medium size and moderately bushy but may be smooth and half curled also.

Forequarters: The shoulders are broad and strong. The forelimbs are bonny and almost perpendicular. The pasterns are relatively shorter and less supple.

Hindquarters: The thighs are compact and muscular. Angulation is moderate and shannon bones are strong.

Feet: These are compact with close set toes rounded in front and moderately arched. The foot pads are thick and well cornified.

Coat: The coat is coarse and smooth. Coat colour varies from black roan to black but face, distal part of limbs, greater part of face, inner aspects of limbs and under side of tail are mostly brown.

Size and Weight: The breed has not yet been standerdized for the show purpose. The males are as usual heavier than the females. The height of dogs at withers may range from 75 to 85 cm and that of bitches from 70 to 80 cm.

THE SPITZ TYPE

Several dog breeds of mostly small to

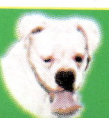

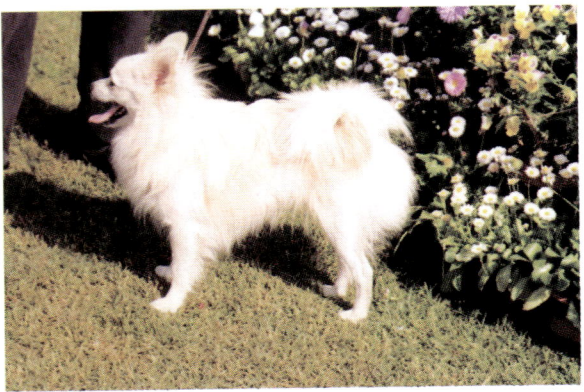

Fig. 110a White Pomeranian Spitz

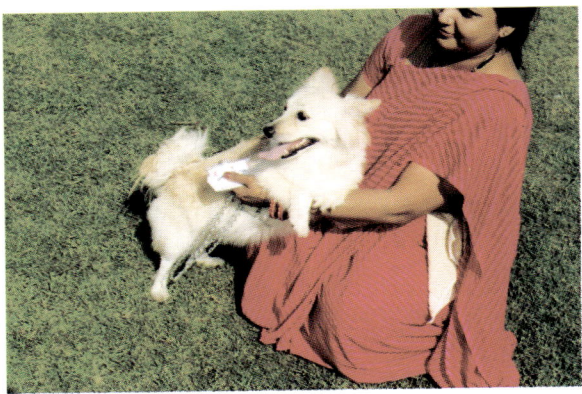

Fig. 110b Golden Pomeranian Spitz with Owner

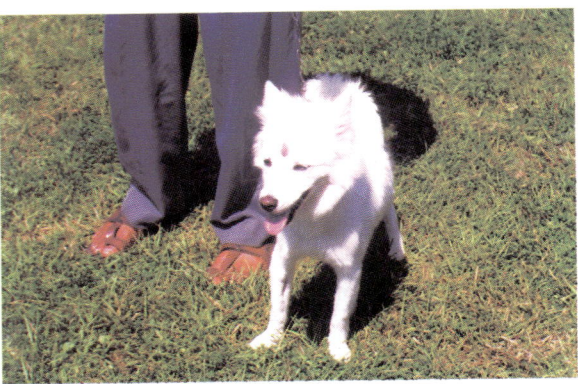

Fig. 110c Samoyed Spitz

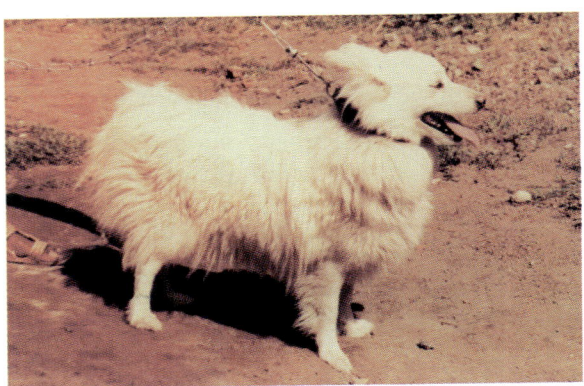

Fig. 110d Japanese Spitz

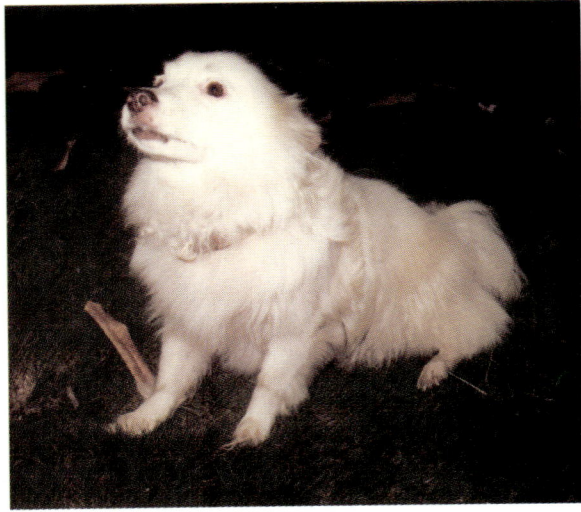

Fig. 110e Japanese Spitz

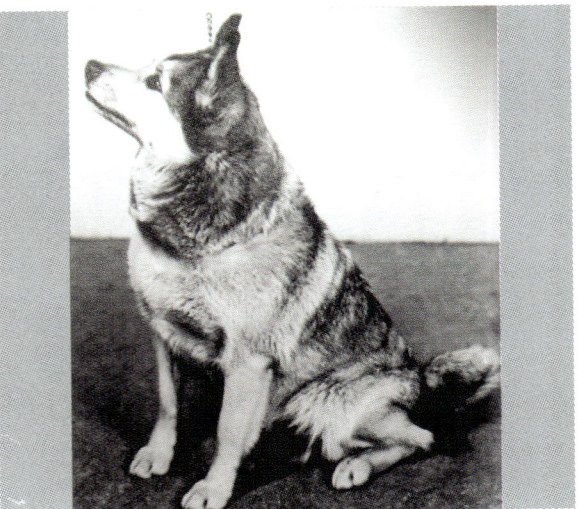

Fig. 110f Icelandic Sheep Dog (Spitz)

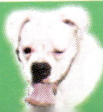

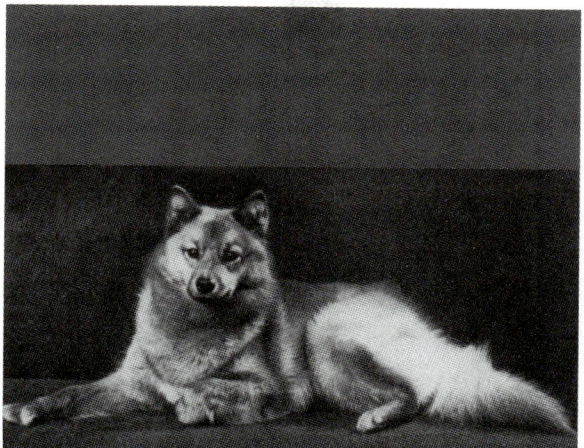

Fig. 110g Finish Spitz

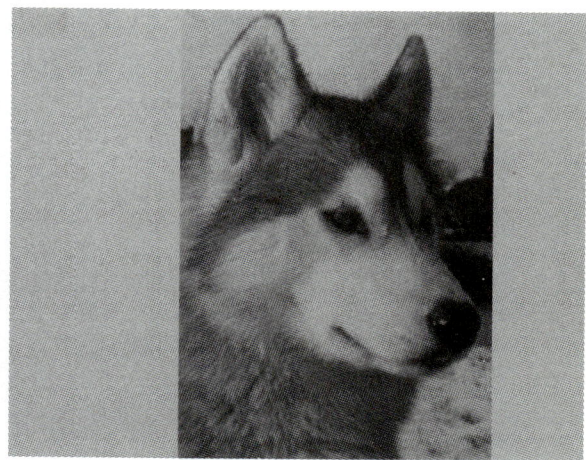

Fig. 110h Siberian Husky (Spitz)

medium size with a square outline (almost equal height at withers and body length from shoulder joint to pin bone) have been clubbed together in a separate class known as Spitz. Unlike common impression among the people unaware of the characteristics of dogs the Spitz are not toys but have been evolved for performance as a good working dog. Most of the breeds are affectionate and intelligent. Generally spitz are an excellent companion as well as working dogs capable of adapting highly variable climatic conditions but find cold climate more comfortable. Most of them like to live and play with children. They like cleanliness and may take bath and groom themselves. These are the dogs of great stamina and generally do not exhaust even after playing or working in difficult areas for several hours.

Common Physical Characteristics

The morphological appearance of most of the spitz breeds is a square outline (Figs. 110a to 110h) being height and length almost equal. The head is wedge shaped with broader skull and nerves faces tapering to somewhat rounded

nose. The face is generally short and ears are pricked with tips rising above the level of occiput. The ears are highly mobile and becomes attentive even with commonly unnoticed sound and may turn even towards the tail. The muzzle is short and jaws are strong. Normally strong teeth are arranged in a scissors bite fashion. However, incidence of parrot mouth or over shot bite and hog mouth or under shot bite is frequently recorded in some of the breeds.

The highly feathered bushy tail is curled over the back in almost all the breeds except a few. Most of the Spitz breeds are covered with double coat. Pashmina like dense and very fine woolly under coat provides perfect insulation for protection against the harsh cold climate. The outer cover of long and relatively rough coat provides protection to under coat from rains, storms, frost and snow fall. Growth of fine under coat is seasonal and shed off annually at the end of winter season and removed while combing the dogs.

The Spitz dogs include the following internationally recognized breeds and also some locally known breeds.

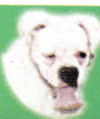

A.   *Internationally Recognized Spitz Types*

1.   Alaskan Malamute
2.   Basenji
3.   Chow Chow
4.   Elkhound
5.   Eskimo Dog
6.   Finnish Spitz
7.   Icelandic Sheep Dog
8.   Keeshound or Wolf Spitz
9.   Norwegian Buhund
10. Pomeranian or Zwerg Spitz
11. Samoyed
12. Schipperke
13. Siberian Husky
14. Swedish Vallhund

B.   *Locally or Regionally Recognized Spitz Types*

1.   Akita

2.   Deutscher Spitz
3.   Finnish Laphund
4.   Giant Spitz
5.   Groos Spitz
6.   Karelian Bear Dog
7.   Klein Spitz
8.   Laiki
9.   Lapland Reindeer Dog
10. Lundehund or Norwegian Puffin
11. Mittel
12. Nordic Spitz or Norbotten Spitz
13. Russo- European
14. Russo-Furnish
15. Samoyed
16. Sanchu
17. Shiba
18. Shika
19. Siberian Lapponian Herder
20. Swedish Elkhund or Jamthund
21. Swedish Lapphund

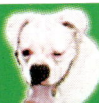

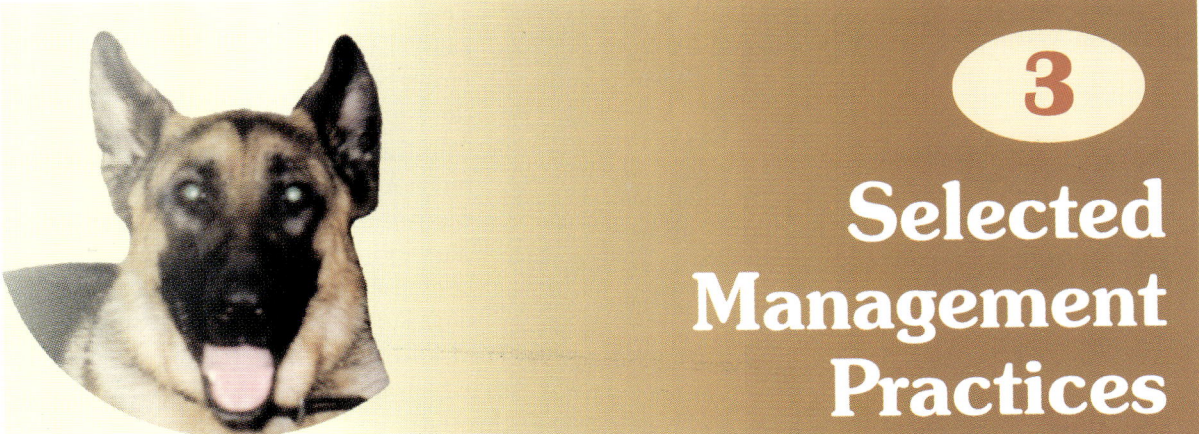

Selected Management Practices

Although keeping of dog as a pet is increasing in India but in want of facilities for the guidance of owners the dogs are reared as per the suggestions of the different persons having some experience of dog-keeping in their own style. Such suggestions have little impact on new owners mostly due to contradictions in the suggestions offered from different corners. Large number of dog owners do not follow any kind of management routine and in most of the households a pet dog is kept as a show piece and with new owners a pet receives too much undesired attention in beginning which faints gradually after the pups become 5-6 months old. Such changes in the treatment of owners bring significant change in the behaviour of pet dogs. The most unwanted change in the behaviour of a dog is the development of aggression due to neglect. Initially such changes occur for drawing the attention of master and if not corrected in a short time these become habits of the dog, and due to such reasons most of the pets in Indian households are carefree and indisciplined. The other reasons for the development of undesired habits in pet dogs are the non-availability of a suitable separate living space in the small flats and houses where

accommodation of even small size family members is often difficult, different treatment received from different family members which frequently infuses confusion in the pet and under such situation it develops more closeness with the dominant person of the family or one who gives more time and better treatment to the pet.

The common vices encountered in dogs are jumping on people, begging, playing with furnitures, soiling the furnitures including beds, digging the ground of lawn, over protectiveness, chewing wood, aggressiveness and repeated escape. Some of these vices gradually disappear with the advancement of age and control of the owner upto six months to one year of age. However, if not controlled strictly, tendency of begging increases. This is highly unwanted and such dogs may not be loyal for their master and develop habit to oblige the persons offering them foods of their liking. Some of these vices are inherent like intense activities of playing, jumping and carelessness in early life, which decrease with the increase in age, while acquired habits once established hardly corrected. Begging is one of such vices in the dogs, that is why it is suggested to follow feeding routine strictly and dogs should be trained to eat foods offered by the family members only.

Behaviour of Dogs

The behaviour of dogs is assessed on the basis of their common activities and reaction with the other subjects. These may be grouped broadly as:

1. **Reactivity of the dogs:** This comprises the followings:
    i. Demand for affection.
    ii. Excitability.
    iii. Continuous or interrupted excessive barking.
    iv. Snapping at children and other subjects.
    v. Chasing human and animals passing through the street or lane.

2. **Aggressiveness:** It is an inherent character of the dog which was developed due to circumstances faced by wild ancestor in the process of evolution. This behaviour of dog is mostly regulated in the pet dogs to meet the requirements of their utility. Aggressiveness of dogs has been generally differentiated as follows:

    (i) Aggressiveness for territory protection: Dogs mark their surrounding by frequent urination at different prominent points of their territory and do not allow stranger dog to enter or inhabit. The initial reaction is generally offensive but may turn defensive, if other party is stronger. but offensive aggressiveness is continued, if dog is with his owner.

    (ii) Barking by watch dog: It is a desired trait in the dogs kept for guarding. They convey message for the arrival of some subject by barking. However, pitch and intensity of barking are different for known persons and strangers.

    (iii) Aggression on other dogs: Almost all dogs do not tolerate the entry of other dogs in their territory and aggressive expression develops on first site. However, fighting occurs only between the same sex.

    (iv) Dominance over owner: Although rare but not uncommon particularly among the hunting breeds, which attempt to disobey the instructons of master. Such behaviour is also observed among the dogs kept as pet in small flats and houses.

3. **Trainability:** Although all breeds of dogs may be trained for different performances through rigorous coaching but it will be wise step for the owners to find a breed that has better record for the activities expected from the pet. The most common trainings required in almost all pet dogs are the:

    (i) Obedience training for proper handling and controlling the pet.

    (ii) Training for house breaking is required in the dogs kept for specialized performances like searching and guarding etc.

4. **Other behavioural traits:** Almost all toy breeds and puppies are playful and like to play with young children. However, some dogs develop the habit of spoiling household and other goods. Such vices can be corrected by

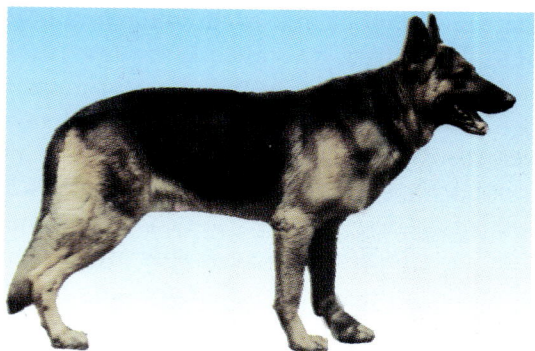

Fig. 111a German Shepherd Obeying Order for Standing

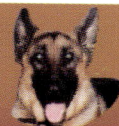

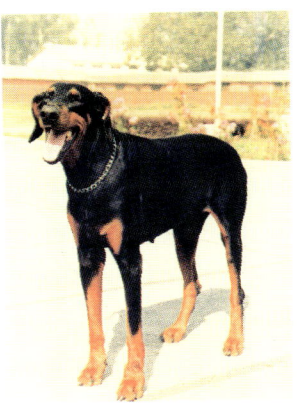

Fig. 111b Doberman Pinscher Obeying Order for Standing

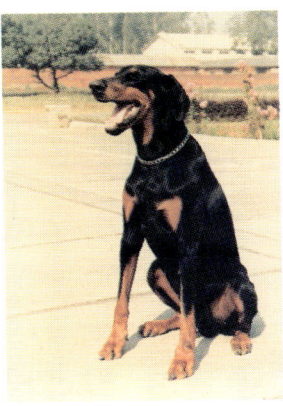

Fig. 112 Doberman Pinscher Barking on Order

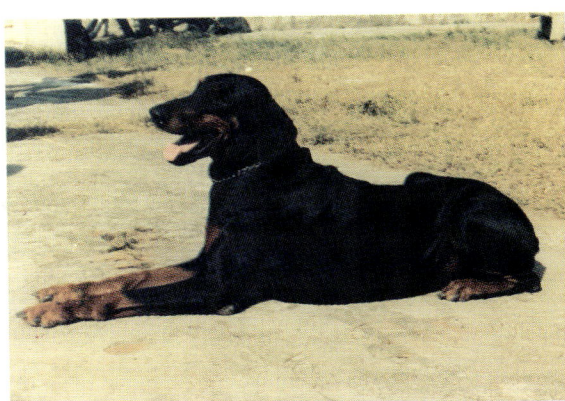

Fig. 113 Doberman Pinscher Sitting on Order

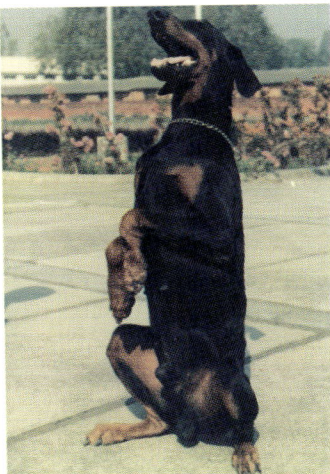

Fig. 114 Doberman Pinscher Lifting Fore-legs on Order

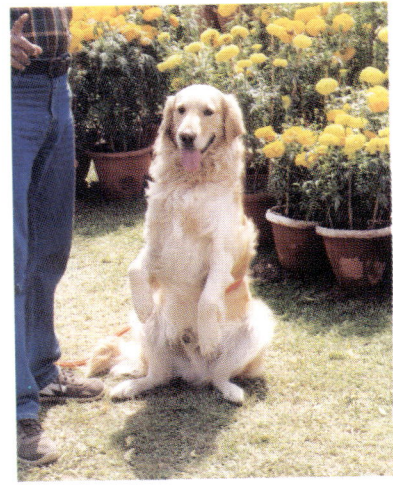

Fig. 115 Labrador Lifting Fore-legs on Order

appropriate punishment at initial stages but it may be difficult to correct aged dogs.

Some Special Intra Species Behaviour of Dogs

In India it is quite common to observe aggressiveness among the dogs on trespassing the territory. Fight among opposite sexes and with puppies is very rare. However, during breeding season almost all eligible dogs of a locality and often from neighbouring locality move behind the bitch in oestrum, but hierarchy on the basis of physical strength and aggressiveness of males is observed. In very rare cases some bitches prefer a particular dog and do not allow others for mating. The litters in such cases are almost uniform even in stray bitches.

Pen Size, Furnishing and Housing of Dogs

Standard providing requirements of space and furnishing depends on the size, age and breed of the dogs.

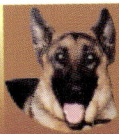

1. **Toy or small breeds:** A pen of 100 cm x 75 cm x 70 cm cubical covered with wire gauze when placed indoor will be adequate. Front door should preferably be made of vertical or horizontal bars with adequate space between the bars so that animal can see through but can not escape out of the pen.

2. **Medium breeds:** The size of pen should be 150 cm x 100 cm x 100 cm cubical with fittings as per pens for toy breeds.

3. **Large breeds:** Appropriate size of pen would be 250 cm x 200 cm x 150 cm and should be made of strong building materials. A separate place from the living area of household would be much better. Construction adjacent to car garage may be more convenient.

Covered space for brood bitches should be almost double than the given size. There should be also space for putting a box for the puppies. In each pen one wooden bench of appropriate size and about 15 cm height should be provided for retiring. A blanket may be required to cover the dog in winter season.

It would be better to provide an open run at least equal to the size of pen. The run should be fenced and height of walls should be high enough to prevent the jumping. For preventing sporting breeds and during breeding season when animals become very active and acrobatic a height of about 2.5 m should be raised.

Bedding

The climate in tropical countries is not comfortable for the dogs as temperature remains high for about eight months and discomfort further increases due to high humidity in the hot rainy season. Stray dogs and yard dogs rest at a dry place on the ground after cleaning it with tail. However, confined dogs may be provided a smooth bench of wooden plank. A blanket or rug may be required in winter season when atmospheric temperature falls very low. Young puppies are kept clustered by the dam and receive reasonable heat from the contact of mother and clustering.

Routine Outing

Adult dogs should be taken out for urination and defaecation after about 6-8 hours of feeding. However, for convenience it would be better to train the pets for defaecation between 6 to 8 hours in the morning and 18 to 20 hours in the evening. During these period some member of the family is expected to be present in the house. Most of the dogs are quite cooperative but in few cases outing may be required in mid day for urination. The place of defaecation and urination should be fixed and away from the public places.

Handling

Handling of dogs is a routine one and required for restraining the animal for cleaning and manipulations. In routine handling the pets are taken out preferably chained for out door routine activities like urination, defaecation and exercise. The dogs should be taken away at an isolated place for exercise. The animals of heavy and hunting breeds need more rigorous exercise than the lighter breeds. The dog must be under control during the exercise and should not snap, bark or jump on people passing through the place of exercise. If the pet is not properly trained and lacks obedience, then exercise should be provided by restraining with a long rope or on a treade mill.

For clinical examinations the dogs are restrained by one of the following methods.

1. **Use of muzzle tape:** A strong cotton tape of about 2 cm width and one meter length is used for restraining the dogs from biting during handling.

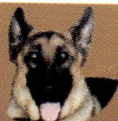

Two half hitches of appropriate size are made in the middle of tape. The owner is guided to slip the half hitches over the nasal bridge and pulled fairly tight. The free end are kept on the ventral aspect of the muzzle and then tied behind the ears. In short blunt faced dogs with small nose bridge an additional tape may be required for securing the muzzle tape and it is pulled along the frontal bone and tied with the collar.

2. Use of muzzle: The perforated muzzles of leather, plastic string and wire gauze are available in different sizes. Restraining with application of muzzle is quite easy. These muzzles are also suitable for harnessing for longer period even 10-12 hours for preventing licking of harmful drugs applied topically for the removal of ectoparasites and curing of skin lesions.

3. Handling of unruly and restless dogs: A collar with shoulder harness connected with a lead or chain is used for handling an unruly and restless as well as ferocious dog.

Registration of Pet Dog(s)

In most of the big towns and cities of India offices of Indian Kennel Club are available for the registration of pet dogs. Besides this it is also essential to obtain a license for keeping a pet dog in the urban limits of some big Indian cities. Registration of the dog with Kennel club makes it eligible for participation in shows.

Grooming

Grooming is important for keeping the dog clean and healthy. During grooming skin and coat problems, if any, are also detected and it also provides an opportunity to assess the soundness and physical condition of the dog.

A good grooming kit includes a partitioned small box carrying a dandy brush, a long bristle brush, a short bristle brush, a common comb with broad and fine teeth, one or two small and clean pieces of linen, a washed towel of about 30 cm×45 cm size or similar one along with a mild antiseptic lotion and topical cream.

Grooming of dog should be a routine practice and it should be done at a fixed place and time at a distance from the households. However, it is not possible in small flats and in such situations, care should be taken to make necessary arrangements for the collection of debris to avoid the spread of dust and fallen coat. It would be better to perform grooming out door after holding the pet on a mat in balcony or other places like back verandah, garage or a clean slab placed at a corner near the boundary wall etc.

The grooming starts with the picking of extraneous large size hairs. This is followed by removal of dirt and dust with a dandy brush or other brush suitable for the type of body coat. After this coat is combed in the natural direction of hairs for extracting ectoparasites, if any. The external orifices are cleaned with the soft linen soaked in a mild antiseptic lotion. The teeth and gum are examined. At the end entire body is wiped with a wet clean towel starting from face to end at the foot pads.

Bathing/Washing

All dogs, except the young puppies, delicate specimen and very old one, should be allowed bathing or washed regularly in the climatic conditions of tropical countries. Young ones may be washed after 8-9 weeks of age but should be protected from chilling in winter season. After washing puppies should be wiped dry with a clean and soft towel and kept confined at a dry place for complete drying.

Bathing of dogs may be required daily during the hot climatic condition with higher than 40°C ambient temperature otherwise washing at weekly interval during hot season,

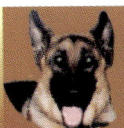

bi-weekly during comfortable climate and monthly or bi-monthly during cold season would be adequate, if regular grooming is carried. A good quality bath soap or shampoo should be used for cleaning the coat and body of the dogs. The animal should be rinsed thoroughly to remove soap/shampoo completely. A mild antiseptic may be used occasionally to keep the skin healthy. Wet dog should not be let loose as they are in habit to rub the body on ground when wet.

Care of Feet

Dewclaws do not have any use rather these are prone to create injury when hooked with any object. This is commonly encountered in sporting breeds. It is better to remove them in early life with the help of a pair of sharp scissors. Tincture iodine should be applied for a minute to facilitate the sealing of wound. At the time of grooming, all the four feet should be thoroughly examined and cleaned off any extraneous material and parasites as many species of ticks have affinity for the inter toe space and root of the nails. Clipping of nails may also be required in dogs exposed to little or no exercise. A special nail nipper is used for the cutting of nails and use of scissors may spoil the shape of nails by splitting or cracking.

Hair Dressing

Special hair dressing is required in a few breeds like Poodles and other similar toy and small breeds of long hair. Hair dressing of dogs is more popular among the lady owners of Western countries and specific hair dressing saloons are working in many European countries, particularly in France. So far there appears to be no such facility in India and in big cities some helpers at veterinary clinics have acquired the skill of hair dressing. In case of all hairy breeds a minor plucking or removal of

some odd hairs is required which is done by the owners themselves or with the help of a skilled person.

Docking

Amputation of tail is done in early life, as it is necessary for the registration of some of the breeds with the Kennel club. The operation is simple and performed under the cover of local anaesthesia. Antiseptic dressing for 6-7 days is required for the healing of cut wound. Some times docking is also required for the treatment of an injured tail for checking the spread of infection.

Ear Cropping

Clipping of external ear (Pinna) is known as ear cropping. It may be required to give erect shape to the ear. In a few breeds with very long hanging ears, cropping is used to protect the dog from the injury of ear and to avoid complications associated with the injuries. Ear cropping also makes the grooming and cleaning easier but induces deformity in the normal appearance. In some of the breeds long, drooping, fleshy and feathery ears are the main attractions and adds to the beauty of the breed as in Golden Retriever.

Spaying

Spaying is the surgical removal of ovaries and performed to suppress sexual activities and stop the puppies bearing ability of the bitches. The spaying of bitches should be done on the onset of puberty, i.e., just after the recession of first oestrus.

Castration

The process of induction of surgical sterility in males (dogs) is known as castration. This is

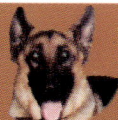

done at the age of puberty. Castration at prepubertal age may reduce the masculine behaviour of the dog.

Transportation

Often need arises for the transportation of pet dogs for various purposes, viz., the change of place of owner (inland and abroad), for participation in a show at other place and some-times (rarely) for the treatment of a complicated disease. The transportation of pets within the country does not pose any serious problem. A pet dog can be transported via public and private transports, provided the animal is secured as per the norms of the transport company. Pet dogs may be transported in a special cage provided in passenger trains, in steamer, in motor vehicles and for short distance (local movement within in 10-12 km) even on cycle rickshaw and in rural areas animal driven carts are used. Nomads quite often carry entire litter on the back of a pack animal (pony or buffalo), after properly restraining in a close but ventilated basket of appropriate size. For transportation in public vehicles, application of wire muzzle or leather muzzle may be compulsory. For international transportation several formalities according to the rules of the two countries are required. Some of these are: (i) health certificate, (ii) vaccination certificate, (iii) entry permit from the embassy and (iv) complete address of the parties responsible for sending and receiving the dog.

For all kinds of transportation of pet dog(s), following actions and precautions are required:

1. The dog(s) should be vaccinated against rabies and where required against other infectious diseases also [specially several kinds of vaccinations may be necessary for exporting dog(s)].

2. The animal should be secured properly.

3. A tag containing necessary details, viz., name of the dog, colour, sex, owners name and address, and destination should be attached with the collar of the dog. The tag should be made of good cord and should be well protected to avoid damage.

4. The dog should be muzzled. The muzzle should be reasonably loose to facilitate eating and drinking but prohibit biting.

5. A training for obeying the instructions for certain activities like get in and come out and also handling and leading may be advantageous for transportation.

6. Aggressive dogs should be mildly tranquilized and should be well secured with a strong collar and chain.

7. In travel requiring more than 12 h, arrangements should also be made for their watering, a light meal (preferably dry biscuits) and for release of natural urge. i.e. urination and defaecation. Normally these are not required if journey time is less than 12 h and all these activities are completed before loading the dog(s) in the vehicle.

Care of Teeth

The teeth of dogs are made to handle cadaver of animals and birds for feeding in natural habitat but domestication has made considerable changes in their diets and in most of the feedings, dogs do not get opportunities for adequate exercise of teeth and gums and also their cleaning. For this purpose fresh bone without spicule should be offered occasionally for chewing. Now-a-days artificial bones are available for the dogs of vegetarian families. Alternative of bones are reasonably hard fruits and vegetables like carrot, cucumber, apple, pears, peaches, guava and mango with stone.

Some of the modern owners are using tooth-paste with a soft brush for keeping the teeth

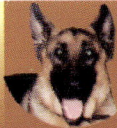

and gum clean and healthy. However, such practice may not be applied by all owners and there appears to be no specific advantage over the offering of bone or alternates for the bone.

Use of Deodorants

Normally deodorants are not required for the working and sporting breeds because mostly they are housed away at a separate place. But for the toy breeds and lap dogs mostly living in the home as a family member use of suitable deodorants is required to keep off the characteristic odour of the pet dog. Almost all common deodorants used by family members can also be used for the dogs.

Teeth Eruption and Age Estimation

The dogs are one of the most variable species in shape, size, growth, maturity and other configuration, which affect the eruption of teeth. The estimation of age from the sequence of teeth eruption is difficult to make accurate. Indeed, it gives some approximate values which may be used for a crude estimation of age as follows:

1. The deciduous incisors erupt at 4 to 5 weeks of age and these are replaced by permanent incisers at 4 to 5 months of age.

2. The deciduous canines erupt at 3 to 4 weeks of age and are replaced with permanent canines at about 3-4 months of age.

3. However, among the pre-molar teeth only first, second and third pre-molars are deciduous and erupt at about one month of age and these are replaced by permanent pre-molar teeth at 5-6 months of age.

4. The fourth pre-molar and first molar teeth erupt permanent at 4-5 months of age. This is followed by the eruption of second permanent molars at 4.5 to 6 months and third pair at 6 to 7 months of age.

Thus, the following two dental formulae are:

(i) Dental formula for deciduous/temporary teeth

2(I-3/3 C-1/1 P-3/3 M-0/0) = 28

(ii) Dental formula for permanent teeth

2(I-3/3 C-1/1 P-4/4 M-3/3) = 44

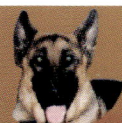

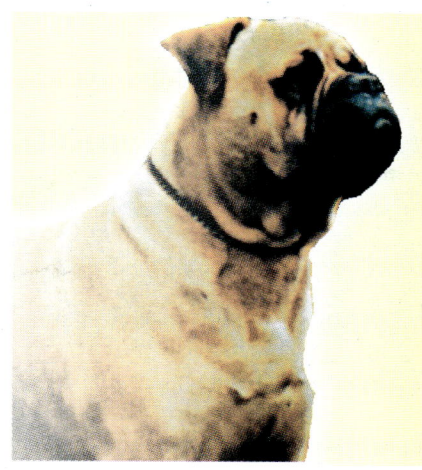

Foods and Feeding of Dogs

4

Selection of foods and feeding of dogs to supply optimum quantity of different essential nutrients to meet the requirements for normal physiological functions is an art of the application of the scientific basis of nutrition. Being simple stomached and carnivorous in feeding habits, the natural food of dogs is flesh and bone, but feral as well as wild dogs have been seen to eat some roots, leaves and fruits although occasionally and in small quantity. Domestication for several thousands of years has made the dogs omnivorous and in many cases in India, pet dogs are reared on exclusive vegetarian foods supplemented with milk and milk products but without the feeding of any kind of meat, fish, eggs and bone. The diets of dogs should be designed to satisfy the hunger and meet the optimum nutritional requirements. The various nutrients required in the diets of dogs are as usual the carbohydrates, lipids, proteins, minerals and vitamins as required in the diet of other mammalian species including the man. The feeding of pet dogs becomes easier due to close resemblance with the human foods.

Nutrients Required for the Feeding of Dogs

These, may be grouped as follows:

1. **Carbohydrates:** The dogs are able to digest starchy foods and their ability to digest fibrous carbohydrates and most of the simple sugars is very little.

2. **Proteins:** There is very little scope of microbial digestion in the dogs and they require intact proteins containing adequate quantity of essential (non-dispensable) amino acids in correct ratio for supporting growth, repair of the wear and tear of the tissues and also for the normal reproductive performances.

3. **Lipids:** The fats and oils are also essential in the foods of dogs and they are capable to digest more than 10% fat in the diet. However, for all practical purposes concentration of fats in the diets of dogs should not be less than 5% on dry matter basis and it should supply at least 1 per cent essential fatty acid (linoleic acid).

Very high fat content in the diet may cause back flow of some bile in the stomach. This is probably a natural manipulation for facilitating resumption of normal passage of digesta from stomach to intestine.

4. **Minerals**: Dietary essential minerals have been classified into macro and micro minerals.

   (a) Macro minerals: The minerals requirement at 0.1% or more on dry matter basis in the diets are known as macro minerals and most of these are required for the development of structural organs specially the skeletal system and maintenance of acid levels in body fluids. These are calcium, phosphorus, magnesium, potassium, sodium, chloride and sulphur.

   (b) Micro minerals: These are dietary essential but required in minute quantity, and deficiency of most of these micro elements in the body may produce different production, reproduction and health problems. These elements are iron, copper, cobalt, zinc, iodine, manganese and selenium. There are also some other dietary essential micro elements found to be associated with different functions in the body. However, most of them are highly critical and excess may be often harmful. These are molybdenum, fluorine, chromium, nickel, tin, silicon and vanadium.

   Higher dietary concentration and intake of some of the trace elements like copper, molybdenum, fluorine and selenium may be hazardous and some times fatal also.

5. **Vitamins**: Only few vitamins are synthesized in the body of the dogs and most of the essential vitamins need to be supplemented in the diet. Sometimes parentral administration of some vitamins in much higher doses may be required for the management of clinical conditions. The vitamins are placed in (i) fat-soluble and (ii) water-soluble vitamins.

   (i) Fat-soluble vitamins are A, D, K and E, and dogs are capable of synthesizing vitamin K by gut microflora. All the other fat-soluble vitamins A, D and E are dietary essential but vitamin D may be made available for physiological functions in the body from synthesis in skin of the dog itself provided the skin get adequate exposure to solar radiation. Rancidity destroys fat-soluble vitamins specially the vitamin E which is essential for the maintenance of normal health of muscles and nerves.

   (ii) Water-soluble vitamins include all the members of B-complex and vitamin C. Adequate vitamin C is made available to the host from the synthesis of gut flora. Important water soluble vitamins for the dogs are thiamine (B_1), Riboflavin (B_2), niacin, pyridoxine (B_6) pantothenic acid, folic acid and cyanocobalamine (B_{12}). Choline is although controversial but its deficiency has been reported to be associated with the development of fatty liver syndrome in dogs.

6. **Energy**: It is the calorific value of feeds which liberates on metabolism of organic nutrients, i.e., dietary carbohydrates, proteins and lipids. In deficient conditions caused by under-feeding and starvation, tissues like muscle proteins and lipids are metabolized for the liberation of energy by the process of gluconeogenesis.

7. **Water**: Water is the main constituent of body tissues and it ranges from almost 85

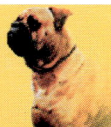

percent in new born puppies to 65 percent in the body of aged and obese dogs. Daily supply of wholesome drinking water is essential for the normal vital functions of the body and survival of the animal.

Feed additives: During the last few decades several feed additives and nutraceuticals have been developed for improving the performance of animals. These are mostly used as a supplement in small quantity. Few enzymes like sucrase lack in the digestive juices of dogs due to which dogs are unable to handle higher level of sugar in the diet. Similarly probiotic, lactic acid producing bacteria have been found to control infant diarrhoea by suppressing the proliferation of most of the enteric pathogenic microorganisms.

Common Foods of Dogs

Though carnivorous by food habit the domestication has made the dogs effectively omnivorous. The dog's diets are composed of different combinations of various foods eaten by human being as follows:

1. Cereal grains: These are the main sources of carbohydrates including crude fibre, e.g. wheat, rice, maize, sorghum, pearl millet, pearl barley, pearled oats and various minor millets.

2. Pulses: These are the sources of carbohydrates as well as proteins, e.g. gram, green gram, urad, moth, kidney bean, lentil, peas, etc.

3. Oilseeds: A few oil seeds are also used in small quantity. These are soyabeans, sunflower seeds, safflower seeds, gingly seeds and linseed.

4. Oilcakes: Mycotoxin free oil seed cakes are incorporated in the complete feeds of dogs. The common oilseed cakes are soyabean meal, groundnut cake, sesame cake and dehulled sunflower meal.

5. Fresh meat, bones, adipose tissue and glands.

6. Fishes and various edible aquatic species like lobster and crab etc.

7. Milk and milk products.

8. Roots and tubers – Carrot, potato, sweet potato, cassava and artichoke etc.

9. Fruits: Apple, pears, mango, guava, peaches, apricot and berries.

10. Nuts: Groundnut, cashew nut and roasted seeds of melons and pumpkin.

11. Dry fruits – Almost all kinds of dry fruits.

12. Green vegetables: Cabbage, cauliflower, ladies finger, bottle guard, snake guard, ridge guard, radish, capsicum, tomato and different leafy vegetables.

All kinds of foods except the fruits, nuts and dry fruits should be cooked before feeding and should be fed fresh cooked.

Processed Foods

Different kinds of processed packed, and canned foods or food supplements are now available in the markets of big cities.

These may be:

1. Dry biscuits, wafers and crumbles.

2. Semi moist canned foods

3. Moist canned foods.

Almost all packed foods are expensive and common pet dogs can be easily adapted to foods available in the owners kitchen with some rare occasions for supplementation.

Precautions in Dog Feeding

1. Young pups should preferably be offered foods in liquid or slurry form.

2. The foods should be fresh, wholesome and cooked.

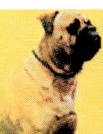

3. The place and time of feeding should be almost fixed.

4. Dogs should not be forced for eating, rather cause(s) of rejecting foods should be investigated, if fasting exceeds 24 hours.

5. Wholesome drinking water should be offered and changed after 6-8 hours interval. Cold water should be offered in hot season.

6. The utensils used for feeding and watering should be cleaned properly.

7. The diets should be prepared from the variety of items for providing all the nutrients in optimum quantity and proper ratio.

8. A piece of fresh long bone of sheep or goat with open ends should be offered for chewing which is required to keep the teeth and gums clean and healthy. The bone should be steamed.

9. In vegetarian families fresh carrot, radish, apple, pears or other fruits may be offered in place of bones.

10. Small and sharp pointed bones and splints in meat and spicule in fish pieces should not be included in dogs foods.

11. As far as possible meat of hormone treated animals should be avoided in the diets of growing and breeding animals.

12. A limited amount of low fibre diet should be fed to dogs during transit to avoid frequent defaecation and urination.

13. Ingredients of diets should be changed at a reasonable interval so that dogs do not develop liking for a particular food.

14. Raw eggs should not be fed because raw eggs contain an anti-nutritional factor avidin, which interferes in the digestion of protein.

15. Spoiled food should not be fed to dogs.

16. Over-feeding should be avoided. This can be achieved by decreasing fat content and increasing fibre level in the foods.

17. Tinned foods must be fed before the expiry of date and empty tin, cash memo as well as shop number must be kept until the supply is finished without any diet related problem.

18. The dogs should be taken out for natural urge like urination and defaecation about 1 to 2 hours before offering foods.

19. Each dog should be fed in his own utensils and feeding of two or more dogs in a single utensil should be avoided.

20. Lactating (nursing) bitches should be fed high energy, high protein and mineral rich diets for supporting optimum milk secretion.

21. Stud males should not be fed high energy diets to avoid development of obesity.

Food (Dry Matter) Requirement for Maintenance

The diets of adult dogs should be compounded incorporating several food items together or separately for supplying balanced nutrients. A moderately balanced diet for the maintenance of adult dogs should contain about 18-20% protein, upto 10% fibre and 3000 to 3300 Kcal ME per kg dry matter of the complete diet. The dogs upto 5 kg body weight should be fed to supply about 30-35 g dry matter (DM) per kg metabolic body size (body weight, $W^{0.75}$ kg); and DM supply per kg $W^{0.75}$ should be reduced gradually to supply about 25, 20, 18 and 15 g between 5-10, 10-20, 20-35 and beyond 35 kg body weight. These feeding rates are applicable to dogs for routine activities including a light exercise. Care should be taken to regulate the

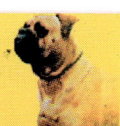

food composition and feed supply to control obesity or excessive thinness.

The requirements of protein and energy for the performing dogs are higher and diets for such dogs should contain 20-22% protein and 3500 to 4000 Kcal ME per kg dry matter of complete diet. The growing dogs may require about 100% more nutrients in early life which is gradually reduced to maintenance level at 12-15 months of age. Sporting dogs may require upto 50% more energy depending on the intensity of sports. The energy requirements of pregnant bitches during last fortnight may increase upto 450 Kcal ME per kg $W^{0.75}$ and during lactation (nursing) may be upto 500 Kcal ME per kg $W^{0.75}$.

Feeding of Pups

At birth although the puppies are blind but find teats by inherent natural instinct assisted by the dam and start suckling with in a short time. Normally bitches secrete enough milk to meet the requirements of puppies in early life. However, young pups start nibbling of dams food at about 2 weeks of age after opening the eyes. There is no fixed schedule for weaning and pups are weaned at 4, 6 and 8 weeks of age. However, 6 week age may be considered more suitable for both pups and the dam as by this

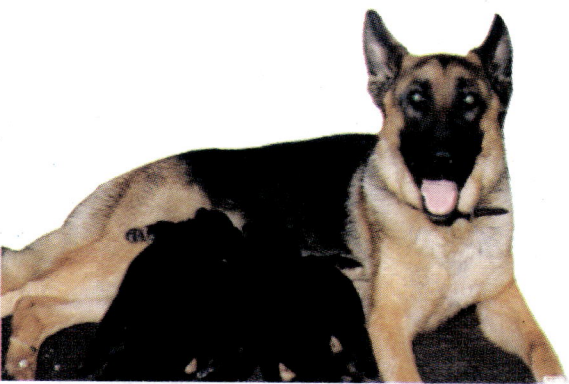

Fig. 116 A nursing German Shepherd Bitch

time pups learn to eat considerable amount of semi-solid and solid foods and milk secretion of dam is significantly decreased which normally does not pose any clinico-pathological problems like mastitis and engorgement followed by plugging due to coagulation in teat canal.

Milk secretion in nursing bitches is affected by breed, age and body condition at first breeding, litter size, stage of lactation and foods offered. Average milk production is about 2.4, 2.7 and 2.8 percent of body weight in first week of whelping in small, medium and large size animals respectively. These rise to about 3.4, 4.6 and 3.6 percent at peak (4 weeks) in corresponding types and then gradually fall to cease at 6 to 8 weeks of nursing period. In some exceptional bitches milk yield as high as 7.3 per- cent of body weight has been recorded.

Artificial Foods for Weaned Pups

Although good quality commercial foods for weaned pups are available but these are not accessible in small towns and at remote places. A satisfactory milk replacement diet for the feeding of pups, weaned even at birth or orphaned due to demice of dam or agalactia, can be prepared from the common food items available in home or local market. A few examples of formula foods for young pups are given in Table 4.1.

Method of Feeding the Pups

The formula foods are diluted with sterile water to contain about 20 percent almost uniformly distributed dry matter. The diets should preferably be fed at body temperature or when it is tolerated by fingers dipped in it. Feeding by bottle may be necessary in early life upto 2 weeks but pups should be simultaneously encouraged to eat by licking from shallow bowel with smooth edge.

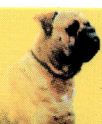

Table 4.1: Formula Foods for Weaned Pups				
Ingredients (g)	1	2	3	4
Liquid, whole milk	200	-	-	-
Cow	-	700	-	-
Buffalo	-	-	800	-
Goat	-	-	-	700
Fresh cream (30% fat)	200	200	100	200
Egg yolk	-	50	50	50
Rice gruel/Wheat flour gruel	200	50	50	50
Boiling water	400	-	-	-

(i)   N.B. (+) Supplements are to be added per kg of prepared foods are vitamin A 2000 IU, vitamin D_3 500 IU and citric acid 4 g.

(ii) Tetracycline or other recommended antibiotic @10g per kg food should also be mixed for providing protection against bacterial infections, if any.

Feeding Schedules

Normally pups should be fed at 2 hours interval in first week. In the second week feeding interval may be increased to 3 h in day and 4 h in the night. During 3rd and 4th week day time interval may be 4 h and only one feeding at 6 h interval in the night. From fifth week onwards the pups should be fed at 6 h interval and feeding time should be adjusted in a manner to avoid late night feeding. Night feeding can be escaped if last food is offered between 6-9 pm.

Feeding of Growing Dogs

At 8 weeks of age complete change in feeding schedule is required which should preferably be a twice daily feeding schedule synchronizing with the time of break-fast and dinner for the family members i.e. between 6-9 and 18-21 h respectively. The diets of growing dogs are made of cereal grains, pulses and nuts and their products and some of the by-products. This is fortified with milk and milk products (in vegetarian foods) and meat and various edible carcass offals, eggs and fish etc. in the common foods.

In addition to these, dogs should also be fed boiled tubers and starchy roots, cooked green vegetables and fresh fruits. Some breeds are very selective and do not like vegetables and fruits. In such cases green vegetables and fruits should be processed to make them acceptable. Cooking with meat has been found to increase the intake of green vegetables and fruits. Dogs during active growth phase upto about 6 months of age should be fed a balanced palatable diet to ensure about 50-55 g DM intake per kg body weight, which is gradually reduced to about 38-40 g DM intake per kg body weight at about one year of age. A guide-line of feeding schedule for actively growing dogs of different size is shown in table 4.2.

Feeding of Adult Dogs for Maintenance

Companion and non-performing working or sporting dogs require about 132 Kcal ME per kg metabolic body size. Optimum nutrients

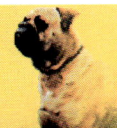

Table 4.2: Daily Foods for Growing Dogs

Body Wight (kg)	Cereals (g/d)	Meat (g/d)	Milk (g/d)	Remarks
5	200	50	100	One fresh metacarpal, metatarsal or
10	400	100	100	humerus of goat or
15	500	150	100	sheep with open ends
20	600	200	100	should be offered once
25	700	250	100	in a week for chewing.

N.B. (i) About 50-100 g boiled green vegetables and fruits should be fed.

(ii) Meat can be replaced with double the amount of milk.

(iii) In absence of milk and meat an egg may be fed daily or diets should be balanced with the incorporation of other ingredients for protein and amino acids supply.

(iv) For the dogs on complete vegetarian diets (including milk) half boiled whole carrot, beat, turnip or raw cucumber and fruits are offered for keeping the teeth and gums clean and healthy.

can be supplied by feeding a diet containing about 20 percent protein and 3000 Kcal ME per kg dry matter. Small and toy breeds have been found to like milk. As usual, meat should be replaced with milk and milk products in a vegetarian diet. A tentative feeding schedule for adult dogs is given in the following Table 4.3.

Feeding of Working Dogs

Working dogs engaged for guarding the house and flocks or herds of domestic animals on pasture or in yards require 25 to 50 per cent more energy than the maintenance requirement. This increased intake is frequently compensated by higher intake of a food containing 3000 to 3200 Kcal ME per kg DM.

Feeding of Hunting (Game) Dogs

Hunting dogs are mostly engaged in strenuous exercise in chasing and searching of the game with their hunter master, and often run for 50 to 100 km in a day. The energy requirement of such dogs is 3 to 4 times higher than the maintenance requirement. Such a high amount of energy is rather difficult to obtain by eating a low energy diet due to limitation of the stomach capacity. Thus, a diet containing about 20-22 percent protein and 4000 Kcal ME per kg DM of the diet should be fed. This is achieved by the replacement of cereal grains with edible fat or oil at the rate of 1 gramme lipid for every 2 grammes of starch. Tentative rations of game dogs have been given in Table 4.4.

Feeding of Pregnant Bitches

Pregnant bitches compensate additional nutrients requirement during first four weeks of pregnancy by increasing the intake of feeds offered for maintenance. However, due to considerable increase in the uterine mass, greater part of the abdominal cavity is occupied by the gravid uterine horns and during the last trimester of gestation period, bitches require a high protein (20-24% on DM basis) and high

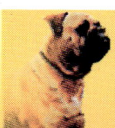

Table 4.3: Feeding Schedule of Adult dogs for Maintenance and Light Routine Activity

Body weight, kg	Food items (g/day)			
	Cereals	Meat	Green vegetables and legume pods	Milk
5	100	50	50-60	100
10	150	50	50-60	100
15	200	100	80-100	100
20	300	100	80-100	-
25	400	100	100-150	-
30	450	150	100-150	-
40	500	150	150-200	-
50	600	150	200-300	-
60	700	150	200-300	-
70 & more	800	150	200-300	-

N.B. In absence of meat double amount of milk should be offered or 1-2 eggs may be fed.

Table 4.4: Rations of Hunting Dog

Body weight, Kg	Foods requirement (g/d)			
	Cereals	Meat	Vegetables	Others
30	1400	500	300	One steamed
40	2000	500	300	humerus / femer or
50	2500	600	300	other long bone of
60	2800	600	400	sheep or goat
70 & more	3000	600	400	should be given for chewing

N.B. Hunting dogs mostly feed on fresh carcasses while on trail.

energy (4000 Kcal ME per kg DM) diet properly balanced for the optimum supply of essential amino acids, minerals and vitamins. The daily ration schedule has been given for different body weights in the Table 4.5.

Feeding of Stud Dog

Male dogs for breeding are selected at an early age of 6 to 9 months when reflexes are developed. The dogs are fed as per the schedule given for growing dogs upto one year of age. After this they are put on 10 to 15 percent higher diet upto 15 month of age when they are used for breeding. Adult dogs should be fed maintenance ration alongwith plenty of boiled green vegetables and fresh fruits. However, a little higher level of feeding, i.e. 20-25 percent

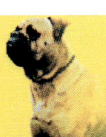

Body weight kg	Food ingredients (g/d)				Steamed bone
	Cereals	Meat	Milk	Greens/Fruits	
5	100	50	100	100	Fresh femer/
7.5	150	50	100	100	humerus/meta
10	200	100	100	150	carpal/metatasus of
12.5	25	100	100	150	sheep or goat with open
15	250	100	100	200	ends. If not available
20	350	100	100	200	soup of long bone of
25	450	150	-	200	buffalo may be given.
30	550	150	-	200	
40	600	150	-	250	
50	700	200	-	250	
60 and more	800	200	-	250	

Table 4.5: Daily Diet of Pregnant Bitches

N.B. (i) Vitamins and minerals may be supplemented, if bones, glands, vegetables and fruits are not fed.

(ii) Some bitches suffer from pregnancy naucea and they should be given some suitable salt for controlling naucea and acidity.

more than the maintenance requirements should be fed alongwith supplementation of additional vitamins A, E and B-complex about 3-4 weeks prior to the expected breeding season. Covering of a single bitch once daily for six days in a week may be allowed without any problem after 18 months of age.

Feeding of Obese (Fatty) Dogs

Obesity is an abnormal condition, which reduces the performance of dogs and increases the risk of systemic diseases, particularly that of the cardio-vascular system. However, obesity can be controlled and rectified by the manipulation of the diet composition and feeding schedule. A tentative feeding schedule has been given in the Table 4.6 for obese dogs. However, this may be modified according to extent of obesity and also to keep the animal physically presentable. The energy content of diets should be reduced to contain about 2800 Kcal ME per kg DM with minimum 3 percent lipids but fibre level may be raised upto 10-12 per cent through the replacement of starchy grains and fatty muscle with bran rich flour and lean meat.

Grass Eating Habits in Dogs

There may be several reasons for grass eating by a dog. It is commonly believed that dogs eat grass for stimulating vomiting. It is also true to some extent, particularly for expelling the alimentary tract nematodes which have entered the stomach. The other reasons are just for a change or when dogs are fed high meat diet continuously for several days.

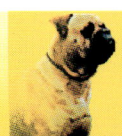

Table 4.6: Feeding Schedule of Obese Dogs

Body weight, Kg	Feeds offered (g/d)		
	Bran rich cereal products	Lean meat	Green beans and vegetables (steamed fresh)
10	50	100	150
20	50	100	200
30	100	150	300
40	150	150	500
50	150	150	500
60	200	200	600
70	250	200	600
80 and more	300	200	600

N.B. (i) Minerals - vitamins supplement should be given weekly or fortnightly or as per need.

(ii) Diets may be further modified as per body condition of the dogs as per the advise of the dietitian.

Special Foods for Sick Dogs

Selection of foods for sick dogs is very important and foods differ due to disease, breed and condition of the patient. The preparation of foods is very important for the feeding of sick dogs and as far as possible, freshly cooked foods should be offered for feeding within 3-4 hours. The different kinds of foods required for the feeding of patients in various kinds of diseases are:

1. Soup of long bones – Fresh long bones with open ends or broken in two or three pieces are boiled on slow heat for 5-6 hours to obtain a good and palatable soup rich in minerals and protein.

2. Whole rabbit meat: Entire dressed carcass along with liver and kidneys are boiled in equal amount of water, for 600-700 g carcass and 1 kg carcass respectively, for 2-3 hours. The meat cum soup is fed after cooling. Quantity may vary from 800g to 1500g.

3. Meat tea: It is prepared by boiling fresh pieces of meat of edible carcass for 3-4 hours and then strained. The strained liquid is offered to the patients for intake by licking. This is very nutritious and hastens recovery.

4. Fresh bran boiled with milk is a nutritious food.

5. Soup made of pancreas in skimmed milk is considered good for the dogs suffering from diabetes melitus.

6. Fish soup in milk is easily digestible and nutritious.

7. In cases of gastritis when foods are not

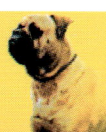

retained in the stomach, rectal feeding is applied. The patients are given warm peptonized milk or soup with the help of an enema jug. The quantity of milk, soup or meat tea may be 10 to 100 ml, depending on the size of the dog and repeated at 3-4 hours interval.

8. Parenteral feeding of synthetic liquid preparations may be necessary in serious illness, specially during severe dehydration and oral obstructions. Normal saline, glucose saline and nutrient mixture are infused intravenously as per the advise of the veterinarian.

Feeding of Sick Dogs

It will be always better to seek the advice of a Veterinary Doctor or a Veterinary dietician. However, some common precautions required for the selection of foods for different systemic and inflammatory diseases are described briefly.

Cardiac Insufficiency

Quantity of common salt should be reduced significantly or excluded, and foods with low sodium contents should be used. Some of such feeds are fresh water fishes, lean meat, egg yolk and white rice.

Diabetes Mellitus

The proportion of starchy and sugar containing foods is drastically cut while that of fibre rich and low fat feeds like skimmed milk, green vegetables and high bran chapati is increased.

Diarrhoea

The foods should be selected to retain water and electrolytes and should be prepared from easily digestible ingredients like curd, paneer, eggs and liver with wheat flour or rice. Heavy foods should be avoided. Diets containing high level of paneer or egg should be balanced for the supply of potassium. Oral administration of powdered chalk, caolin and catechu has been found useful for controlling diarrhoea.

Dysentery and Gastroenteritis

All kinds of irritant and bitter foods should be avoided while mucilagenous foods like linseed tea, egg white beaten with milk or barley water should be fed. Thicker diets made of peptonized milk and arrowroot flour or sago may be fed as slurry or gruel. Parenteral administration of glucose saline may be required, in severe dehydration, for the restoration of body water level.

Ascites

Depending on the severity of the condition common salt should be restricted or even removed from the diet. Feeding of liquid diets should be avoided.

Fever (Pyrexia)

Since loss of energy during fever is increased, this should be compensated for by the feeding of easily available energy sources. Increased supply of energy will be 6-7 kcal ME per kg body weight for each degree rise in body temperature above the normal value. Energy should preferably be supplied by incorporating pasteurized cream or butter, boiled eggs and edible oil in the diet.

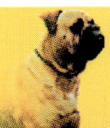

Hypoglycaemia

In acute hypoglycaemic condition, glucose should be administered immediately per os or if necessary by intravenous route. This should be supported by the feeding of digestible starchy foods. Working dogs should be put to light work only during the recovery period.

Flatulence

Flatulence is the symptom of many gastro-intestinal disorders associated mainly with dyspepsia, constipation and gastro-enteritis. In such conditions all easily fermentable foods should be avoided from the diets of patients. A mild laxative diet should be fed alongwith the treatment of the ailments.

Renal Insufficiency

An easily digestible low protein diet of high biological value should be fed. A diuretic with such diet would be helpful in the treatment of renal insufficiency.

Urolithiasis

The diet of dogs suffering from urolithiasis should be made of low protein and low mineral ingredients and highly digestible starch and many vitamins. The level of salt with high water intake may help the clearance of smaller uroliths. Composition of uroliths may also be helpful in the formulation of suitable diet for the removal of uroliths.

Diseases of Liver

Easily metabolizable foods like simple sugars, rice gruel and sagoo gruel along with protein of high biological value are fed. The supply of protein should be limited to less than 4 g per kg body weight. The diet should contain plenty of B vitmains and vitamins A, C and E as supportive therapy.

Stress

The dogs exposed to harsh and hostile environmental conditions, viz., extreme cold or heat will require the feeding of high-energy foods at short intervals of 2-4 hours depending on the severity of exposure. An oral administration @ 1 to 2 g per kg body weight but minimum 10 g of glucose at an interval of 3-4 hours dissolved in water is effective in stress management. The administration is continued until recovery of the patient.

Depraved Appetite (Pica)

Earlier phosphorus deficiency was considered to be the cause of pica but later on many other deficiencies were found responsible for the occurrence of the symptoms of pica. In case of pica the cause(s) should be identified and feeds should be selected to balance the diet or it should be supplemented with deficient ingredient.

Feeding of Aged (Geriatric) Dogs

The dogs over 10 years of age in case of heavy breeds and 12-13 years of age in small breeds are considered aged dogs. Most of the vital and sensory organs weaken and such geriatric animals often require special care. The common signs of geriatric stage are the weakness of sight and locomotory organs, considerable loss of hearing, decreased appetite and digestibility and general weakness due to rejection of common heavy foods. The teeth become weak or worn out, due to which animals are unable to eat hard and stiff foods.

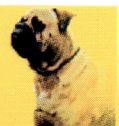

Thus, for the feeding of geriatric dogs, foods should be selected carefully and prepared in such form to facilitate easy intake. The foods should be easily digestible. The diets made of rice gruel, wheat flour gruel or slurry prepared in milk and supplemented with vitamins may be used. Well cooked boneless minced meat, liver and fishes without spicules should be satisfactory for omnivorous dogs. Curd, paneer and puddings with very little or without sugar may also be fed. Vegetable soup and citrus fruit juice may be given once or twice in a week.

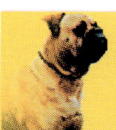

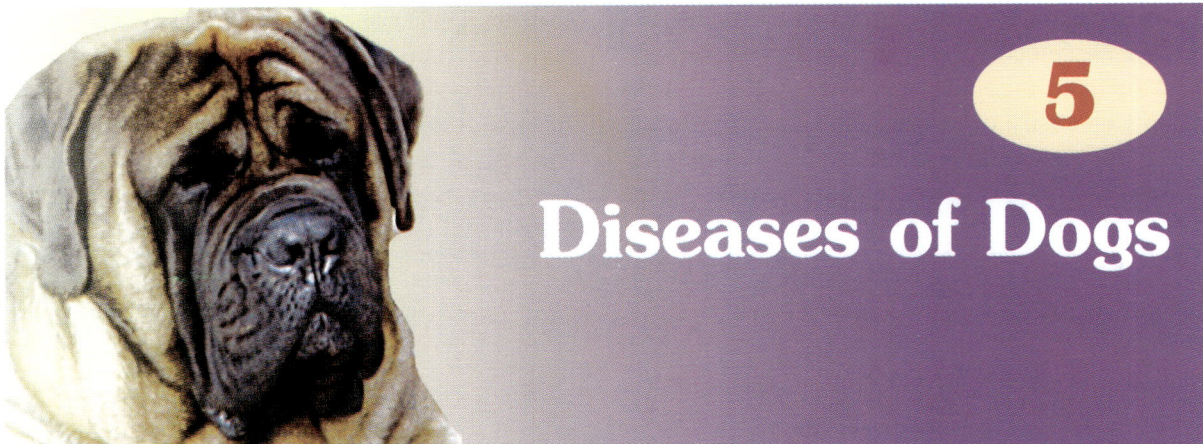

Diseases of Dogs

5

Sometimes due to lack of care, environmental stress, improper managemental practices or nutritional imbalances, the dogs, young and adult suffer from several diseases. These diseases may be categorised into-infectious and non infectious diseases. Infectious diseases includes different viral, bacterial, fungal and parasitic diseases and the non-infectious category includes different systemic diseases, metabolic and deficiency diseases. This chapter deals with the various diseases of the dogs along with their etiology, clinical findings, diagnosis, prevention and cure.

COMMON SYSTEMIC DISEASES

In general veterinary practice the system of treatment at most of the veterinary clinics starts with the registration of patient along with the owner, recording of history of the sickness in detail. Many times persons bringing the patient at clinics may not be fully aware with sequence of events that happened during the previous few days before the ailment was noticed. So, the person actually responsible for handling and caring the pet should be asked to narrate the history. This is followed by the physical examination of the sick pet for making tentative diagnosis. The line of treatment in most of the cases is decided on the basis of history and physical observations, which usually changes, if necessary on the basis of patho-biochemical examination of the patients. A brief account of common systemic diseases and also the manifestation of diseases has been given as guide line for seeking veterinary aids.

1. Halitosis (Foul Breath)

Halitosis in the manifestation of clinico-pathological conditions and inadequate oral cavity hygiene. This condition may be produced by any kind of inflammatory condition in the oral cavity, decay of food particles retained in the mouth and may be due to some of the digestive disorders.

Aetiology: The primary causes are the subclinical or clinical inflammatory changes to infection of gum, teeth and oral cavity, pharyngitis, bronchitis, rhinitis, hepato-biliary disorders, chronic indigestion, cough etc.

Line of treatment

1. The cause is identified and removed.

2. Antiseptic mouthwash is used.
3. Infection is treated.
4. Digestive disorders are treated.
5. Respiration tract ailments are treated.

2. Stomatitis

The general inflammatory condition of the entire buccal cavity is called stomatitis and this includes cheilitis (inflammation of lips), gingivitis (inflammation of the gums), glossitis (inflamation of tongue) pharyngitis, tonsilitis, odontitis, etc.

Clinical Signs: Excessive ropy salivation, reddish and tender oral mucosa, difficulty in ingestion of food causing inadequate food intake and halitosis. The pets suffering from cheilitis lose hair due to rubbing of the lips and muzzle.

Line of treatment

1. Topical application of pain relieving and antiseptic ointment or lotion on the lips and muzzle for reducing the irritation.
2. Cleaning of oral cavity with mild and non-irritant antiseptic lotions.
3. Use of antiseptic toothpaste for cleaning the teeth and gums.
4. Removal of foreign bodies.
5. Use of antibiotics for the treatment of injections.
6. Feeding of non-irritant and laxative liquid or semi-solid diets.
7. Administration of vitamins B complex.
8. Ulcerative lesions should be cauterized with 10% silver nitrate sticks.

3. Gingivitis

Inflammation of gums is known as gingivitis and it is also called periodontitis.

Aetiology

Deposition of tartar on the teeth provides places for the establishment of pathogenic microorganisms causing inflammation of the gums.

Clinical signs

The gums are tender, sensitive, swollen and painful. There is halitosis, decrease or refusal of food intake, drooling of the saliva, toothache and often loss of tooth, if inflammatory condition prolongs.

Line of treatment

1. Removal of the foreign body, if any retained between the teeth and/or gums.
2. Application of non-irritant antiseptic lotion on gums.
3. Removal of tartar from the teeth followed by painting with antiseptic lotion.
4. Administration of antibiotics for the treatment of infections.
5. Feeding of laxative diets.
6. Supplementation of vitamins A, C and B complex.

4. Sialocele

The accumulation of saliva beneath the skin is called sialocele. It may be due to trauma but some time due to obscure reasons.

Aetiology

1. Obstruction of one or more salivary ducts.
2. Flow of saliva through the ruptured salivary duct and its accumulation in the subcutaneous tissue.

Clinical signs

1. Oedematous swelling below the tongue and lower jaw which may sometime extend upto pharynx.
2. Dysphagia in case of oral sialocele.

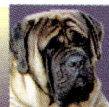

3. Difficulty in breathing in case of large sialocele in the pharynx.
4. Traumatic injury causes anorexia due to pain.

Line of treatment

1. The sialocele is drained out and infused with antiseptic solution.
2. This is coupled with anti-inflammatory drugs.
3. Repair of rupture, if any, and treatment with antibiotics.

5. Pharyngitis and Pharyngeal Dysphagia

It is the inflammation of pharynx. This is a disease of mostly aged animals.

Aetiology

The causes may be mechanical, chemical or thermal injuries due to eating of coarse or hot foods and administration of drugs. The other causes are microbial infections and inflammation of adjoining organs and parts of the body.

Clinical signs

1. Difficulties in swallowing of food and water
2. Coughing and oozing of frothy secretions.
3. Loss of appetite due to inability of ingestion.
4. Halitosis.
5. Thick greyish deposit on the tongue.

Line of treatment

1. Removal of the foreign body, if any.
2. Use of non-irritant and mild mouth, wash.
3. Painting with boroglycerol or gentian voilet lotion 3 or 4 times daily.
4. Feeding of liquid diet at body temperature.

5. Administration of antibiotics or sulpha drugs through parenteral route.
6. Removal of any growth obstructing the passage.

6. Oesophagitis

The inflammation of oesophagus is known as oesophagitis. It is rarely an independent ailment and generally it is the extension of oropharyngeal inflammation or ascending extension of gastritis.

Aetiology

1. Primary cause is mostly the gastroesophageal refluxes.
2. Frequent vomiting of acidic fluid from the stomach.
3. Obstruction caused by foreign bodies.
4. Injuries caused by food or foreign body.
5. Consumption of too cold or too hot food.

Clinical signs

1. There may be regurgitation.
2. Swallowing is painful due to which patients are reluctant to eat solid foods.
3. The oral cavity may be also inflammed due to intake of irritant substance.

Line of treatment

1. Withholding of food.
2. Administration of astringent fluid.
3. Parenteral administration of antibiotics.
4. Feeding of medicated liquid food.
5. Administration of antacids and laxatives.
6. Soft diet and parenteral fluid therapy.

7. Gastritis

It is inflammation of stomach.

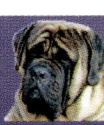

Aetiology

1. Intake of spoiled and decayed foods.
2. Intake of contaminated foods. The contaminants may be chemicals or microbiological agents.
3. Microbial infections.
4. Parasitic infestation.
5. Consumption of mouldy food and poisonous plants.

Clinical signs

1. Vomiting of foul smelling contents.
2. Halitosis.
3. Reluctance to eat.
4. Dehydration and exhaustion due to prolonged vomiting.
5. Anaemia due to prolonged under-feeding and indigestion in chronic gastritis.

Line of treatment

1. Removal of dietary cause and foreign body.
2. Control of nausea and vomiting.
3. Administration of oral antacids in small doses but for shorter interval.
4. Gastric lavage, if required.
5. Feeding of non-irritant foods.
6. Administration of antibiotics, sulpha drugs or treatment for gastroenteric parasitism (if positive for parasitism).

8. Constipation

Delayed evacuation and compact digesta in gastrointestinal tract is called constipation.

Aetiology

1. Faulty feeding.
2. Depraved appetite.
3. Lack of exercise.
4. Excessive feeding and unscheduled feeding.
5. Feeding of low fibre diet and low water intake.
6. Inflammation of gastrointestinal tract.

Clinical signs

1. Difficult defaecation after straining.
2. Very hard faeces which may be bolus form in certain disorders.
3. Various degree of loss of appetite.
4. General weakness.
5. Dehydration.
6. Loss of condition.

Line of treatment

1. Feeding of wheat bran gruel and other fibrous food in case of mild constipation.
2. Administration of laxatives and if required, the oleogenous purgative.
3. Enema for the evacuation of bowel and restoration of motility.
4. Administration of physiological fluid I/v for restoring fluid volume and rehydration.
5. Deworming in parasitism.
6. Coccidiostat in case of Coccidiosis.
7. Administration of vitamin B complex or liver extract parenterally.

9. Vomiting (Emesis)

The expulsion of gastric contents and rarely even proximal intestinal contents through mouth is known as vomiting. It is manifestation of different kinds of gastrointestinal and hepato-biliary disorders.

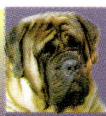

Aetiology

1. Different gastrointestinal disorders.
2. Consumption of spoiled, decayed foods, mouldy food and extraneous materials.
3. Inflammatory conditions of the gastro-intestinal tract.
4. Pyloric stenosis.
5. Dilatation of oesophagus.
6. Ingestion of irritant chemicals.
7. Hepato-billiary inflammatory conditions.
8. Miscellaneous inflammatory conditions, viz., Nephritis, uremia, pyometra, otitis, diabetes mellitus, encephalitis, gastro-intestinal parasitism and poisoning.

Clinical signs

The sequence of events leading to vomiting are nausea, retching and expulsion of gastric contents through mouth. The vomitus may contain ingested materials mixed with saliva, bile and gastric juice. Smell of vomitus is foul. There is dehydration of various degree and depression.

Line of treatment

1. Oral administration of astringent drugs.
2. Appropriate fluid therapy for replacement.
3. Removal of the cause, if possible.
4. Administration of antiemetic drugs.
5. Use of antibiotics in inflammatory conditions.
6. Treatment of the diseases stimulating emesis.

10. Enteritis (Diarrhoea and Dysentry)

The inflammation of intestine is known as enteritis. It may be infectious or non-infectious and exhibited by diarrhoea, dysentry, dehydration and vomiting.

Aetiology

1. Sudden change in the diets.
2. Feeding of spoiled foods.
3. Ingestion of chemical agents.
4. Enteric parasitism.
5. Enteritis causing viral infections.
6. Enteritis causing bacterial infections.

Clinical signs

1. Occurrence of diarrhoea.
2. In some cases there may be vomiting also.
3. Various degree of dehydration.
4. Fever due to stress, exhaustion or infections.
5. Anorexia.
6. Abdominal pain is exhibited by crying and in severe cases rolling or lying prostrate with spread limbs and belly pressing the ground.
7. Hypoglycemic condition may occur in very young pups and weak animals.

Line of treatment

1. Removal of the cause of enteritis.
2. Administration of antibiotics for preventing secondary microbial infections.
3. Parenteral or oral in mild cases of diarrhoea administration of fluids containing electrolytes for rehydration.
4. Administration of oral astringents and if necessary, some mild sedative also.
5. Administration of enzymes, yeast, liver extract and vitamin B complex as per requirements determined by a physician.
6. Feeding on non-irritant liquid diets.

11. Exocrine Pancreatic Insufficiency (EPI)

It is digestive disorder associated with the insufficiency of pancreatic enzymes specially

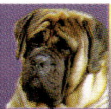

the lipase. EPI is also suspected to have hereditary linkage, as greater numbers of patients are the Alsatian dogs.

Aetiology

1. Atrophy of acinar cells of exocrine gland part of the pancreas.
2. Pancreatitis.

Clinical signs

There appears to be lack of clinical signs applicable for the diagnosis of the condition. There may be chronic diarrhoea of intermittent nature, which mostly subsides spontaneously when non-irritant diets are fed. In many cases diarrhoea does not occur.

Line of treatment

The disease EPI is suspected only when common treatment for diarrhoea do not respond. The line of treatment for EPI has been suggested as:

1. Oral administration of a mixed enzyme preparation as for exocrine pancreatic enzymes.
2. Feeding of low fat diets.
3. Treatment of secondary microbial invasions, if any.
4. Rarely there may be need of Parenteral fluid therapy in case of patients suffering from excessive dehydration due to delayed diagnosis of the ailment.

12. Colitis and Proctitis

The inflammation of the colon and rectum parts of the large intestine are known as colitis and proctitis respectively. The conditions are routinely treated as enteritis.

Aetiology

1. Traumatic injury by some foreign matter.
2. Infections.
3. Feeding of less digestible diets producing larger volume of faeces.

Clinical signs

It is rather difficult to suspect a clinical condition as most of the affected dogs behave normal.

1. Diarrhoea and sometimes dysentery are observed.
2. There may be vomiting also, but rarely and infrequent.
3. Constipation may be followed by haematochezia or dyschezia.

Line of treatment

1. Symptomatic treatment is rendered initially.
2. Laxative and non-irritant (bland) diet should be fed, if defaecation is delayed for more than 24 hours.
3. Eroded skin around anal opening should be painted with non-irritant antiseptic ointment.
4. Suitable antibiotics should be administered for the treatment and also for the prevention of bacterial invasion.

13. Anal Saculitis

The inflammation of the anal sac mostly causing the formation of abscesses. The incidence is more in toy breeds.

Aetiology

It is mostly due to infection of pyogenic bacteria.

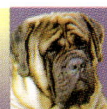

Clinical signs

The common signs are rubbing the anal region on ground due to irritation. The dogs are restless and frequently bite the affected part. There is often bleeding from anal sac during the passage of faeces. In severe cases constipation may occur. The volume of faeces is also more in many patients due to longer holding. In extreme severity there may be formation of fistula.

Line of treatment

1. Infusion of antibiotics along with corticosteroid in the sac is an effective treatment.
2. Fasting for a day or two, or feeding of only liquid diet is advantageous for the treatment of lesion.
3. Abscesses are drained out, cleaned and then packed with topical antiseptic preparations. This is supported with the Parenteral administration of antibiotics (preferably broad-spectrum antibiotics) or sulpha drugs.
4. Laxative diets are fed during the recovery period.
5. In chronic cases and frequently occurring cases the gland is removed surgically.

14. Hepatitis

It is the inflammation of hepatocytes and liver as a whole.

Aetiology

1. Ingestion of intent and toxic chemicals and drugs.
2. Nutritional deficiencies specially of vitamins and micro minerals.
3. Feeding of high fat diets with low fibre.
4. Various infectious diseases caused by bacteria, viruses and parasites etc.

Clinical signs

1. Various degree of anorexia.
2. Constipation followed by diarrhea.
3. Flushed visible mucous membranes due to jaundice.
4. Dullness and depression.
5. In severe cases there may be hyper-excitability and convulsions.
6. Frequent vomiting.
7. Ascites.
8. Hyperthermia in infectious hepatitis.

Line of treatment

1. Parenteral administration of glucose.
2. Use of liver tonics for stimulating the multiplication of hepatocytes for the replacement of damaged cells.
3. Administration of liver extract and vitamin B complex.
4. Specific treatment like administration of antibiotics in bacterial infections and parasiticidal drugs in parasitic hepatitis.
5. Feeding of carbohydrate rich diets low in fat with moderate protein of high biological values and fibre content.
6. Provide complete rest.
7. Diuretics to treat ascites.

15. Ascites

Excessive accumulation of fluid in the peritoneal cavity manifested by abnormal increase in the circumference of the abdomen is known as ascites.

Aetiology

1. Chronic hepatitis of extended duration.
2. Secondary occurrence in hypoalbuminemia, renal retention of salt and water.

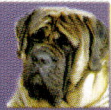

3. Ascites occurs in some of the internal parasitism and infectious diseases.
4. Increase hydrostatic pressure and cardiac insufficiency.

Clinical signs

1. Enlargement of abdomen.
2. Palpation reveals accumulation of fluid.

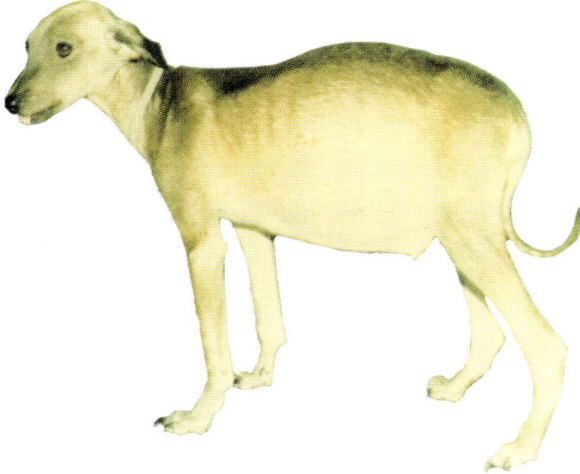

Fig. 117 A Case of Ascites in Dog Showing Extensive Swelling of Abdomen

Line of treatment

1. Feeding of low sodium (salt) diets. In severe cases salt feeding should be completely stopped.
2. Administration of diuretics for the removal of accumulated fluid in urine, however, use of diuretics should be controlled otherwise excessive use may cause dehydration.
3. The cause of disease is identified and treated.
4. Mechanical removal of the fluid by means of:
   a. Paracentesis aspiration – It is done slowly when fluid pressure causes dyspnea and discomforts due to failure of fluid removal by drugs. Ascites should not be allowed to prolong, otherwise there may be acute dilatation of blood vessels leading to subsequent failure of peripheral circulation.
   b. Aspiration with the help of pressure activated valve – By this system ascites fluid is circulated through its draining in jugular vein by a connecting shunt.
   c. Through portal system venous shunt.
5. Liver tonics may be used as supportive therapy.

16. Jaundice (Icterus)

It is a clinical manifestation of various kinds of hepatobiliary disorders in which visible mucous membranes and different excretory products turn yellowish due to the excess of either haemobilirubin or cholebilirubin or both in the blood circulation. The yellow discolouration is prominently visible in the sclera. Following three types of jaundice are more common in the dogs:

1. Pre hepatic (Haemolytic) jaundice,
2. Intra hepatic (Toxic) jaundice, and
3. Post hepatic (Obstructive) jaundice.

Aetiology

The common causes are the damage of hepatobiliary tissues by bacteria, viruses, parasite, chemicals, drugs, toxicants and incompatible blood transfusion.

Clinical signs

1. Irregular digestion.
2. Decreased appetite and animals show lethargy.

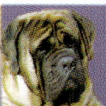

3. Vomiting of greenish yellow tinged digasta.
4. Constipation and diarrhoea.
5. Exhaustion and depression.
6. Yellow colouration of visible mucosa and skin.
7. Enlarged liver (in obstructive jaundice there may not be enlargement of liver).
8. Abdominal pain may occur.

Differential diagnosis

The three types of jaundice can be differentiated on the basis of clinical symptoms and biochemical tests as shown in the Table 5.1.

Line of treatment

1. Complete rest at a comfortable place.
2. Feeding of diets without salt and fat, and reasonably low in protein.
3. Prevention of the causes of haemolysis in haemolytic jaundice.
4. Removal of parasitism.
5. Antibiotics therapy of bacterial jaundice.
6. Management of viral jaundice.
7. Fresh boiled liver should be fed or liver extract may be given Parenterally.
8. Oral administration of vitamin B complex is useful in the treatment of toxic jaundice.
9. Obstruction removal is essential for the treatment of obstructive jaundice.
10. Certain Ayurvedic drugs have been found to be very useful for the restoration of normal functions of liver and biliary system.
11. Fluid therapy particularly with dextrose, should be given orally or Parenterally which is very much essential in all the types of jaundice.

17. Chronic Bronchitis

Long duration inflammatory conditions of bronchi with some non-repairable damage is known as chronic bronchitis.

Parameters	Haemolytic jaundice	Toxic jaundice	Obstructive jaundice
Table 5.1: Differential Diagnosis of Different Jaundice			
Colour of faeces	Pigmented	Normal	Hypopigmented
Consistency of faeces	Normal	Normal	Greasy (fatty)
Colour of urine	Light yellow	Intense yellow	Intense yellow
Icterus index	Low to moderate	Moderate	High
Van den bergh reaction	Indirect	Bi phase	Direct
Total serum cholesterol	Normal	Decreased	Increased
Blood prothrombine time	Normal	Prolonged	Prolonged
Colour of the mucous membranes	Slight to moderate yellow	Slight to moderate yellow	Intense yellow
Colour of serum and plasma	Slight to moderate yellow	Slight to moderate yellow	Intense yellow

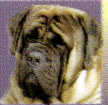

Aetiology

1. Fibrosis of the air passages at certain places.
2. Hyperplasia of epithelial layer.
3. Hypertrophy of glands and inflammation.
4. Air passage contains excess mucous and smaller passages are obstructed and some are collapsed.
5. Irritant gases and other substances, allergic constituents and infectious. Infection can be secondary to chronic bronchitis.
6. The potential complication of chronic bronchitis is the permanent dilation of the air passages.
7. Another complication is recurring infection and overt pneumonia.

Clinical signs

The patients are mostly middle aged and older dogs of small breeds. The clinical signs are:

1. Gradual and slow progressing cough during several months a longer time. However, there is no sign of weight loss, weakness and loss of appetite.
2. There is distressful coughing which is dry in nature.
3. Patient gets tired easily.
4. The irritant or any distress may intensify coughing.
5. Bronchovesicular sounds are intensified.
6. Crackles are heard during auscultation of the cervicothoracic areas.
7. In advanced stage of disease a prominent cardiac sound may be heard.

Line of treatment

The disease takes long time before diagnosis because the patients are usually brought late in the clinics. In such cases physician first treat the symptoms for providing immediate relief. Each patient requires separate management practice because their conditions are different when brought to the hospital.

The common drugs used are bronchodilators, glucocorticoids, antibiotics and cough suppressants. The air passage is hydrated and exposure to irritants and allergens causing stimulation of cough is avoided. Animal should be kept in hygienic and warmth condition.

18. Pneumonia

Inflammation of the lungs is known as pneumonia. The extension of inflammation to bronchioles is called bronchopneumonia.

Aetiology

1. Inhalation of irritant factors like dust, pollen grains, gases and exposure to cold.
2. Dirty housing and bad hygiene.
3. Different infections.
4. Respiratory parasitism.

Clinical signs

Coughing with or without nasal discharge and sneezing along with increased respiration rate and different breathing in stress are the common clinical signs. In severe cases there is abdominal respiration and stress. There is increase in temperature, loss of body condition, nasal discharges are mucoid and the animals are reluctant to move.

Line of treatment

1. Housing of patient at clean, dry and well-ventilated place.
2. Patient should be protected from chilling.
3. Cause of the disease should be identified and removed (wherever possible).

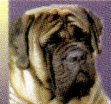

4. Inhalation of soothing vapours of essential oils.
5. Oral administration of expectorants.
6. Parenteral administration of antibiotics and parasiticidal drugs in case of parasitic pneumonia.
7. Administration of antispasmodics.
8. Feeding of non-irritant liquid diets.
9. Administration of vitamin C.
10. Fluid therapy is required in dehydration.
11. The side of lying should be changed at short intervals of 1.5 to 2.0 hours in recumbent animals.
12. Use of bronchodilators is required in chronic pneumonia.

19. Aspiration Pneumonia

The pneumonia caused by aspiration of a small quantity of fluid alone or contaminated with irritants and microorganisms is called aspiration pneumonia.

Aetiology

1. Aspiration of liquid alone or along with solids into the lungs. The aspirated materials are generally stomach contents or food or water.
2. There appears to be some predisposing factors, viz., megaoesophagus, regurgitation and rarely severe vomiting.
3. Neurological or neuro-muscular conditions interfering with the swallowing reflexes of the larynges or pharynx.
4. Congenital anomalies like cleft palate or other anatomical changes (growth of any kind in the air passage).
5. Forced feeding by unskilled person to depressed sick animals.
6. Incorrect introduction of stomach tube into the trachea.

These may be followed by obstruction and infections due to inhalation of infected contents.

Clinical signs

1. Occurrence of acute and severe respiratory disorders specially the stressful and continuous coughing.
2. Vomiting and regurgitation, administration of some unpalatable drug or passage of stomach tube may have preceded before the occurrence of the condition.
3. The patients are brought in shock at the veterinary clinic.
4. The other signs are pyrexia, inappetence and depression.
5. Auscultation of the distant dependent parts of the lungs reveals abnormal sounds like crackles and wheezes, moist rales.
6. The disease mostly found ending fatally.

Line of treatment

Recovery occurs in most of the cases of small aspiration but in excessive aspiration prognosis is generally grave. The therapy includes:

1. Suction of aspirated material where facility is available.
2. Parenteral administration (i/v) of physiological saline with glucose.
3. Oxygen supply to lungs.
4. Administration of bronchodilators and corticosteroids.
5. Preventive administration of antibiotics.
6. Corticosteroid therapy and vitamin C therapy is also found beneficial.

20. Pulmonary Oedema

The excessive accumulation of fluid in the lung parenchyma causing distension is known as

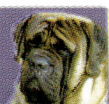

pulmonary oedema. It is the manifestation of many disorders responsible for increased vascular permeability and lymphatic over-load.

Aetiology

1. Fall in osmotic pressure of plasma.
2. Vascular over-load due to engorgement of the vessels.
3. Obstruction in lymphatic vessels.
4. Increased permeability of pulmonary vessels.
5. Irritant drugs and toxins.
6. Hepatic diseases.
7. Excessive hydration.
8. Inhalation of harmful gases.
9. Various inflammatory conditions of pancreas and renal system.

Clinical signs

1. Respiratory disorders are cough, distress and exhaustion.
2. Crackles heard in advanced cases.
3. Increased breathing.
4. Acute respiratory distress.

Line of treatment

1. Animal should be provided complete rest in comfortable position under conformant.
2. Oxygen therapy should be provided, if needed.
3. Use of bronchodilators may be required.
4. Administration of diuretics is helpful in removal of considerable amount of fluid in most of the oedematous conditions.
5. In case of hypoalbuminemia, plasma or blood infusion is used.
6. Supportive treatments are administration of antibiotics, vitamin B complex and corticosteroids.

21. Epistaxis

Bleeding from the nose is called as epistaxis.

Aetiology

The common causes of epistaxis are traumatic injury, sudden change in climate, high blood pressure, nutritional deficiencies and hereditary factors, Nasal granulomma and ulceration etc.

Clinical signs

Sudden bleeding of fresh blood is the only sign.

Line of treatment

1. Application of ice cold pack on the nasal and frontal bones.
2. Application of cold bentonite (yellow soil) mus on the nasal and frontal bone.
3. Surgical repair of injury.
4. Removal of cause.
5. Administration of vitamin K.
6. To stop bleeding haemostatic drug should be administered.

22. Common Cold

Drainage of fluid from the nares is known as common cold or nasal catarrh.

Aetiology

Irritants like foreign body, pollen grains and other allergens, dust, gases, flumes, exposure to chilling breeze, dampness, darkness and lack of ventilation in the animal house are the common causes.

The condition is complicated by the invasion of bacteria, viruses, fungi and parasites.

Clinical signs

1. Watery mucous discharge from the nares.

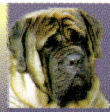

2. High fever
3. Sneezing
4. Muscular pain, influenza etc.
5. Pharyngitis
6. Dysphagia
7. Restlessness
8. Loss of appetite

Line of treatment

1. Removal of the aetiological factor.
2. Administration of antibiotics and sulpha drugs in infectious catarrh.
3. Antimycotic drugs in fungal infestation.
4. Inhalation of tincture bezoin and essential oils, viz., Eucalyptus oil.
5. Administration of analgesic, anti-pyretics, vitamin C and A and drugs for reducing the congestion.

23. Haematuria

The passage of blood in urine is called haematuria. Haematuria may be gross or occult. In occult urine, RBC per high power field is not more than 5. It occurs in many diseases of the urinary tract.

Aetiology

The causes of haematuria may be pre-renal or post renal.

1. Pre-renal causes are toxaemia, septicemia and trauma etc.
2. Renal causes are acute glomer-ulonephritis, embolism of renal artery, renal infarction, pyelonephritis, tubular injury caused by calculi or tumours in kidney and trauma. Some parasites like *Capillarisa plica, Dioctophyma renale* and *Dirofilaria imitis*, and bacteria like Leptospira etc. are also associated with the occurrence of haematuria.

3. Post renal causes are cystitis, urolithiasis, urethral trauma, and injury in urinary bladder, faulty passage of catheter and tumours (specially the venereal granuloma), post renal causes are mostly due to obstructions.

Clinical signs

The colour of urine is deep red or brown due to the presence of red blood cells. The RBC can be separated by centrifugation of the urine sample, which are packed in the bottom of the centrifugation tube. In mild cases occult blood test is carried in urine sample and in positive cases of haematuria blue colour reaction occurs.

Line of treatment

1. Removal of the cause when identified.
2. Symptomatic treatments are used for providing immediate relief.
3. Administration of drugs like haemostatics, alkalizers (if urine is acidic) and urinary antiseptics gives satisfactory response.
4. Antibiotic therapy is also essential.

24. Haemoglobinuria

The passage of haemoglobin in urine is exhibited by coffee colour appearance of urine. The condition is usually a symptom of some haemolytic diseases.

Aetiology

1. Babesiosis
2. Prolonged phosphorus deficiency
3. Torsion of the spleen

Clinical signs

Coffee colour appearance of urine. The intensity of colour depends on the damage of the erythrocytes.

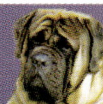

Line of treatment

Almost similar to that suggested to the treatment of haematuria.

25. Uremia

The abnormal increase of blood urea nitrogen (BUN) is called uremia. The catabolic products associated with the uremia are urea, reacting phenolic compounds and guanidine.

Aetiology

The causes of uremia can be differentiated into the following three categories:

1. **Pre renal causes:** There are dehydration due to excess loss of blood of any origin, decreased cardiac output, decreased osmotic pressure, shock and hypoadrenocorticism. Septicemia may be also responsible for uremia.

2. **Renal causes:** These are nephritis, nephrosis and jaundice the main causes while salt toxicity and sulphanilamides are the predisposing factors.

3. **Post renal causes:** Rupture of urinary bladder, obstruction of bladder and urethra and bilateral urethral obstructions are the main causes of disorder.

Clinical signs

1. The common symptoms are abdominal gripping pain, tremors, pruritus, pallor, petecheal pigmentation, dullness and comatose condition.

2. Gastrointestinal disorders are loss of the appetite, dry vomition, and dry mouth due to dehydration and haemorrhagic diarrhoea.

3. There is respiratory distress and bradycardia.

4. Urinary tract disorders are polyuria, anuria and oliguria, and also smell of ammonia may be felt from the month.

5. The other signs are conjunctivitis, keratitis and anaemia.

Line of the treatment

1. Removal of the primary causes of the disease.

2. Restoration of the renal function.

3. Removal of the toxic substances to release the renal strain and also the normalization of pH and electrolytes level.

4. Use of laxative, fluid therapy for the removal of toxic factors.

5. Administration of alkalizers for controlling the acidosis.

6. Catheterization for removal of urine in severe cases.

7. Administration of respiratory stimulants in comatose condition.

8. In patients of oligouria dietary protein should be least and main constituent is carbohydrate. Fluid infusion should be restricted.

9. Haemadialysis may be needed in acute dehydration.

26. Cystitis

The inflammation of urinary bladder is known as cystitis and it is characterised by painful vomition, dysuria, frequent urination, mild fever and stress.

Aetiology

The main causes are the infections of ascending order from the lower part of the urinary tract and also from the kidneys. Bacterial infection of urinary bladder via haematogenous route is

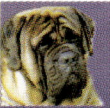

very rare. Infection in the upper urinary tract may serve as contributing factor of recurrent infection. The various bacteria associated with the condition are *Escherichia coli, Proteus* spp., Staphylococci, streptococci and Klebsiella spp. are more common.

Predisposing factors are urinary tract stasis due to trauma, abnormal urine composition, calculi, neurological dysfunction and certain metabolic disorders.

Clinical signs

The condition may be acute or chronic in nature. The characteristic signs are frequent and painful micturition, straining, occasional haematuria, and pain on abdominal palpation, stiffness of hindquarter and emesis. The last portion of urine may be dark cloudy or red. The diseases is diagnosed on the basis of clinical signs and urine examinations for debris and infections agents.

Line of treatment

1. The primary causes of disease are removed.
2. Suitable drugs are administered for correcting the pH.
3. In mild and chronic cystitis administration of a combination of urinary antiseptic and alkalizer is more effective and useful.
4. In infectious cystitis suitable antibiotic should be administered.
5. Adequate fluid supply is necessary for flushing.
6. Antispasmodic therapy is required for pain relief.

27. Nephritis

The inflammation of kidney is called nephritis.

Aetiology

1. The diseases associated with nephritis are viral infections, bacterial infections and parasitic invasions.
2. Inflammatory causes are immune mediated diseases, pancreatitis and systemic lupus erythematous.
3. Other causes are diabetes mellitus, hereditary factors and extended use of high dose of corticosteroids.

Clinical signs

1. Pain, tenderness in the loin region and arched back.
2. Increased thirst.
3. Depression and lethargy.
4. Gradual loss of appetite and vomiting.
5. Renal pain and frequent micturition.
6. Increased respiration rate.
7. Oedema of dependent parts.
8. The other symptoms associated with nephritis are the systemic hypertension, hypercoagulability. The former is probably due to accumulation of sodium and scarring of glomerular capillary and arterioles, decreased renal production of vasodilators, glomerulosclerosis and amyloidosis.

The hypercoagulability and thromboembolism are the secondary effects of nephritis. A mild thrombocytosis occurs and hypoalbuminemia linked thrombocytic hypersensitivity produces platelet adhesion and collection to raise proportional to the intensity of hypoalbuminemia.

Line of treatment

1. Removal of the causes of nephritis.

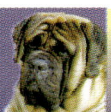

2. Complete rest at a comfortable hygienic place.
3. Feeding of carbohydrate rich, low protein diet.
4. Parenteral fluid therapy for controlling dehydration.
5. Administration of diuretics.
6. Administration of antibiotics in case of bacterial infections and parasiticidal drugs in parasitism.
7. Surgical removal of renal and cystic stones.
8. Sodium (salt) intake should be drastically cut.
9. Treatments for the inflammation and resolving the anticoagulability syndrome.

28. Acute Renal Failure

Urinary disorders developed due to severe damage (>70-75%) of the nephrons of both kidneys resulting in the ceasure of the functions. Acute renal failure occurs suddenly due to sudden damage of nephrons at a very fast rate.

Aetiology

Intoxication is the main cause of acute renal failure. This is favoured by the special feature of physiological function of the urinary system. Almost 20% of the blood pumped out from the heart passes through the kidneys daily. The results in the filtration of toxicants in blood that causes severe damage of the nephrons causing acute renal failure.

1. Almost 20% of the cardiac output of blood passes through the kidneys daily, and 90% of this passes through the renal cortex.
2. Voluminous endothelial surface area of the glomerular capillary.
3. Hypoxia of the proximal tubule and thick ascending loop of the Henle cells.
4. Tubular secretion and resorption may help in accumulation of toxic substance in the cells.

Some of the most harmful toxicants are listed as follows:

1. Heavy metals like lead, mercury, cadmium, chromium, arsenic, bismuth etc.
2. Organic substances –Ethylene glycol carbon tetrachloride (CTC), chloroform, other, herbicides, pesticides, paints, and solvents etc.
3. Haemoglobin and myoglobin.
4. Chemotherapeutic drugs.
5. Anaesthetic drugs.

Clinical signs

1. The clinical signs are generally non-specific and characterized by anorexia, depression, lethargy, emesis, diarrheoa and dehydration.
2. Sometimes smell of ammonia is felt.
3. In some cases oral ulcers may be seen.
4. Decreased cardiac output.
5. Oliguria leading to retention of urea.

Line of treatment

1. Removal of the cause.
2. Administration of plenty of physiological fluid and diuretics for flushing out the toxic substances accumulated in the kidneys.
3. Gentamicin administration and providing high protein diet (about 23-24%) has been found to be more useful than the (13-14%) and low protein (8-10%) diets, as the high protein diets help in retention of gentamicin at the site of action for longer duration.
4. In case of suspected renal damage, the administration of nephrotoxic drugs should

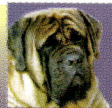

be stopped and fluid therapy should be started to flush out the tract.

5. Prolonged administration of antibiotics may be required.

6. The treatment is supported with the administration of vitamin A, C and B complex.

7. To correct acidosis, sodium bicarbonate orally can be given.

29. Chronic Renal Failure

The destruction of renal parenchymal cells at a slow rate is the chronic form of renal failure and it is detected after very long period.

Aetiology

It is very difficult to ascertain the aetiology of chronic renal failure. However, the long list of suspected or actually involved factors are as follows:

1. Retention of urine for longer period.
2. Administration of nephrotoxic drugs for the treatment of other diseases.
3. Ischemic condition of kidneys.
4. Presence of inflammatory factors, viz., disease like pyelonephritis, leptospirosis and renal calculi formation etc.
5. Tumours.
6. Hereditary abnormalities.

Clinical signs

The duration of pathogenesis of chronic renal failure varies from several weeks to even a year and its diagnosis is delayed due to occurrence of much milder symptoms like azotemia. The common clinical signs of the disease are the progressive loss of body weight, polyuria, polydipsia, decreased body condition, and progressive and non-regenerative anaemia. Radiography reveals the presence of smaller and irregular shaped kidneys.

Line of treatment

1. Chronic renal failure is generally a non-reversible pathological condition but suitable therapy can provide relief. The line of treatment is designed to reduce ammonia generation in the kidneys, systemic hypertension and mineralisation of the soft tissues.

2. Infectious and other renal conditions like pyelonephritis and urolithiasis should be treated.

3. The level of dietary protein is reduced in case of high blood urea concentration, rather carbohydrate rich diet should be provided.

4. Dietary phosphorus level is reduced in case of hyperphosphatemia.

5. Vomiting and gastroenteritis are treated, when present.

6. Anaemia is treated.

7. Parenteral feeding of nutrition fluid may be required in case of frequent vomiting.

8. Adequate energy should be supplied through the administration of highly metabolizable sources.

9. Dehydration should be controlled and over-hydration should be avoided.

30. Urolithiasis

The formation of stones in the urinary systems is urolithiasis. The uroliths may be found at any place in the urinary tract but the common sites are the kidneys and the urinary bladder. Several types of uroliths isolated from the dogs are listed as follows:

1. Struvite uroliths are formed of magnesium ammonium phosphate impregnated with a small amount of calcium.

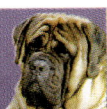

2. Calcium oxalate uroliths are usually the monohydrate or whellite form. Although the causes are not yet fully known, high concentration of urinary calcium either due to high intake and greater absorption or due to decreased tubular resorption.

3. Urate uroliths are mostly formed of ammonium acid urate.

4. Silicate uroliths contain silicate of dietary origin.

5. Cystine uroliths are formed of cystine and some other amino acids crystallized and deposited with minerals.

Aetiology

The formation of foci in the kidneys or urinary bladder and high concentration of depositable minerals are responsible for the formation of uroliths. The common causes are:

1. High concentration of salts in the urine.
2. Longer retention time of urine.
3. Favourable urine pH for the crystallization and precipitation of the salts.
4. Presence of a nidus in the system on which salts are deposited.
5. Intake of high protein and minerals rich diets.
6. Decreased resorption of calcium, cystine and uric acid by the tubules.

Clinical signs

The quantity, quality and location of the stones in the urinary system generally determine the nature of clinical signs.

1. In case of cystic uroliths the common signs are that of cystitis, viz., haematuria and dysuria, stranguria. Mucosal irritation is much severe with jack shaped uroliths.
2. In male dogs passage of smaller uroliths may sometime cause obstruction resulting in the distension of urinary bladder, dysuria, stranguria and post renal azotemia exhibited by anorexia, emesis and depression. The uroliths create obstruction due to lodging in the urethra at the posterior aspect of the penis. In severe cases there may be rupture of urethra and/or urinary in the abdomen or gut cutaneous fluid accumulation in the perineal region which causes post renal azoturia.

3. In animals with unilateral urolithiasis in many cases there may not be any notable symptom whereas in some of the cases haematuria and chromic pylonephritis are observed.

4. Abdominal pain is often intense and unbearable due to which patients are restless, roll on the ground and cry.

5. Unilateral obstruction of ureter may produce unilateral hydronephrosis with many apparent signs of fall in renal functions.

Line of treatment

1. Surgical removal of the uroliths.
2. Repairs of the ruptured part, if any.
3. Aspiration of fluid accumulated in the abdomen or perineal region due to rupture of the urinary bladder.
4. Administration of drugs for dissolving the stones.
5. Administration of antibiotics for controlling secondary microbial infections.
6. Administration of analgesics and antispasmodic drugs.
7. pH of the urine should be altered.

31. Anaemia

The decrease in the number and mass of the erythrocytes coupled with the decrease in haemoglobin concentration is known as anaemia.

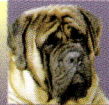

It is the manifestation of different clinico-patho-logical disorders. The different kinds of anaemia observed in dogs are the haemolytic anaemia, iron deficiency anaemia, anaemia due to chronic diseases, hypoproliferative anaemia and anaemia due to renal diseases.

Aetiology

1. Chronic wasting diseases, viz., tuberculosis, brucellosis, etc.
2. Malnutrition and deficiency of iron, copper and protein (globin).
3. Infectious diseases.
4. Parasitic infection and infestation.
5. Ingestion of toxic chemicals, drugs and other substances.
6. Endocrine disorders.
7. Hypoplasia or aplasia of bone marrow.
8. Myelophthisis, myelofibrosis and myelo-dysplastic syndromes.

Clinical signs

1. Pale discolouration of visible mucous membranes.
2. Animals get tired even on mild exercise.
3. Lethargy and weak.
4. Gradual loss of appetite or in some cases other may be pica.
5. The activities of the patient is significantly reduced.
6. Increased precordial beats.
7. Reduction in packed cell volume (PCV).
8. Haematuria and haemaglobinuria.
9. Dyspnea.
10. Jaundice.
11. Oedema of the dependent parts.

Line of treatment

1. Removal of causes.
2. Treatment of infections and infestations.
3. Correction of nutritional deficiencies.
4. Administration of haematinics along with vitamin B complex and liver extract.
5. Feeding of highly digestible nutritious diets.
6. If necessary, whole blood transfusion is recommended.

32. Heart Failure

The failure of ability of heart to maintain the circulatory equilibrium is known as heart failure. It is characterized by the congestion of venous side accompanied by dilatation of blood vessels, oedema of lungs, enlargement of heart and increased heart rate. Heavy and over-weight (obese) dogs are more susceptible to heart failure. Two types of heart failure occur in dogs, i.e., acute heart failure and congestive heart failure.

A. Acute Heart Failure

Acute heart failure is manifested by the sudden loss of consciousness and falling with or without convulsions. There will be pallor of mucous membrane followed by either recovery or termination of the life.

Aetiology

1. Myocardial infarction.
2. Massive pulmonary embolism.
3. Paroxysmal tachycardia and myocarditis.
4. Rapid I/V injection of calcium containing fluid.
5. Severe trauma.
6. Anaphylactic reaction.

Clinical signs

1. Shock either due to peripheral circulatory failure or cardiac failure.

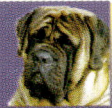

Peripheral circulatory failure occurs due to excessive haemorrhage, trauma, excessive burns, neurogenic disorders, anaphylaxis and other factors responsible for the liberation of histamine, septic shock and infections. Cardiogenic shock is characterized by cardiac oedema tachycardia, ventricular fibrillation, muscular dystrophy and deficient pumping ability of myocardium.

Line of treatment

The condition is so sudden that treatment may not be possible in most of the cases. However, anti shock drugs and oxygen therapy are used to save the patient. This followed by the administration of cardiac stimulants.

B. Congestive Heart Failure

It denotes a chronic heart failure associated with congestion in the circulation.

Aetiology

The causes of disorder may be pericardial, endocardial or myocardial disorders alone or in combination.

1. The pericardial disorders are produced by cardiac tamponade, pericarditis, haemopericardium and hydropericardium. It may be unilateral or both sides may be involved. Left-sided cardiac failure is manifested by respiratory problems, respiration at the base of the lungs, coughing, pulmonary oedema, and alteration of pulse and enlargement of the heart. The right-sided cardiac failure is manifested by oedema, hydrothorax, pneumothorax, ascites, albuminuria, jugular pulse and cyanosis.
2. The endocardial disorders are produced by endocarditis and valvular defects.

3. The myocardial disorders are caused by myocarditis, myocardial dystrophy, cyst in the heart, neoplasms and acute drug toxicity.
4. Congenital disorders may also be involved.

Line of treatment

1. Complete rest at a wellventilated, clean dry and comfortable place.
2. Exercise is completely stopped.
3. Salt free digestible diets are fed.
4. Potassium sparing diuretics are used orally.
5. Respiratory stimulants are given in associated respiratory problems.
6. Digitalisation may be necessary.

33. Conjunctivitis

The inflammation of conjunctiva is known as conjunctivitis.

Aetiology

The various causes of conjunctivitis are the different kinds of irritants like pungent gases, dust, microbial infections (viral, bacterial, mycotic), parasitic infestation, corrosive chemicals and injuries etc.

Clinical signs

The common symptoms of conjunctivitis are the painful irritation, epiphora, profuse lacrymation, redness of the conjunctiva, mucopurulent discharge in advanced cases or in delayed treatment and rise in temperature etc.

Line of treatment

1. Removal of the causes.
2. Irrigation of inflamed eyes with cold normal saline.

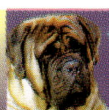

3. Application of antiseptic and astringent eye lotions.
4. Eye lotions of sulpha drugs.
5. Antibiotic eye ointment.

34. Keratitis

The inflammation of cornea is known as Keratitis and it is mostly associated with conjunctivitis as keratoconjunctivitis.

Aetiology

The causes may be infections of virus, bacteria and fungi, and infestation of parasites. The other causes are trauma, irritants and climatic factors. The latter are generally pre-disposing cases.

Clinical signs

Excessive lacrymation, congestion of the cornea and mucosal surface of eyelids and photophobia. Impairment of vision may be caused in chronic cases and prolonged duration may result in the development of corneal opacity.

Line of treatment

1. The affected eyes are washed 3-4 times with mild eye lotion.
2. Antiseptic eye ointments or medicinal eye drops are applied after washing the eyes.
3. In some cases topical drugs containing steroids are applied.
4. In some rare prolonged cases sub-conjunctival causes are removed wherever possible
5. Trauma is repaired surgically, if necessary.

35. Coma

Coma is the terminal stage of unconsciousness. It is manifestation of the conditions affecting the depression of the cerebrocortical function.

Aetiology

1. Encephalomyelitis.
2. The diseases causing intracranial pressure.
3. Cerebral anoxia.
4. Hypoglycaemia.
5. Uremia.
6. Heat (Sun) stroke or *chill blain*.
7. Several kinds intoxication affecting the brain.
8. Electrolytes imbalance.
9. Drug introxication due to hepatic failure.

Line of treatment

1. Removal of the causes(s) of disorder.
2. Appropriate fluid therapy.
3. Administration of cardiac and respiratory stimulants.
4. Complete rest in a hygienic atmosphere at a comfortable place.

36. Ataxia

It is the incoordination of gait either due to neuro-muscular disorders or abnormal cerebellar function. This is a complex of defects in the rate, range and direction of movements.

Aetiology

1. Due to primary diseases of nervous system.
2. Lesions in the bone or brain.
3. Pain in joints, muscles, skin and abdominal organs.
4. Pain in the urogenital organs.
5. Neurological disorders like lesions in the cerebellum, upper motor neuron, hemiplegia, spastic paraplegia and chorea as a sequel to distemper (common in young dogs).

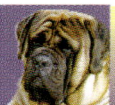

Clinical signs

1. In mild cases affected animals stand with legs placed wide apart.
2. Sway occurs on irritation of movement and patient may fall on any side.
3. Oscillation of head and neck.
4. Limbs do not move in unison.
5. Grossly staggered movement.
6. Weakness of muscles and nerves.

Line of treatment

1. Treatment for the removal of cause.
2. Use of tranquilizers for relief of the symptom.
3. Fluid therapy with dextrose.
4. Administration of vitamins B_1, liver extract and B complex.

37. Epilepsy

The epilepsy is the sequel of a complex clinico-pathological reactions characterised by tonoclonic convulsions accompanied by loss of consciousness. The epileptic seizures are the clinical manifestation of an active, cerebral, bizarre neuronal irritative process involving billions of cortical neurons.

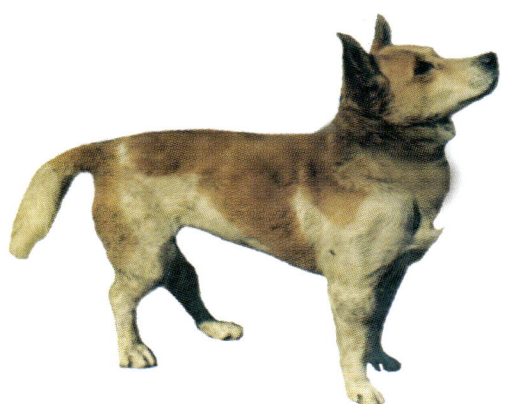

Fig. 118 Dog Suffering from Epilepsy

Each epileptic event has the following five components

1. Prodrome or aura: Signs preceding the epileptic event.
2. Ictus the actual seizure lasting from few seconds to several minutes, which may be generalised, partial or non-motor.
3. Post inctus or post seizure phase: The period of confusion, depression, coma, blindness and encircling after the seizure.
4. Interictal phase: This is the period between seizures lasting from few seconds to months. The behaviour during this period ranges from normal to mild or severelly abnormal.
5. Status epilepticus: There are the seizures that run together and do not have normal period in-between.

Classification of epilepsy

The following two systems of classification of epilepsy are more common:

A. Classification on the basis of aetiology

These are of two types. The causes of idiopathic epilepsy are listed as follows:

(i) Grandmal (major)
(ii) Petitmal (minor)
(iii) Status epilepticus (continuous).

The causes of symptomatic epilepsy are:

(i) Space occupying lesions.
(ii) Inflammatory process of the central nervous system (CNS).
(iii) Distemper and cryptococcosis.
(iv) Congenital defects in cranial regions.
(v) Uremia and hypocalcaemia.

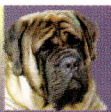

B. Classification on the basis of the clinical form of seizure

(i) **Major motor seizure:** Tonoclonics are the most common and easiest to observe.

(ii) **Minor motor seizure:** This is a partial, non generalized seizure which originates in one part of the brain and reflected by movement of only the affected part of the body.

(iii) **Behavioral seizure:** This is a non-motor seizure characterized by periodic and paroxysmal events of behaviour. This is exhibited by a wide variety of clinical manifestations including staring, growing, vomiting, retching, fly snapping and viciousness.

Dog breeds susceptible for epilepsy

Certain breeds susceptible for epilepsy are the German Shepherd, Belgian Tervuren, Keeshond, Beagle and Dachshund. The relatively less susceptible breeds are the Cocker Spaniel, Irish Setter, Boxer, Saint Bernard, Labrador Retriever, Miniature Poodle, Golden Retriever, Siberian Husky, Wire Haired Fox Terrier, Alaskan Malmute, Border Collie and Springer Spaniel.

Diagnosis

Many other diseases or disorders can result in seizures. That is why blood tests, radiographs, electroencephalography, physical examination, and history leading up to the seizure are necessary for accurate diagnosis.

Line of treatment

1. Symptomatic treatments according to cause(s) of the condition.

2. Administration of vitamin B complex, A and E.

3. Use of CNS depressants for the control of gradual epilepsy and epileptics.

4. Administration of dextrose saline and electrolytes.

5. Body temperature should be maintained through warming or cooling, as per requirement.

6. Housing should be comfortable and free from sharp edged fittings etc. to avoid injury.

7. Castration and ovario–hysterectomy are considered beneficial for the management of epilepsy in dogs and bitches respectively.

Prevention

The purpose of using anticonvulsants is completely to stop occurrence of seizure activity. However, actual success of treatment is often dependent upon the events which bring on an epileptic seizure are unknown, episodes can be initiated by periods of stress or excitability. It is, therefore, recommended that dogs afflicted with the disorder abstain from sources of stress which may include sporting competition events and breeding.

38. Paralysis

It is a condition of the failure of nervous control on any part of the body. The failure may be partial or complete, and may be either sensory of motor or both in origin, the paralysis is characterized by an inability to make purposeful movements. But in paresis contracting ability of muscles becomes weaker than the normal. The origin of paralysis may be either cerebral, peripheral or spinal.

Aetiology

1. **Cerebral paralysis:** Encephalitis, cranium fracture and the compression of brain due to formation of tumour, cyst or bases.

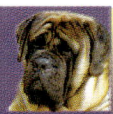

2. **Peripheral paralysis:** Injury to the nerve trunk, rheumatic condition of muscles and nerves, and deficiency of vitamin B_1, B_6 and B_{12}.

3. **Spinal paralysis:** Traumatic injury to spinal cord, vertebral fracture, abscess in the cord, hernia of the intervertebral disc, analysis of the vertebrae, meningitis, myelitis and concussion of the spinal cord.

The causes of paralysis classified on the basis of the affected motor nervous are as follows:

1. **Monoplegia:** Paralysis of one region caused by the failure of functions of one nerve.

2. **Diplegia:** Paralysis of both sides of the body.

3. **Hemiplegia:** Paralysis of one side of the body.

4. **Quadriplegia:** The paralysis of all the four quarters.

5. **Paraplegia:** Paralysis of hind quarters.

6. The causes and classification of a paralysis on the basis of the part of the motor nervous affected are as follows.

    i. **Spastic paralysis:** It is due to the lesions of the upper part of the motor neurons characterized by loss of voluntary movement and decreased tone of limb muscles and increased tendon jerks.

    ii. **Flaccid paralysis:** Its causes are the lesion of lower motor nerons and it is characterized by loss of voluntary movement and decreased tone of limb muscles, absence of tendon jerks and washing of the affected muscles.

Line of treatment

1. Correction of the diet and supplementation of the micronutrients associated with the repair of neuro muscular damages.

2. Removal of the causes(s) resulting in compression of the nerves/neurons.

3. Feeding of digestible and nutritious laxative diets.

4. To provide comfortable bed at a dry, clean and well ventilated place.

5. Patients should be turned frequently at 3-4 hours interval for avoiding the occurrence of bedsores.

6. Application of liniments.

7. Parenteral administration of pain relevers.

8. Supporting therapy of vitamin B complex and vitamins B_1, B_6 and B_{12}.

9. Administration of anabolic steroids and stimulants.

39. Polyneuritis

Inflammatory condition of the sensory or motor nerves is called polyneuritis or peripheral neuritis.

Aetiology

1. Deficiency of vitamins, B_1, B_6 and B_{12}.

2. Metabolic diseases like diabetes mellitus.

3. Infectious conditions like pyemia, septicemia, meningitis and myelitis.

4. Rheumatoid disease.

5. Neurotic drugs, viz., streptomycin nitrofurazone, antimony, arsenic and copper etc.

Line of treatment

1. Removal of the cause(s)

2. Symptomatic treatment

3. Administration of therapeutic doses of vitamins B_1, B_6 and B_{12} orally or Parenterally.

4. Treatment of primary causes like diabetes mellitus and infectious diseases.

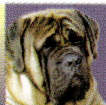

40. Eczema/Eczematous Dermatitis

It is an allergic dermatitis of various intensity. Eczema is a superficial inflammation of skin which may be produced different kinds of external and internal materials against which cells are sensitized. It mostly involves a local or general predisposition.

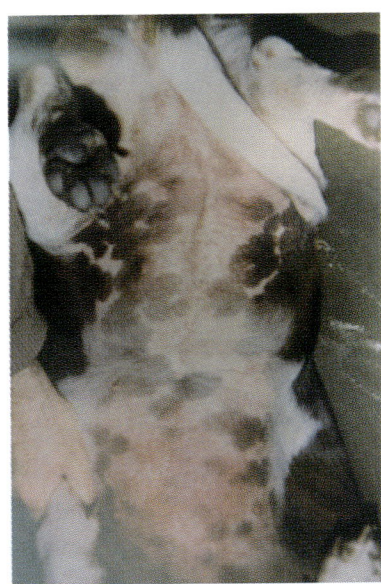

Fig. 119c Dog Suffering from Bacterial Dermatitis

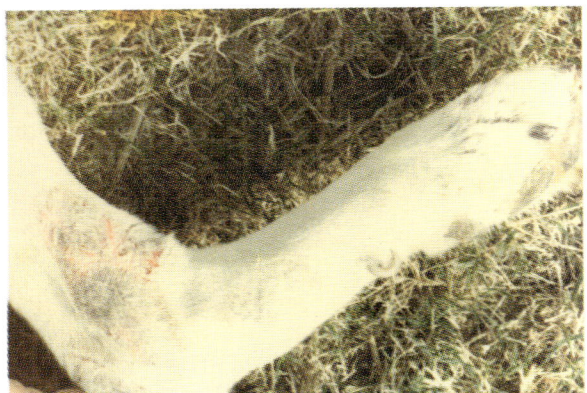

Fig. 119a Eczematous Dermatitis on the Hind Limb of Dog

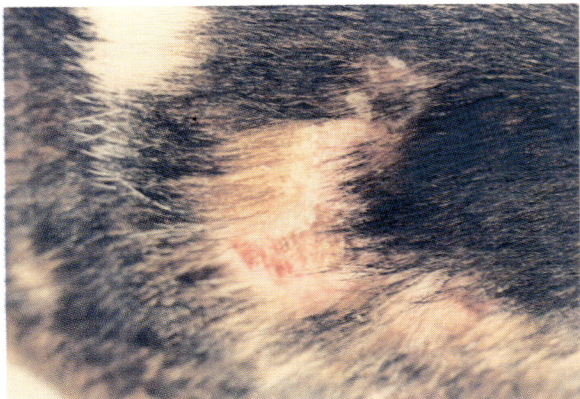

Fig. 119b Allergic Dermatitis Showing Extensive Lesions

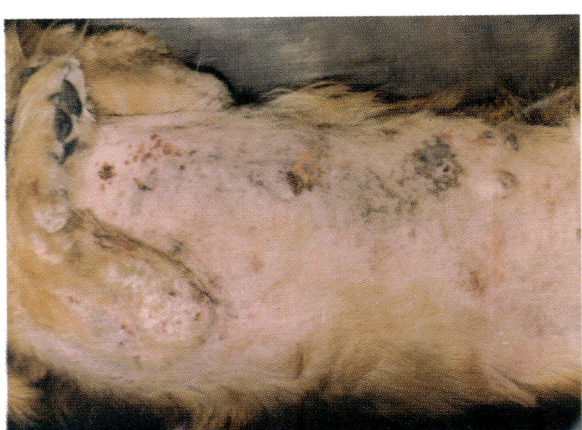

Fig. 119d Extensive Eczema Showing Exudation

Aetiology

Different kinds of aetiological factors may be differentiated into endogenous and exogenous allergens.

A. Endogenous allergens

a. Food allergens, viz. Vegetables, meat, eggs, lettuce, milk and milk products, rice, fishes, spinal, tomato, wheat and several other foods.

b. Protozoan allergen, viz. Leishmaniasis.

c. Bacterial allergens, viz. Tuberculosis and leptospirosis.

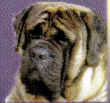

d. Mycotic allergens, e.g. trichophytosis.

e. Helminthic allergens, viz., Ascaris, hookworm, tapeworm and whipworm etc.

f. Allergic skin conditions caused by sera, vaccines and other proteins.

g. Allergic reactions of drugs, viz., Potassium iodide, potassium bromide and phaenothiazine.

h. Exogenous allergens.

i. Ectoparasites like fleas, lice, ticks and mites etc.

j. Antiseptics and disinfectants.

k. Miscellaneous factors, viz,. Paints varnish, bedding materials, rubber or plastic balls, dyes, synthetic fibres, pollen grains etc. either alone or mixed.

Predisposing factors: Interlude susceptibility, hepatic disorders, hormonal imbalance and climatic factors etc.

Clinical signs

Clinical pictures are complex and varied but these always take the form of superficial dermal changes. Initially small reddish spot appears on the skin due to allergic reaction, these may often progress to papule formation and further inflammatory changes producing vesicles of different size. Along with these changes there will be swellings which may be either diffuse oedema or localized urticarial oedema of the superficial layer of skin. The condition may be acute or chronic depending on the duration of the eczema. The nature of eczema may be dry or moist. In case of moist eczema there is exudation of serum and often pus formation due to secondary causes. In chronic cases the lesions turn dry, thickened and hyperkeratotic along with almost constant pruritus.

The definite diagnosis of eczema is rather difficult due to problems of differentiating eczema from other dermatitis. Eczematous lesions are normally superficial unless complicated by the secondary bacterial or mycotic invasions.

Line of treatment

1. Removal of the aetiological factor(s).

2. Need-based treatments for the external and internal allergens.

3. Highly digestible balanced diets should be fed and foods containing allergens should not be used.

4. The diets should be free from meat and eggs.

5. Milk, milk products and soup should be fed.

6. Administration of antihistaminic drugs.

7. Steroids are helpful in early recovery.

8. Topical application of antibiotic ointments for checking secondary complications.

9. Use of enzymes and antiproteinases.

DISEASES OF NEW BORN PUPPIES

Fading Puppies Syndrome

This is an important disease of the puppies in which puppies start to die at about 4 or 5 days, losing their desire to suckle and becoming blue. Some puppies, despite adequate feed, do not thrive and grow poorly. They often suffer from a variety of digestive and respiratory problems.

Aetiology

Beta haemolytic Streptococci (BHS), Staphylococci, and Eschericia coli cause Fading Puppy Syndrome. Canine Herpes Virus, a flu-like virus, can also cause Fading Puppy Syndrome.

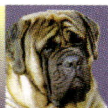

Transmission

The most common way for the bitch to pick up BHS is by direct contact of the external genital organs, particularly during her season when her cervix is dilated, as she sits to urinate and the vulva comes in contact with the contaminated ground. The stud dog can act as a carrier. BHS can survive on his penis for about 48 hours.

Clinical findings

The bitch will become distressed by the crying, puppies and she will still be carrying milk-causing discomfort. These puppies, born healthy, are infected by suckling infected milk. Affected young puppies are generally less active, lack vitality and often fade away, and finally die within 2-3 weeks of birth. Body weight gain in affected puppies is much less than their litter mates, despite appearing to suckle well and consume part of their special puppy food. In most cases, fading puppies will suffer a lowgrade infection with a virus or bacteria.

Treatment

They can be saved by antibiotics and being hand-reared or fostered. The importance here is obviously early diagnosis and treatment. A course of antibiotics over 5-7 days can help to delay the onset of secondary bacterial infection of viral damaged tissue in the lungs, gut or liver. However, the most effective supportive therapy is to give an injection of blood serum from another healthy animal. Collection of blood and preparation of serum is strictly a job of vet. Alternatively, a dog of full vaccination course with regular annual boosters against the common viral infections can be used as a donor. The bitch herself can be used as a serum donor, if she has been vaccinated during pregnancy. Now-a-days, with a wide range of excellent vaccines available, a planned vaccination programme carried out during pregnancy, can help to boost the immunity passed in the colostrum, against common viruses. Most puppies that suckle strongly will take in enough colostrum antibodies to protect them against minor viral infections during the first 2-3 weeks of age.

EMERGENCY CONDITIONS

Different kinds of emergency may be encountered in the life of pets, which require immediate attention on priority. These are shock, fracture, internal haemorrhages, profuse bleeding, burns, accidents, heat stroke, pyrexia and pain etc.

1. Shock

In a state of shock, the pets generally collapse in a short time. The gums are flushed, pupil is dilated, breathing is shallow and rapid and temperature is generally sub normal. Sometimes the temperature of the extremities is low even though the internal body temperature is higher. The pulse is weak and thready.

Line of treatment

1. Patient is placed at a clean and well ventilated place, and if necessary, artificial respiration may be required.

2. I/m or I/v administration of corticoster-oids.

3. The patient is kept warm by wrapping in a blanket at a clean and dry place.

4. Administration of broad-spectrum antibi-otics.

5. Blood infusion may be needed when PCV is low.

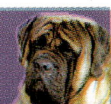

6. The patient should not be disturbed and should be kept calm and comfortable.

2. Fracture

In case of a fracture of leg, the broken leg swings and can not bear weight. In fracture of back bone the rear legs limp extension of forelegs is rigid. In pelvic fracture, the patient is unable to use the hindlegs, drooping tail and pain on the back portion of the body.

The patient of fracture should be kept restrained for avoiding further damage and necessary appliances should be used as early as possible for the repair of fracture. The patients are provided relief from pain with the administration of analgesic. The wound(s) is treated aseptically.

3. Internal Haemorrhages

The internal haemorrhage is exhibited by flushed mucous membrane and weakness. Appearance of blood in faeces, urine and cough is noticed depending on the involvement of the organs(s).

The internal haemorrhage is mostly fatal because it is not easy to diagnose the injury. Indeed, attempts are made to save the patient with the use of the line of treatment used for the shock.

4. Profuse Bleeding

Severe trauma causes profuse bleeding often leading to shock.

Line of treatment

1. Repair of the trauma for stopping the bleeding.
2. Infusion of blood for compensating the loss
3. Supportive therapy with vitamin B complex and nutrient therapeutic fluids.
4. Antiseptic treatment of the injured part.

5. Burns

Damage of tissue by direct or indirect heat and it is classified on the basis of the extent of tissue damage as first, second and third degree burns. In first-degree burns only the superficial layers of skin are burnt but not eroded. Such burns are painful but healing is rapid. In second degree burns blisters are formed and deep layers of tissues are damaged causing significant fluid loss. In the third degree burn there is complete loss of action of skin and inner layers are involved. The wound does not heal, unless the dead tissues are removed.

Line of treatment

1. The imposed first-degree burn is treated with demulcent and antibiotic lotions.
2. Sedatives, tranquilizers and i/v fluid therapy is used as per the requirements of the patient.
3. Topical antiseptic lotion or ointment is applied to control secondary infections.
4. Antibiotics are administered parenterally.
5. Anti tetanus injection is given shortly after the injury.
6. Antihistaminics are administered.
7. Corticosteroids are helpful in enhancing the recovery.
8. Parenteral administration of therapeutic fluids may be necessary.

6. Accidents and Injuries

Accidents and injuries are of varying intensity and may involve one or more tissues and organs.

Line of treatment

Treatment depends on the extent of damage, involvement of the body part and after-effect of the damage. The line of treatment may be:

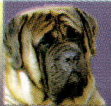

1. Administration of physiological fluid.
2. Immediate application of ice cold water preferably normal saline for blunt injuries.
3. Topical application of soothing ointments containing antibiotics.
4. Topical application of local anaesthetics.

7. Heat Stroke or Sun Stroke

The unbearable hyperthermia caused by the exposure to sun generally during the summer. The condition is complicated by severe dehydration due to delayed water intake.

Aetiology

1. Sudden and excessive exposure to hot sun.
2. Dehydration and unusual delay in water supply.
3. Excessive exercise in hot dry climate.
4. Obesity and lack of heat tolerance.

Clinical Signs

Exhaustion, dullness, depression, high fever panting, prostration and coma followed by death in unattended animals.

Line of treatment

1. Administration of coramine
2. Frequent cold bath to bring down temperature to normal
3. Administration of plenty dextrose saline through I/v route.
4. Administration of febrifuge.
5. Use of tranquilizers, if animal is restless.
6. Feeding of cold milk.
7. Control of diarrhoea, if occurs.

8. Pyrexia (Fever)

An increase in body temperature by any reason is pyrexia. It is body reaction of many diseases.

Aetiology

1. Excessive exposure to sun/heat.
2. Dehydration and lack of water supply.
3. Various infectious diseases, viz., Bacterial, viral etc.
4. Toxicosis due to ingestion of certain chemicals.
5. Food poisoning and associated diarrhoea and dysentery.

Clinical signs

1. Abnormally higher body (Rectal) temperature.
2. Dehydration evident from dry nose.
3. Increased respiration rate or even panting.
4. Cardiac asphyxia in very high temperature exceeding 105 °F. It may lead to brain damage and death.

Line of treatment

1. Application of cold pack on head and body.
2. Administration of therapeutic fluid for the restoration of body fluid, energy supply and balancing of electrolytes,
3. Administration of therapeutic febrifuge drug.
4. Administration of antibiotics or sulpha drugs may be used only after reduction of fever to near the normal level.

9. Pain

It is difficult to judge and skill of diagnosing pain is acquired by experience. The pain is exhibited by unusual postures, abnormal vocalization, and defensive reaction to palpation, autonomic responses and muscular splitting of the affected area of the body. The reaction of to pain depends on the severity of

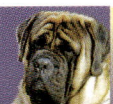

the pain, causes and temperament of the individual animal.

Line of treatment

1. Administration of analgesics.
2. Removal of cause if identified.
3. Administration of narcotics in case of the involvement of muscles and internal organs.
4. Use of steroids and anti inflammatory drugs in cases of identified caused, viz., Dental injury, gum inflammation, gastro enteritis, renal pain cystitis, arthritis etc.

REPRODUCTIVE DISORDER

1. Infertility in Bitches

Infertility can be defined as inability to conceive or to carry a pregnancy to term. Infertility in female dogs (bitches) includes abnormalities of the heat cycle (oestrus), failure of breeding (copulation), failure of becoming pregnant (conception), and pregnancy loss. To know the reason of failure of breeding in bitches is important because they get only few chances to get pregnant.

There are three main types of infertility:

1. **Delayed oestrus:** Normal time of oestrus is 6 months to 1 years. Possible effect of season and effect of pheromones in some bitches are the cause of delayed oestrus. Equine chorionic gonadotrophin can be used to induce oestrus (20 IU/kg sc).
2. **Improper timing of mating:** Generally bitches are mated in between 10 and 14 days after the onset of prooestrus. One or two mating two days apart is usually allowed. Deviation from this schedule may result in infertile matings.

3. **Infection of non-specific bacteria:** Bacteria like Beta-haemolytic streptococci and E. coli have been found to be associated with disorders of oestrus.

Other conditions causing infertility in bitches:

1. Disorders related to psychology of the bitches.
2. Physical inability of the bitches.

Causes of infertility

The most common cause of infertility in bitches is insemination at an improper time in the estrous cycle. Problems with the female reproductive tract may lead to infertility. Other causes include uterine infection, male infertility, thyroid gland insufficiency. Infection with *Brucella canis* should be considered and eliminated as a cause in all infertile bitches.

Diagnosis

Infertility in female dogs (bitches) is diagnosed by a good clinical history including breeding management and a physical examination. The serum progesterone concentration is an important diagnostic tool. Progesterone, a female hormone, prepares the uterus for pregnancy and maintains the pregnancy. Measurement of progesterone during the pre-heat and heat cycles (estrous cycle) can predict ovulation time and optimize breeding management.

The veterinarian may perform a serologic test for Brucella canis in dogs. Bacterial cultures of the reproductive tract may be used for determining the infection of the uterus. Other tests include adrenal gland hormone or thyroid hormone testing to determine hyper-adrenocorticism or hypothyroidism and serological testing for canine herpes virus.

The normal ovaries and uterus are not visible on radiographs (X-rays); therefore, large

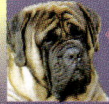

ovaries and a visible uterus on a radiograph indicate some type of abnormality in the infertile female. Ultrasound may reveal disease of the ovaries or uterus. Ultrasound is also used for diagnosing pregnancy as early as 2 to 24 days after ovulation and for documenting pregnancy loss.

Treatment

Improper breeding is often at the root of perceived infertility. If improper breeding techniques are not the problem, the veterinarian will treat the underlying cause of the infertility. Antibiotics may be given for infection of the uterus. Thyroid hormone is given to dogs with hypothyroidism. A hormone called "gonadotropin" can be given to induce ovulation in bitches with ovulation problems.

Surgical considerations include surgical correction of abnormalities of the vagina, repair of an obstructed reproductive tract, drainage of ovarian cysts, and removal of a cancerous ovary.

2. Infertility in Dogs (Male Studs)

Infertility is more pronounced in male animals and can be investigated more easily than in females. Generally, infertility in male dogs refers to diminished or absent fertility. It does not imply sterility.

Aetiology

The causes of infertility in male dogs are divided into two main groups, i.e. congenital infertility and acquired infertility. Congenital infertility is caused by genetic abnormalities which is present at birth. Affected dogs cannot produce sperm. Acquired infertility develops during the dog's lifetime. It has several causes, viz., unfamiliar surroundings, slippery flooring, absence of a female dog in heat, presence of a

dominant pet guardian or female dog, obstruction due to inflammation, infection, hormonal abnormalities like hypothyroidism, hyperadrenocorticism and drugs and toxins.

Diagnosis

Infertility is diagnosed by a good clinical history including breeding management and physical examination. To determine infertility, hormonal (endocrine) profile may be performed. Measurement of several hormones can help in the identification of the cause of infertility. One of the hormones is testosterone, the male hormone. Ultrasound helps in identifying the abnormalities of the male reproductive tract and evaluation of the prostate gland.

A breeding soundness examination is performed. Few sperm samples are collected and evaluated for volume, number or concentration of sperm, motility of the sperm, and other characteristics. Microscopic examination and bacterial culture of sperm and urine also are performed. Other tests may be performed, based on the veterinarian's assessment of the cause of infertility. Testicular biopsy may be necessary to obtain a definitive diagnosis for infertility in dogs.

Treatment

The treatment for infertility in male dogs depends on the underlying cause. No treatment is available for congenital infertility. Most perceived infertility is actually incorrect timing of breeding or poor breeding conditions. Supportive treatment includes reducing heat or other stress and ensuring balanced diet including mineral supplementation. Antibiotics are administered to treat infection. Usually, a minimum of 3 to 4 weeks of treatment is recommended to allow adequate and sustained concentrations of antibiotics within the reproductive tract. Other treatment will depend

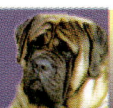

on the identified cause of the infertility. The testicles will require at least 60 days time to return to function. Treatment of infertility requires longer duration of medication.

Prognosis

The prognosis for infertility in male dogs depends on the underlying cause. Since most perceived infertility in male dogs is actually incorrect timing of breeding, the initial prognosis is good. However, if breeding management has been ruled out as the cause, the prognosis is determined by the cause of infertility. Dogs with congenital infertility will not produce sperms in most of the conditions. Many causes of acquired infertility can be corrected.

AUTOIMMUNE DISORDERS

When a body encounters something foreign in its environment, it reacts to produce an immune response against that substance to protect itself from potential harm. In order to do this effectively it must be able to recognise what is self in order to respond to non-self or foreign. In autoimmune diseases there is a failure to recognise some part of self. Such autoimmunity may be restricted to a single organ, a localized region or the whole animal. The consequences may vary from minimal to catastrophic, depending on the extent to which the body is affected. In autoimmune disease pathologic signs are seen as a result of the autoimmune response. Frequently more than one autoimmune disease will be seen in the same animal, as well as an increased susceptibility to bacterial infection. There are four basic mechanisms underlying autoimmune disease.

1. **Antibody mediated diseases:** A specific antibody exists targeted against a particular antigen (protein) which leads to its destruction and signs of the disease.

Examples are: auto-immune mediated haemolytic anaemia, where the target is on the surface of the red blood cell; myesthenia gravis where the target is the acetylcholine receptor in the neuromuscular junction; and hypoadrenocorticism (Addison's) where the targets are the cells of the adrenal gland.

2. **Immune-complex-mediated diseases:** Antibodies are produced against proteins in the body, which combine into large molecules and circulate around the body. In systemic lupus erythematosus (SLE) antibodies are formed against several components in the cell's nucleus (hence the anti-nuclear antibody test (ANA) for SLE). Most notably antibodies are made against the body's double stranded DNA, and form circulating soluble complexes of DNA and antibody, which break down in skin causing an increased sensitivity to ultraviolet light and a variety of signs. As the blood is filtered through the kidneys the complexes are trapped in the glomeruli and blood vessels, causing the kidney to leak protein - glomerulonephritis. They also cause leakage in other blood vessels, and there may be hemorrhage, as well as accumulating in synovial fluid causing signs of arthritis and joint pain. Rheumatoid arthritis results from immune complexes (IgM class antibody called rheumatoid factor) against part of the animal's own immune. These form complexes which are deposited in the synovia of the joint spaces causing an inflammatory response, joint swelling and pain. The collagen and cartilage of the joint breaks down and is eventually replaced by fibrin which fuses the joints causing ankylosis.

3. **Antibody and T cell-mediated diseases:** T cells are one of two types (the other being B-cells) which mediate immune reactions. Upon exposure to a particular antigen they become programmed to search for and

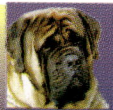

destroy that particular protein in future. Once an animal has been exposed to an antigen it will be able to mount a much faster response in next encounter. This is the basis of vaccination. Thyroiditis (autoimmune hypothyroidism) seems to be of mixed etiology. Several target antigens have been identified, including thyroglobulin the major protein made by the thyroid. Autoantibodies to antigens in the epithelial cells of the thyroid have also been found. The thyroid becomes invaded by large number of T and B cells as well as macrophages which are cells that engulf and destroy other cell types. T cells specifically programmed for thyroglobulin have been identified.

4. **Diseases arising from a deficiency in complement:** Reaction between antigen and antibody may activate a series of serum enzymes (the complement system) resulting in either the lysis of the antigen molecule or to make it easier for phagocytic cells like macrophages to destroy it. Animals with deficiencies in enzymes are activated early in the complement system and develop autoimmune diseases like SLE.

5. **Autoimmune mediated anaemia (AIMA):** Auto-immune mediated anaemia (AIMA) also called autoimmune haemolytic anaemia (AIHA) and immune mediated haemolytic anaemia (IMHA); and antibodies formed against antigens in the red blood cell membrane cause these cells to burst open. The resulting anaemia reduces the dog's ability to provide sufficient oxygen for cell function in the body.

6. **Immune-mediated thrombocytopenia (ITP):** It is a dangerously low level of platelets, either due to an increase in antibody and complement-mediated phagocytosis of platelets in the spleen, bone marrow and liver, or decreased production due to antibody and/or complement mediated phagocytosis of

platelet stem cells (megakaryocytes) in the bone marrow. The low platelet levels lead to spontaneous bleeding, often nose bleeding or petechiation (bleeding just under the skin and mucous membranes) are seen. Blood in the stool, urine or vomitus is less common.

7. **Autoimmune thyroiditis (hypothyroidism):** It is generally found with the other autoimmune diseases or may occur by itself. Loss of thyroid hormones is manifested early by behavioural changes - aggression, hyperactivity, anxiety/fear, compulsive behaviours, phobic behaviours; allergies and reduced resistance to bacterial, viral, fungal and protozoal infection - often manifested as skin and respiratory disorders. Seizure disorders are often related to low thyroid levels. As the disease progresses letharginess, obesity, alopecia and infertility are more common signs.

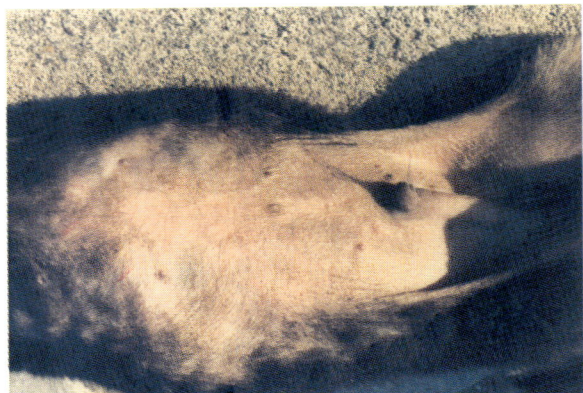

Fig. 120 A Case of Hypothyroidism in a Dog

8. **Hypoadrenocorticism (Addison's disease):** The adrenal gland produces hormones which regulate the level of sodium and potassium (mineralocorticoids) and mediate the body's response to physiologic and psychologic stress (corticosteroids). The former are needed to maintain proper cell function and their loss is seen to cause muscle weakness and eventually heart failure as the

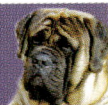

heart's muscle cells can no longer produce the nervous impulses needed for the heart to contract. Gastrointestinal function is also usually impaired and weight loss is frequently seen. Animals are less able to cope with mild, everyday occurrences, refuse to eat and show other symptoms of stress.

9. **Pemphigus foliaceus:** It is a skin disease in which pustules are formed. They seem to be more common on the feet but may be restricted to the face or appear patchily all over body of the dog. After the pustules burst, the skin appears crusty or scaly and hairs are lost. The dog may chew on or scratch the lesions increasing the damage and ulcers resulting in serious skin erosion. Although the antigen has not been specifically identified, pemphigus is a result of autoantibodies directed against the cell membrane of epithelial cells, causing them to become round and separate instead of forming a solid sheet.

10. **Myasthenia gravis:** This disease results in a loss of muscle function due to obstruction in transmission of nerve signals. Disuse muscular atrophy causes weakness and dogs are reluctant to move. Enlargement of the esophagus (megaoesophagus) may result. This is often seen as regurgitation of food as soon as it is swallowed and frequently results in aspiration of food into the lungs. Even when treated, dogs are liable to die of aspiration pneumonia due to megaoesophagus. Untreated dogs eventually lose the use of swallowing and respiratory muscles and suffer from extended illness and die ultimately in a pitiable state.

11. **Lupus Erythematosus:** There are several forms of lupus erythematosus that are recognized in people and two of these have been identified in dogs. Lupus is an autoimmune disorder, meaning that the body mounts an inappropriate immune response to some part of itself.

Systemic lupus erythematosus (SLE) is an uncommon but severe disorder in which the inappropriate immune response is wide-spread in the body, and can cause arthritis, kidney disease, anaemia and skin disease. Cutaneous lupus erythematosus (CLE) is thought to be a milder variant of SLE and the problems are confined to the skin. CLE is also called discoid lupus erythematosus.

Breeds Affected by Lupus (Erythematosus)

CLE is seen more often than SLE, although both conditions are uncommon. There is a breed predisposition for the Collie, Shetland Sheepdog, and German Shepherd, as well as crosses of these breeds.

For many breeds and many disorders, the studies to determine the mode of inheritance or the frequency in the breed have not been carried out, or are clinical findings inconclusive.

SLE most commonly affects joints, muscle, skin, blood, and/or kidneys. The condition tends to wax and wane, so dog will have periods of remission and flare-up. The kinds of problems noticed include shifting lameness, weakness and pale gums (due to anaemia), and/or increased drinking and urination (kidney disease). The face and the feet are most often affected areas of the skin, with ulcers and loss of pigment on the nose, and ulceration and thickening of the footpads. With CLE, most likely lesion are red, scaling areas of inflammation on dog's face, and loss of pigment from the nose. There may also be lesions on the ears and thickening of the footpads. Affected dogs are otherwise healthy. Nasal scarring is common with both SLE and CLE. Exposure to ultraviolet light is a factor (especially in CLE), and so the condition is seen more often and is more severe in the summer and in sunny parts of the world.

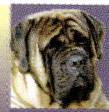

Diagnosis

Since SLE can affect different body systems, diagnosis is challenging. Once suspected, diagnosis is confirmed by specific blood tests and biopsy for examination by a veterinary pathologist. CLE is diagnosed through examination of biopsy samples.

Treatment

Treatment for SLE generally requires relatively high doses of steroids in combination with chemotherapy. In general, dogs with joint, muscle or skin disease seem to respond better to medication, and have longer periods of remission than those with severe blood or kidney problems. Unfortunately, many dogs with SLE die or euthanized within a year of diagnosis, either due to the disease itself, the inability to control it, and/or unacceptable drug reactions. In many dogs, the disease can be well-controlled with medication for several years. It is treated with relatively lower doses of steroids plus vitamin E and fatty acid supplements. Treatment generally needs to be lifelong, and dogs usually do well on it. Exposure to ultraviolet radiation worsens the skin lesions in both conditions, so sunscreen is advisable and dogs should be sheltered from peak sunlight.

Rheumatoid Arthritis

It is a chronic inflammatory condition which differs from that of arthritis. It is rather a destructive arthritis.

Aetiology

The cause of the autoimmune disease like Rheumatoid arthritis is not known properly, although it may be due to formation of immune complex in the synovium.

Clinical findings

This disease occurs in all kinds of animals irrespective of age and breed. The disease occurs mostly in the animals of age group 4-6 years. The signs are manifested by high rise of temperature, loss of appetite, letharginess and lameness due to which the animal can not walk properly. There is pain in the joints and bilateral symmetrical swelling is also found.

Diagnosis

Diagnosis depend upon history, clinical features like pain, swelling of joints, stiffness of legs, radiographical changes, presence of abnormal synovial fluid, histopathological changes etc. Differential diagnosis with multiple arthritis and infective arthritis play an important role too. Rheumatoid arthritis in dog is detected by modified Rose-Waaler test.

Treatment

Treatment of Rheumatoid arthritis is not so easy. Several NSAID have been used but little benefit is observed. Prednisolone, on the other hand have been found to be better. Levamisole intramuscularly is given to strengthen the immune system. In some cases surgical intervention is useful.

METABOLIC AND MINERAL DEFICIENCY DISEASES

In veterinary medicine, problems with the diets during growth occur especially in giant breeds. Other breeds or/and older dogs also have to be fed in accordance with their requirements. The energy content of a diet seems to strongly affect calcium (Ca) metabolism. A balanced diet is important for an optimal bone health. Furthermore, corrected diet will reduce the occurrence of bone diseases associated with

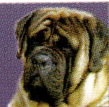

primary and secondary hyperparathyroidism, renal-induced asteomalacia and osteopenia associated with diseases of the gastrointestinal tract.

1. Rickets

This is a disease characterized by interference with mineralisation and consequently with normal resorption of growth plate cartilage. Rapidly growing plates in fast growing bones are most severely affected.

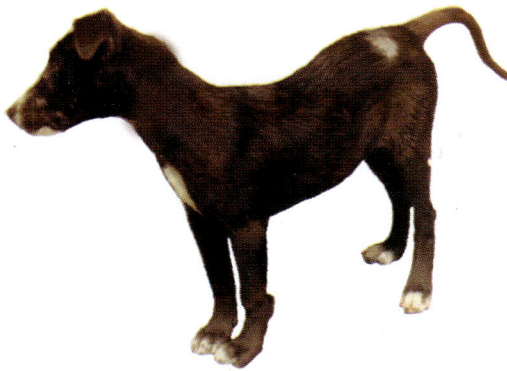

Fig. 121 A Pup Suffering from Rickets

Aetiology

Deficient intake or absorption or both of Ca, P and vitamin D either alone or together are often the causes of rickets in young growing puppies. The low level of phosphorus may result from disease of gastro intestinal tract, liver or kidney which may impair the absorption of phosphorus from the digestive tract. Vitamin D deficiency can be considered in animals, which are housed indoors unexposed from sunlight, or having abnormal metabolism of vitamin D.

Clinical symptoms

The major signs of rickets are abnormal curvature of long bones and increased prominence of bone ends. There is widening of the growth plates (which is present at the end of the bones from where the bone elongates) which is due to the failure to reabsorb cartilage and lack of normal calcification. The outer lining becomes very thin and may appear as a shell. Apparent bowing of bone is more evident.

Treatment

Therapeutic doses of calcium, phosphorus and vitamin D in the proper balance are usually beneficial in rickets. Excess supplementation of vitamin D can cause defects in bony matrix, soft tissue calcification, nausea, diarrhoea and even renal damage.

2. Osteoporosis

Osteoporosis is a non-specific term referring to a condition that is characterized by quantitative loss of bone (atrophy of bone). The bone appears entirely typical, since the organic and inorganic phases diminish in equal proportion. The reduced amount of bone is exhibited by thinning of the cortex or reduced number and caliber of calcareous trabeculae, or more commonly both. Thus, affected bones are thin, porous and brittle. However the volume of bone remains constant but density is reduced.

The cause of osteoporosis is not yet fully known. A lowering in bone mass can be seen in primary hyperparathyroidism, nutritional hyperparathyroidism, renal secondary hyperparathyroidism, pseudo hyperparathyroidism, hyperthyroidism, acromegaly, hepatic toxicity, long-term tetraplegia, multiple myeloma, as a result of the administration of certain anticonvulsant drugs and in hyperadrenocorticism. However, the reduction in bone mass (osteoporosis) is seen only secondary to the primary condition, hence the term secondary osteoporosis should be more appropriate. Primary osteoporosis has not been reported in the dog.

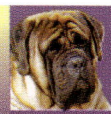

Aetiology

Osteoporosis occurs as a result of an imbalance between bone formation and bone resorption. It may occur, if bone formation fails to keep pace with normal resorptive processes or if bone resorption exceeds bone production. Thus, generalized osteoporosis may be associated with diseases that affect either the organic matrix or the mineralized matrix of bone.

Pathogenesis

Osteoporosis may occur in disorders of mineral metabolism such as fibrous osteodystrophy (hyperparathyroidism) and rickets or osteomalacia, in which the axiomatic pathogenic mechanism is excessive osteoclastic resorption or failure in the mineralization of the organic matrix. However, in these diseases, the osteoporosis is usually accompanied by other microscopic features characteristic of the disease, such as proliferation of fibrous tissue in fibrous osteodystrophy and wide osteoid in rickets and osteomalacia. The radiographic appearance of these conditions can be remarkably similar. Disuse osteoporosis is the term used to describe the type of osteoporosis caused by immobilization of the affected bone. Frequently, this is the result of plaster casts or paralysis. The osteoporosis occurs due to a reduction or cessation of normal muscular activity around the bone, which in turn diminishes the flow of blood through the bone. Osteoporosis often is the earliest lesion detected in fibrous osteodystrophy, in some instances this disparity may be related to early versus late diagnosis. The differences in the lesions observed may also be related to the magnitude of the secondary parathyroid response and the extent of compensation of the hypocalcemia that occurs initially. The age of the animal at the time of the imbalance appears to be a factor in the development of bone lesion.

Diagnosis

The diagnosis of secondary osteoporosis can be made by clinical signs, radiography and association of one of the primary disease conditions may help to confirm. Clinical signs are referable to fractures of the long bones and vertebrae and a reduction in bone mass of the mandible and maxilla. Laboratory findings are referable to the primary disease.

Treatment

Secondary osteoporosis is treated by correcting the primary problem or condition.

3. Osteopetrosis

Osteopetrosis is a rare congenital and genealogical developmental abnormality of skeletal growth of animals. Bone length and shape are relatively normal. There is, however, marked retardation of the remainder of the endochondral ossification cycle which includes bone maturation, resorption of immature bone, bone remodelling and cortex formation beyond the primary trabecular stage. The accretion and persistence of cores of calcified cartilage, osteoid and primitive bone in the medullary cavities results in this.

Aetiology

Investigations in dogs suggest a genetic basis for the condition. The characteristic feature of the disease is excessive accumulation of bone and mineralized cartilage throughout the skeletal system. The most prominent and dense lesions occur in the metaphysis of the humerus, femur and tibia.

Pathogenesis

The basic pathogenetic mechanism of osteopetrosis is aberrant osteoclastic function.

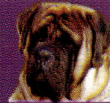

Functional defects that have been observed in osteopetrotic animals include decreased activity of lysosomal and oxidative enzymes and partial or complete absence of ruffled borders. Owing to the failure in osteoclastic remodelling, the mineralized cartilage spicules of the physis and the primary trabeculae of the metaphysis are not resorbed, causing the medullary cavity to be filled with large caliber, cancellous trabeculae containing central cores of cartilage. The possibility of deficiencies of the immune system, such as T-cells, may secondarily affect bone. Attention is also focused on factors that control differentiation of the osteoclast, elucidation of the homing phenomenon and determination of the fate of the osteoclast.

Diagnosis

Clinical diagnosis is difficult to describe. However, osteopetrotic bone is brittle and may result in pathological fracture. The obliteration of normal bone marrow spaces is likely to result in a non-regenerative anaemia. Radiography and histopathological changes may be beneficial to draw a conclusion for the diagnosis of this disease.

Treatment

Because the etiology is unknown, treatment can be directed only for symptomatic correction of problems. The greatest concern in the mature animal is treatment of the anaemia by transfusion.

4. Osteomalacia

In adults, the lack of same minerals as observed in rickets and osteoporosis, causes a similar condition, called osteomalacia. The changes in bone structure are not nearly as obvious or severe because the skeletal system is already completely formed. Bone pains are common in osteomalacia, particularly in the hips and spine. In both osteomalacia and rickets, severe cramps develop as a result of falling blood-calcium levels.

Vitamin D is crucial for the absorption of calcium, the most essential mineral for hard, stable bones. Since calcium is also needed in the blood at all times and fall in blood-calcium levels stimulates mobilization from bones, if supply through feed is inadequate. Without vitamin D, calcium cannot be absorbed from food. Ultraviolet rays in sunlight are also essential for the synthesis of vitamin D in the skin. Vitamin D is also supplied through absorption of nutrients from the intestinal tract. Vitamin D is a fat-soluble vitamin, and deficient dietary lipids reduce its availability disturbing Ca assimilation leading to development of either rickets or osteomalacia. Malabsorption syndrome is caused by fat deficient diets and poor bile production. If a liver or kidney disease prevents the full conversion of vitamin D to its active form, osteomalacia can also occur. Anticonvulsant medications also cause osteomalacia. Occurrence of rickets or osteomalacia due to lack of calcium in the diet is rare.

Supplements and herbs

Although osteomalacia is usually the result of nutritional deficiencies of vitamin D, calcium should also be supplied in ample amounts alongwith optimum quantity of magnesium, silica, vitamin C and bioflavonoids for the formation of strong bones. The silica from horsetail helps to increase calcium absorption by the bones without calcium supplementation. Take 3 cups of horsetail tea, or 3 capsules of aqueous horsetail extract daily or 10-15 drops

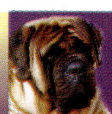

tincture in liquid three times daily. A composite preparation of vitamin D 400 IU, calcium 1,000 mg, Magnesium 500 mg, Silica 1,000 mg, vitamin C, with bioflavonoids 1,000 mg, quercetin 250 mg can also be beneficial.

5. Canine Hip Dysplasia

Canine Hip Dysplasia (CHD) is a misunderstood but painful and crippling disease that results in a weakened hip joint in dogs and causes painful inflammation and decreased flexibility. Canines have historically been given NSAID treatment for this condition, but many vets are now recommending glucosamine for this condition instead. The word dysplasia means improper growth. Canine Hip Dysplasia literally means impaired growth of the canine hip.

Aetiology

The improper growth makes the hip loose and wobbly, leading to increased movement of the hip. This will ultimately result after some time in arthritis and lameness of the animal, if left untreated. CHD is a progressive condition that may manifest vastly different levels of severity in different animals. Hip dysplasia can result from genetic mutations or simply from masked hidden genes that can skip one or more generations. Diet can also contribute to hip dysplasia. Feeding puppies a leaner diet during their formative years may help mitigate the risk of hip dysplasia and make them less susceptible to develop CHD later in life. Large breeds are the most susceptible to Canine Hip Dysplasia, but many small and medium sized animals also suffer from CHD. Labrador, Golden Retreiver, Blood Hound, St. Bernard, Boxers and Rottweilers are some of the more susceptible breeds for CHD hip. Siberian Huskies and Dobermans tend to be at a lower risk for CHD.

Clinical symptoms

Many animals afflicted with hip dysplasia will have problems in walking up stairs, slowness in rising, lameness after exercise and may exhibit personality changes due to their ever present pain. Animals with hip dysplasia are at greater risk of injury through normal and especially through strenuous activity. It is entirely possible for a dog to have CHD but show no symptoms or a dog to have severe crippling symptoms. In Canine Hip Dysplasia the hip joint is not the only affected area, knee, shoulder and spinal joints can also show evidence of changes. The gradual loss of cartilage, joint inflammation, bone spurs and pain can result from osteoarthritis or hip dysplasia.

Diagnosis

CHD is dignosed via a radiographic (X-ray) examination. The interaction between genes and the environment plays a great role in determining, if a dog will develop hip dysplasia. While poor breeding does not always mean the animal will surely be afflicted with hip dysplasia, there is a genetic predisposition for hip dysplasia, especially in larger breeds. For smaller dogs, yowling or grumbling when lifted or handled, lameness, a lack of motivation to move, stiffness, increased sensitivity to touch, a marked change of behaviour, a faint popping sound coming from the hindlegs with each step, difficulty in rising from a lying or sitting position, moving both rear legs in unison, a painful or violent reaction to an extension of their rear legs, reluctance to walk, jump or play, hiding or disappearing from the sight and whining or making noises for no other reason are the signs used for diagnosis.

Treatment

Surgical intervention and the supportive therapy are beneficial in this case. Animal

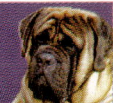

should be kept in rest and provided with soft bedding.

6. Zinc Deficiency Disorder

Zinc is the second most abundant micro-mineral present in tissues. Recommended daily requirements vary between 40 ppm (NRC 1985) and 120 ppm (AAFCO).

The best sources of zinc are meats, fish, whole grain, cereals, legumes, and root vegetables. Experimental studies of zinc deficiency in dogs have found that skin and coat changes are the first clinical signs to develop. Poor growth and development, skin lesions, skeletal defects, and reproductive and congenital defects are also the signs of zinc deficiency. Poorly formulated dry dog foods have been known to cause zinc deficiency in dogs and growing dogs of the larger breeds are more susceptible. Zinc is one of the most important nutrients for determining the appearance of the coat.

Zinc gluconate is a proven nutritional supplement for working dogs (sled dogs, hunting dogs and herding dogs). It helps to promote tougher feet and healthier coats. Its use reduces the occurrence of splits and cracks in dog's feet, as well as nail breakage. Zinc gluconate also helps to toughen dog's pads and speeds up the healing process when an occasional foot problem does occur. Zinc is also extremely important for the proper function of the dog's immune system. Zinc gluconate can be used as a supplement for show dogs, as it will keep their coats in top condition. It should also be fed as a dietary supplement to prevent zinc deficiency, a common condition in northern breeds. For dogs in active training, with chronic foot or coat problems, for competitive show, twice the amount of zinc gluconate (2 teaspoons for 13 dogs/day if the

average weight of one dog is about 50 lb) should be given in diet. Increased dosages can be given without fear of toxicity. The best way to feed zinc gluconate is to put it in dog food and mixed it thoroughly just before feeding. It can be also fed by dissolving it in water and dosing it into drinking water.

Zinc deficiency causes zinc-responsive dermatosis leading to scaling and crusting of the skin. It is not always due to a dietary deficiency of zinc; instead affected dogs appear to have a higher than normal requirement for zinc, perhaps due to abnormal intestinal absorption.

Breeds affected

Alaskan malamute, American Eskimo dog, Samoyed and Siberian Husky are more susceptible. Young rapidly growing Doberman Pinscher and Great Dane sometimes experience a similar condition due to a transient zinc deficiency. For many breeds and many disorders, the studies to determine the mode of inheritance or the frequency in the breed have not been carried out, or are inconclusive.

Clinical symptoms

Signs are usually first seen around puberty. There is reddening, scaling, crusting and hair loss on the muzzle and around the eyes. The footpads as well as the area around the vulva and anus may be affected. The lesions are itchy in about half of dogs with this disorder causing chewing of the feet or rubbing or pawing at the face.

Diagnosis

The diagnosis is made through a skin biopsy. This is a simple procedure done with local

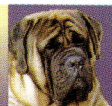

Table 5.2 : Summary of the functions and deficiency disorders of macro and microminerals in dogs

Mineral	Functions	Deficiency Disorders
Calcium (Ca) and Phosphorus (P)	Involved in the structure and strength of teeth and bones. Needed for the normal clotting of blood and for nerve and muscle function. Phosphorus is involved in the storage and transfer of energy in the body. The balance between these two elements is important, as well as the individual concentrations in the diet.	Causes skeletal deformities and lameness in the growing animal. In a lactating bitch there can be hypocalcemia, causing eclampsia with nervous disturbances.
Magnesium (Mg)	Required for healthy bones and teeth, for the normal day to day functioning of the heart, muscle and nervous tissue, and is also involved in many enzyme reactions in the body.	Deficiency can cause muscle weakness, although this is rare in practice. A very high intake has been associated with an increased incidence of lower urinary tract disease.
Potassium (K)	Necessary for energy metabolism, nerve and muscle function and the control of the osmotic balance.	Deficiency is very rare, but could potentially lead to muscle weakness and poor growth, as well of body fluids and kidneys damage to heart
Sodium (Na) and Chloride (Cl-)	Important for the regulation of body fluids water balance,	A deficiency can cause exhaustion, retarded growth, fatigue, an inability to maintain dry skin and hair loss. An excess will cause a greater than normal intake of fluid.
Iron (Fe)	Present in haemoglobin (in the blood) and myoglobin (muscle), as well as in enzymes involved in cell respiration.	A deficiency can cause weakness and fatigue, and anorexia and weight loss in dogs.
Copper (Cu)	Involved in the normal activity of red blood cells and many enzyme systems	A deficiency can cause anaemia due to poor absorption of iron.
Zinc (Zn)	Essential for maintaining a good coat and skin, and an essential component of many enzyme systems. Requirements can be affected by other components of the diet.	A deficiency can lead to poor growth, anorexia, emaciation, skin lesions and testicular atrophy.

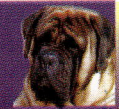

Mineral	Functions	Deficiency Disorders
Iodine (I)	Iodine is an essential component of thyroid hormones, and therefore concerned with the body's metabolism	A deficiency produces the characteristic goitre, but can also affect the skin and hair, causes apathy and drowsiness and affect reproduction
Selenium (Se)	Selenium has important antioxidant properties by protecting the cell membranes, in association with vitamin E in dogs	Degeneration of skeletal and cardiac muscles. Toxic in large doses. There is a fairly fine line between normal and toxic doses
Manganese (Mn)	Required for carbohydrate and fat metabolism and cartilage formation as well as many enzyme reactions	A deficiency can cause defective growth and reproduction, as well as adversely affects fat metabolism.
Cobalt (Co)	An important constituent of the vitamin B_{12} molecule	A deficiency is very unlikely, if the diet contains sufficient vitamin B_{12}

anaesthetic. The biopsy will show changes characteristic of this condition.

Treatment

Temporary zinc supplementation is effective in treating the transient zinc deficiency that may occur in young rapidly growing Great Danes and Doberman Pinscher dogs.

VITAMIN DEFICIENCY DISEASES

1. Vitamin A Deficiency (Hypovitaminosis - A)

Vitamin A is a fat soluble vitamin and the alcoholic form present in carotene does not pass the placental barrier whereas vitamin A in the ester form present in fish liver oil passes through placental barrier and increases vitamin A content of foetal liver. Deficiency of vitamin A usually occurs as a primary disease due to dietary deficiency of the vitamin or its precursor carotenes. It may occur as a secondary disease. Secondary vitamin A deficiency may occur in

chronic diseases of liver or intestines as conversion of carotenes to vitamin A occurs in intestines and liver is the storage organ. Continued ingestion of mineral oils such as liquid paraffin to prevent bloat also causes depression of plasma carotene and vitamin A levels of butterfat is lowered.

Vitamin A is essential for regeneration of visual purple necessary for dim light vision and its deficiency results in night blindness. Vitamin A is necessary for normal growth and shaping of the bones and teeth and maintenance of normal epithelial tissues. Vitamin A deficiency, leads to convulsions and syncope in early stages and atrophy of epithelial cells, which have secretary as well as covering functions. The deficient animals do not grow well and there is reduction in conception rates. Classic effects of vitamin A deprivation are retardation of growth particularly in foetus and young.

Animals showing clinical signs should be treated immediately with vitamin A at the dose rate of 10 to 20 times daily maintenance dose. Usually 440 IU/kg b wt is preferable by

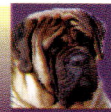

parenteral injections of aqueous than oily solution. The response to treatment in severe and acute cases of deficiency is often rapid and complete but disease in chronic cases may be irreversible. Therapeutic levels given in the initial stage should be continued by oral supplementation.

2. Vitamin D Deficiency Disorder

Vitamin D is synthesized by the body when the skin is exposed to sufficient sunlight. Since it is also involved in regulating the function of specific organs, it is also a hormone. Vitamin D's primary function is to enhance intestinal absorption of calcium and phosphorus. When blood levels of calcium and vitamin D drop, enzyme activity increases in order to produce more of the metabolically active vitamin. Vitamin D also plays a role in the proper mineralization of bone at the site of the bone itself.

Vitamin D deficiency is caused by intestinal malabsorption, gastric surgery and insufficient exposure to sunlight. Several drugs can interfere with the metabolism of vitamin D and cause a deficiency, e.g., liquid paraffin taken as a laxative, anticonvulsant drugs (primidone, phenytoin, phenobarbitone), the hypnotic glutethimide, and corticosteroids such as prednisolone.

In adults, softening of the bones is called osteomalacia. In young, whose bones are still growing, deficiency causes rickets. Vitamin D deficiency during development can also result in thin and irregular tooth enamel.

Vitamin D supplements are available in doses ranging from a few units to several hundred units. Two forms of the vitamin are used, vitamin D_2 and D_3. vitamin D_2 is the synthetic form, and is also called calciferol, or activated ergosterol. vitamin D_3 is the naturally occurring form and is usually obtained from fish liver oils.

3. Vitamin E Deficiency (Hypovitaminosis E)

Vitamin E is fat soluble. The main biological function of vitamin E is to control the rate of tissue oxidation. It enhances the reproductive efficiency in dogs. Feeding on diets deficient in vitamin E and selenium with presence of excessive amounts of polyunsaturated fatty acids in the diet is the major cause of deficiency. Presence of the myopathic agents like fatty acids such as fish liver oils, fish meal, linseed oil, soyabean and corn oil, unaccustomed muscular exercise, prolonged transport and other stress factors alleviate deficiency. The major effects of vitamin E deficiency are muscular weakness and dyspnoea. This is because of true skeletal muscle degeneration and congestive cardiac failure due to myocardial involvement. Acute muscular dystrophy results in liberation of myoglobin into the blood stream but this varies with the myoglobin content in different species.

Combination of vitamin E and selenium is recognized as superior treatment for it. Immediate administration of alpha tocopherol acetate often gives favourable response and signs of deficiency disappear within three days. Subcutaneous injection of 1.0 mg of selenium/kg b wt are recommended. Ideally a mixture of 3 mg selenium (as sodium selenite) and 150 IU of d-alpha tocopherol acetate per ml is a good combination and dose of 2.0 ml/45 kg b wt is recommended.

WATER SOLUBLE VITAMINS
1. Vitamin B Complex

The vitamin B-complex and vitamin C are water soluble. They cannot be stored in the body in large amounts so must be supplied regularly in the diet. When a dog loses fluids by vomiting

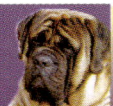

or diarrhoea, water soluble vitamins must be replaced. Overfeeding these watersoluble vitamins does not cause toxicity as excesses are lost in the urine.

1. Vitamin B₁ (Thiamine) deficiency

This is very important to dogs. Dogs differ genetically in their need for thiamine. Metabolic disturbance, exercise and cold housing may increase demand. Only small amounts of thiamine are stored in the body. Treating meat for hydatids (freezing and boiling) reduces thiamine - it is lost in the thawed water and boiling juices. The heat of cooking destroys thiamin. Commercially prepared dog feeds have extra thiamine added to their diets to compensate for cooking losses. Addition of some yeast tablets to feed is beneficial. Brewer's (not live) yeast and wheat germ are valuable sources. Meat and cereals are also good sources. A high fat diet contains less thiamine than a high carbohydrate diet. Dogs should never be fed on raw fish as some species contain an enzyme (thiaminase) which will make thiamine unavailable. Nervous symptoms may develop leading to paralysis. Cooked fish is safe as thiaminase is destroyed.

2. Riboflavin (Vitamin B₂)

Riboflavin is essential for cellular oxidative process in all the animals but its deficiency is rare under natural conditions because actively growing green plants and animal proteins are good sources and some amount is synthesized by alimentary tract microflora in all species. Milk is very good source. In dogs anorexia, poor growth, scours, excessive salivation, lacrymation and alopecia occur.

3. Pantothenic acid deficiency

Pantothenic acid is dietary essential for all species. Dermatitis and patchy alopecia, diarrhoea and incoordination with spastic goose stepping gait are characteristic. Treatment with calcium pantothenate 500 mg/kg b wt per day is effective as treatment and prevention. As feed additive, it can be given @ 10-12/tonne.

4. Nicotinic acid (Niacin) deficiency

Nicotinic acid or niacin is essential for carbohydrate metabolism. In dogs ulcerative stomatitis and bloody diarrhoea and convulsions are the most common symptoms of niacin deficiency which responds to vitamin supplementation treatment quickly. Niacin deficiency is afebrile and should be differentiated from parvoviral haemorrhagic enteritis.

5. Pyridoxine (B₆) deficiency

Deficiency of pyridoxine is not known to occur under natural condition. Dogs on vitamin deficient diet are unthrifty, and have symptoms of central nervous system involvement, such as stiff, jerky gait and convulsions. Deficiency is characterized by anorexia, poor growth, dull coat and alopecia. Some animals may suffer from severe fatal epileptiform fits.

6. Folic acid deficiency

Folic acid deficiency leads to pernicious anaemia. Normally domestic animals produce sufficient folic acid by intestinal synthesis and dietary intake is not necessary.

7. Biotin deficiency

Biotin is also synthesized by ruminal and intestinal bacteria and dietary source is not necessary. Continued feeding of sulpha drugs and antibiotics may induce its deficiency. Deficiency arising from dietary errors may give

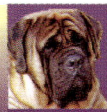

rise to biotin deficiency in dogs, which may suffer from alopecia and stomatitis.

8. Vitamin B$_{12}$ (Cynocobalamine) deficiency

Naturally when cobalt is present as a constituent of feed, the deficiency of cynocobalamine does not occur because rumen microflora synthesize this vitamin. Signs of anorexia, muscular weakness and poor growth may be seen. Daily requirement of 20-40 mg of vitamin B$_{12}$ is necessary.

9. Choline deficiency

Choline is a dietary essential. Deficient young animals suffer from weakness, inability to get up, laboured breathing and anorexia but older ones remain unaffected.

2. Vitamin C

Dogs of all ages suffer with various joint and spinal disorders. Vitamin C is a vital nutrient in bone and cartilage metabolism. Although dogs can manufacture their own vitamin C, they may not produce enough to counter the effects of ageing, stress, inherited dysfunctions, environmental irritants and poor quality or high fat pet foods.

In fact, early studies in dogs suggest that daily vitamin C supplementation might be beneficial in reducing chronic inflammation. Unfortunately, ordinary vitamin C may cause gastrointestinal upsets in dogs. A form of vitamin C that would promote higher levels of intracellular ascorbic acid without negative side effects would be useful. Vitamin C ascorbate/ vitamin C metabolite complex, administered orally, may have application for the reduction of discomfort associated with non-specific, chronic inflammatory disorders of dogs. Vitamin C may act as an immunoresponsive and chrondrogenerative agent. In degenerative (i.e., ageing) or inflammatory conditions, collagen breakdown is excessive, resulting in joint discomfort and skeletal changes.

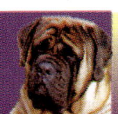

Table 5.3: Showing Functions and Deficiency Disorders of Water-soluble Vitamins

Vitamins	Functions	Deficiency disorders
Thiamin (Vitamin B_1)	Involved in the metabolism of carbohydrates	A deficiency can produce anorexia and neurological disorders
Riboflavin (Vitamin B_2)	Essential for cell growth	A deficiency can lead to skin disorders, eye lesions and testicular hypoplasia.
Pantothenic acid	Essential for carbohydrate, fat and amino acid metabolism.	Deficiency, which is unlikely can lead to depressed growth, fatty liver, gastrointestinal disturbances, convulsions, coma and death
Niacin	Required for oxidation-reduction reactions necessary for the utilisation of all the major nutrients	Deficiency in dogs and cats causes black tongue – inflammation and ulceration of the oral cavity.
Vitamin B_6	Involved with nitrogen and amino acid metabolism	A deficiency can cause anorexia, weight loss and anaemia
Biotin	Important for the skin and hair, and involved in the metabolism of fats and amino acids	Deficiency, which is unlikely can lead to dry, scaly skin, pruritus and skin ulcers. However long term use of oral antibiotics can induce a deficiency
Folic acid	Important for a number of reactions in the body, including the maturation to of red blood cells in bone marrow	Deficiency is unlikely, but can lead to anaemia and leucopenia
Vitamin B_{12}	Involved in the metabolism of carbohydrates and fat, and in the synthesis of myelin	Deficiency can lead to pernicious anaemia
Choline	Essential for the maintenance of cell membranes, and a precursor of acetylcholine, a neurotransmitter chemical	Deficiency is unlikely

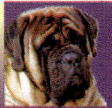

6

Infectious Diseases

A. VIRAL DISEASES

Due to lack of proper treatment, control of viral diseases is done by preventive vaccination and hygienic management. Almost all viral diseases produce hazardous health problems but rabies being zoonotic is very dangerous not only for the dog and his master but for all those coming in contact with the infected dog. A brief account of prevalent viral diseases of dogs has been presented in this chapter.

1. Canine Distemper

It is a highly contagious disease of cosmopolitan distribution. Young pups are highly susceptible and termination may be fatal. The disease is wide spread and almost all domesticated and wild canine species and some other species are highly susceptible and may be carrier also. Thus, it is difficult to eradicate the disease, but it can be prevented by timely vaccination.

Aetiology

The Aetiology of Canine Distemper is a specific paramyxo virus or Morbilli virus which has close resemblance with rinderpest and measle viruses. It is a relatively large size virus of 120 to 300 nm particle size with a single stranded RNA structure in helical symmetry and surrounded by a lipoprotein cover of cell membrane origin. Its multiplication takes place in host cells by budding.

Transmission

The disease is highly infectious and transmitted by aerosol droplets of respiratory exudates. The virus is also present in the other tissues of infected animals. Maximum occurrence of disease has been reported in young dogs between 6 weeks and 6 months of age. Cured dogs acquire lifelong immunity against the disease.

Clinical findings

The development of clinical symptoms depends on the virulence of the infecting strain, environmental conditions, age of the hosts and their health status. Subclinical or very mild form of disease is quite common and it is characterized by fever, restlessness, decreased appetite, oculonasal discharge and coughing with dyspnoea. In many cases respiratory disorders are treated for common cold and cough.

Severe cases

In severe infection with highly virulent strains the disease is characterized by rise in body temperature for 2-3 days followed by second attack after a gap of 7 to 10 days which persists for almost one week or even longer. There may be various degree of conjunctivitis, respiratory disorders, diarrhoea, often dysentery, dehydration and emaciation. The disease may have fatal termination. Careful management and supportive treatment may save the animal. In few patients with neurologic signs the animals suffer from twisting of muscle(s), chorea, flex or spasm and even paralysis of hindquarters. Yellowish white pustules on the abdominal surface particularly in the groin region help nontechnical owners to suspect canine distemper.

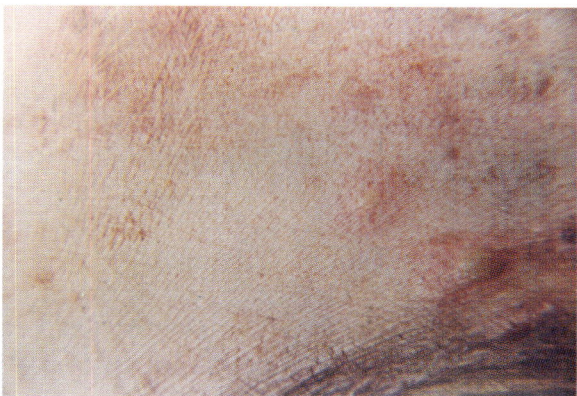

Fig. 122a Vesicles on Abdomen of a Dog Suffering from Canine Distemper

Transplacental infection of canine distemper has also been reported in puppies. This causes the development of neurological signs during 4 to 6 weeks of birth. The pathogenesis may range from abortions, stillbirths or birth of weak

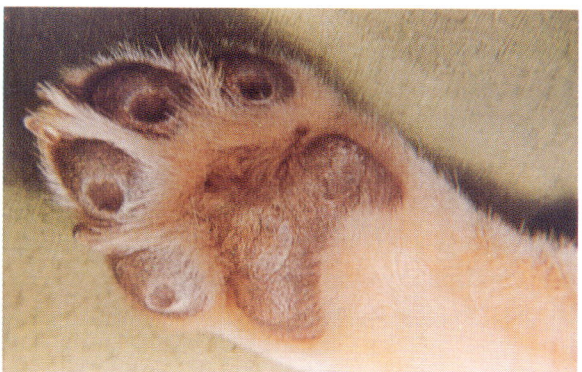

Fig. 122b Vesicles on Footpad of a Dog Suffering from Canine Distemper

puppies and this depends on the virulence and duration of infection.

Infection of canine distemper in neonatal stage before the eruption of permanent teeth causes extensive damage to enamel by destroying the enameloblastic cells. This may be associated with the occurrence of cardiomyopathy and ophthalmic disorders in the pups.

Diagnosis

The disease is diagnosed from the clinical signs along with laboratory examinations to show inclusion bodies in the epithelial cells of the respiratory tract, isolation of virus in susceptible ferrets and serological test. Complement fixation test is applicable in recent infections. Radiography is also used to demonstrate interstitial lung pattern in early infection and alveolar pattern in advanced stage due to secondary bacterial infection.

Therapy

There is no specific treatment for the disease. However, a course of antibiotic for controlling the secondary bacterial infection is supported by neuromuscular tonics like B-complex

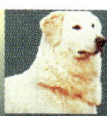

vitamins, antipyretics and other drugs for the management of clinical reactions. Topical antiseptic lotions or cream are used for curing the pustules, when present.

Prevention

It is always advantageous to use preventive vaccination. Young pups should be vaccinated first at 6 to 9 weeks of age and it should be repeated at 3 to 4 months of age. Now-a-days good effective vaccines are available in the market.

2. Infectious Canine Hepatitis (ICH)

This is a contagious viral infection of dogs and other canines. The primary signs of disease are slight elevation in rectal temperature, congestion of visible mucous membranes, marked leucopenia and prolonged coagulation time of blood. The organism was observed in 1930 in the form of intranuclear inclusion bodies.

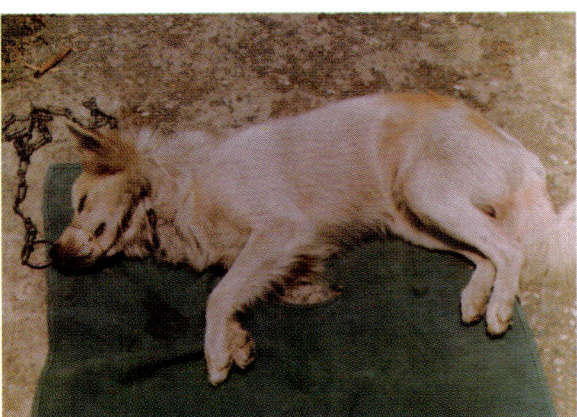

Fig. 123 A Case of Infectious Canine Hepatitis

Aetiology

The disease is caused by canine adenovirus –1 (CAV-1) and this is serologically related with CAV-2. The later causes canine tracheo-bronchitis. It is a DNA virus of an average 75-80 nm diameter. The particles are icosahedral (20-sided) but electron microscopic images are often hexagonal. The virus is highly resistant to environmental inactivation and most of the disinfectants like ether, alcohol, chloroform, formalin and acid solutions are less and virus may survive for 30 minutes in a wide pH range of 3 to 9 at room temperature. It may survive several days in many contaminated articles of the Kennel and for 6 to 8 years in glycerol.

Transmission

The virus is sheded in saliva, faeces, urine and nasal discharge of the infected animals. Sheding of virus may continue in urine upto 6 months of apparently recovered animals. All canine species are susceptible.

Clinical findings

The disease starts usually with nasal exposure and initially localises in the tonsilar crypts and Payer's patches and then spreads to lymphatics and lymph nodes and blood vessels via thoracic duct. Viremia lasts for 4 to 8 days post infection and rapidly spreads to other tissues. The prime targets are hepatic parenchymal cells and vascular endothelial cells of many organs. The initial cellular injury of liver, kidneys and eyes are associated with cytotoxic effects of the virus. After 7 days post infection adequate antibody response clears the virus from the liver and blood, and further liver damage is restricted. Acute necrotic phase of liver damage can be self-limiting. Alongwith recovery, regeneration of liver starts in the surviving dogs. However, the dogs showing partial neutralizing antibody by 4 to 5 days post infection may develop chronic active hepatitis often leading to fibrosis.

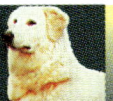

During acute hepatitis, localized renal lesions also develop and initial necrosis of endothelial cells may cause proteinuria due to glomerular damage.

Eyes may be also inflamed due to spread of virus causing uveitis exhibited by conjunctivitis, photophobia and often serous discharge. Recovery may take about 21 days to clear the eye lesions.

Diagnosis

The disease may be diagnosed by elimination of the clinical symptoms of canine distemper, leptospirosis and other diseases. Clotting time of blood is increased, if there is haemorrhage. Hepatic cells exhibit characteristic intranuclear inclusion bodies. Fluorescent antibody test is also useful.

Therapy

The patient is protected from secondary infections with the use of parenteral and topical antibiotic drugs alongwith the use of febrifuge and other symptomatic treatments supported by liquid diet feeding.

Prevention

As usual it is better to provide protection through vaccination in the endemic areas. First vaccination is done at 9 weeks of age and repeated at an interval of 3 to 5 weeks. This is followed by annual vaccination.

3. Rabies

It is one of the most dangerous viral disease of public health importance due to its zoonotic nature. The disease affects all canine species, rodents, human and most of the domestic and wild animals. Incubation period of the disease is normally 15 to 50 days, but in some unusual cases it may be one year or even more. The infection with rabies virus causes acute encephalomyelitis exhibited by furious or dumb form of madness. The term rabies in Latin language probably originated from the Sanskrit word 'rabhas', which means the act of violence and it was first described during 500 B.C. by Democritus and Egyptian scholar Aristotle, the honourable teacher of Alexander The Great, described its transmission from infected to healthy animal by bite.

Aetiology

The cause of rabies is a Lyssa virus of Rhabdoviridae family. It is a large size virus of 60 nm × 175 nm size. It is enveloped, bullet shaped and contains ribonucleic acid. The outer surface of the envelope contains projections of glycoprotein G, which is considered to play role in the attachment of the virus with the host cells. A term 'fixed' rabies virus is used for the strains adapted in secondary hosts for experimental purposes and their characteristic behaviour is reproducible. The virus is highly labile to solar exposure and does not survive more than 24 hours in dead bodies.

Transmission

The disease is mostly transmitted by bite of the infected animals or contamination of open wound with the fresh infected saliva. Infection by inhalation of saliva may also occur.

Clinical findings

The three phases of disease are the prodromal, furious and dumb or paralytic stage. During the first 2-3 days of infection the dog shows anxiety, apprehension and seek solitude. Some degree of shyness may develop in friendly dogs but instability and snapping are not unexpected. A reverse trend of docility and friendship may develop in many furious dogs due to disease.

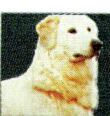

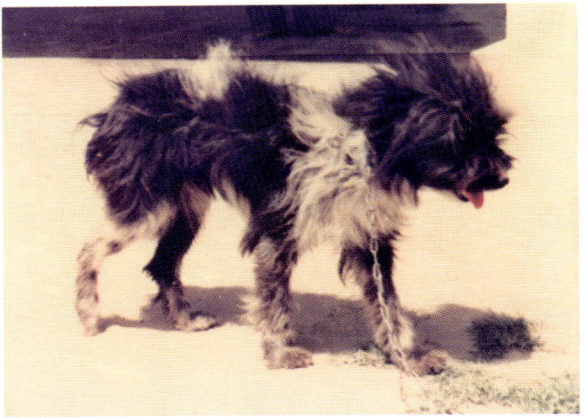

Fig. 124 A Dog Suffering from Rabies

The classical symptom of mad dog syndrome is exhibited by high degree of uncontrolled and vicious aggression. This may last for 1 to 7 days. The animals are alert and anxious with dilated pupils and unprovoked attack is quite common. In India teasing of such dogs is quite common which makes the animal highly furious and aggressive and mostly results in serial list of man and animals encountered in the route of running rabid dog.

The dumb or paralytic form of rabies may develop in about 10 days of infection. It is characterized by the paralysis of throat and masseter muscles, usually excessive salivation and failure of swallowing. Dropping of lower jaw is quite common in advanced stage. The termination of disease is always fatal and may be longer in some very exceptional cases.

Diagnosis

The clinical signs, behavioural changes and history are the only parameters of diagnosis in live animals. The disease is confirmed by the presence of Negri bodies or Lyssa bodies in the cytoplasm of hippocampus.

Therapy

Although there is no specific treatment is rabies however symptomatic treatment to be provided viz., antibiotic ,antiallergic, pain killer, etc. and wound to be clean with soap and water.

Prevention

There should not be any laxity in the timely preventive vaccination of dogs against the disease. Diseased animals should be immediately seggregated at an isolated place inaccessible to man and animals. The premises should be disinfected. It will be always better to use euthenasia in the interest of the pet, owner and society.

4. Pseudorabies or Aujeszky's Disease

This viral disease is also known as mad itch. Its occurrence is sporadic and characterized by mutilation of the infected animal due to continuous biting, chewing and scratching of the affected parts having severe pruritus. The disease is highly fatal in a short course of 2 to 3 days.

Aetiology

The disease is caused by a DNA virus of herpes group of 100 to 150 nm size.

Clinical findings

Clinical signs of the disease are severe pruritus, refusal of food and water, restlessness, continuous scratching and chewing of the affected parts, intense pain, no response to owners call, paresis, convulsions, incoordination of gait followed by coma and death.

Diagnosis

The diagnosis of disease is rather difficult and by the time clinical signs are correlated with the disease, the patient dies.

Therapy

Symptomatic treatments are used to provide

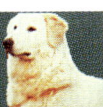

relief from pruritus and pain. Application of topical antiallergic and antiseptic lotions and ointments may provide some relief to the patient.

Prevention

The patients sucumb to infection, so far there appears to be no vaccine in the market for providing protection against the infection. The only measure is to keep the animal under strict hygienic environment.

5. Canine Parvovirus Infection

It is a recently identified disease and parvovirus was perhaps first time isolated from the faecal sample of a clinically normal dog, and it was termed as minute virus of canine. In 1978 a more virulent strain of parvovirus was isolated from the dogs suffering from severe gastroentric illness. The common characteristics of the disease are severe gastro-intestinal disorders exhibited by vomiting, diarrhoea, enteritis and jaundice in young pups.

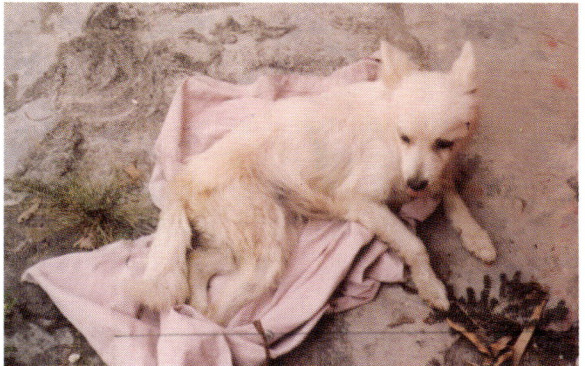

Fig. 125 A Dog Suffering from Parvovirus Infection

Aetiology

The cause of disease is a DNA virus called parvovirus. The virus is small, uncovered and icosahedral and has affinity for the actively multiplying cells. The virus survives in extreme pH and temperature and also exposure to most of the common disinfectants. It can live upto six months in refrigerator (upto - 10°C), three months at room temperature (normally 37°C), 24 hours at 56°C and 15 minutes at 80°C. There is only slight loss in infectivity of the virus after storage for considerable time to be below 30°C and it can survive for many months and years in undisturbed faecal stacks or dumps.

Transmission

Primary source of spread of the disease is faeces. The virus may also be shed in the saliva and vomitus during the acute phase of the infection. Peak faecal shedding of the virus occurs during 4th to 7th day of infection.

Clinical findings

Neonatal pups are highly susceptible. The initial seats of localization of parvovirus are tonsiler crypts and Peyer's patches. This is followed by the infection of gastrointestinal tract in older puppies. Various forms of clinical conditions have been observed, which are generalized disease, myocardial disease, intestinal disease and the affection of bone marrow. Parvovirus infection has been found immunosuppressive in the dogs.

The common clinical signs may or may not be apparent, and may range from non symptomatic illness and mild illness to acute fatal disease. In later two conditions there is loss of appetite, depression, fever (39°–41°C) and vomiting within 48 hours of infection. The vomitus may be clear watery, bile mixed or blood stained. This is followed by the occurrence of diarrhoea of various severity after 6 to 24 hours of vomiting. The secretion of mucus in faeces increases with the passage of the sickness. The diarrhoeal faeces is greyish to yellowish grey in the beginning which may

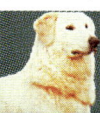

be blood streaked or blood in severely affected patients. In some animals faeces may be only a reddish brown fluid. Diarrhoea is associated with gradual and proportionate dehydration and loss of body weight. Complications usually caused by secondary bacterial invasions are quite common. The other symptoms are the enlargement of tonsilar and superficial lymph glands and mucopurulent nasal discharge.

Myocardial disease is rarely observed after 3 to 7 weeks gap from the recovery of the gastroenteric form of the disease. This is characterized by the occurrence of severe cardiac arrhythmias.

Diagnosis

The disease is diagnosed quite late on the basis of clinical signs, which is confirmed by serological tests and isolation of the organism from the faecal samples.

Therapy

The course of treatment includes the infusion of physiological fluid for controlling dehydration alongwith antibacterial therapy for controlling secondary microbial infections. The other drugs used are astringents and antiemetics. Use of corticosteroids may be needed to prevent enterotoxic shock.

Prevention

Preventive vaccination of weaned puppies at interval of 2-3 weeks upto 18 weeks of age is followed by annual vaccination. In recent years some more effective vaccines have been developed.

6. Canine Herpes Virus Infection

The disease is cosmopolitan in distribution and fatal for young puppies. This is associated with vesicular vaginitis in adult bitches. Almost all canine species are susceptible to infection. This disease was perhaps first recorded in 1964.

Aetiology

The canine herpes virus is morphologically similar to other herpes virus, but its antigenic reaction is closest to that of the human infecting strain.

Transmission

The virus is shedded in the discharges of infected animals and the disease is transmitted by close contact between the healthy and sick animals. In vitro transmission has not been ruled out.

Clinical findings

Dogs of all age are susceptible and clinical manifestations are the fatal termination in young puppies of 1-3 weeks age but in exceptional cases one month old pups also die due to herpes infection. The onset of disease is sudden and most of the infected puppies die within 24 hours. In adult infected bitches abortions, stillbirths, infertility and other associated symptoms are observed. Infected puppies suffer from dyspnoea, anorexia, abdominal pain and vomiting. The faeces is yellowish green without any significant foul odour.

Diagnosis

The disease may be diagnosed from the clinical signs but confirmed only by isolation of the virus.

Therapy and Prevention

So far there appears to be no effective therapy of the disease, and preventive vaccination is the only way of protecting the dogs.

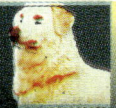

There are few more viral diseases of the dogs and some of these are emerging in India also. Therefore, vaccination against area specific emerging diseases should be followed for providing protection to dogs.

7. Corona Virus Infection

It is a highly contagious disease of dogs of young ages. The disease is characterized by gastroenteritis. The disease occurs in the dogs of any age, which is considered to be an emerging disease in India.

Aetiology

Corona virus is the main organism causing gastroenteritis in dogs. The organism is found to be causing disease in association with other organisms like E. coli, Cryptosporidium and Rotavirus etc.

Transmission

The main way of transmission of the disease is contamination of food and water with the faecal materials. The disease can also be transmitted by contact.

Clinical findings

The clinical manifestations are self-limiting diarrhoea, vomition, weakness, depression and loss of appetite. A diarrhoeic faeces is having foul smell. Apart from the gastrointestinal symptoms there may be signs of respiratory tract affections also, which include nasal discharge.

Diagnosis

As said in the other diseases the diagnosis is based on the history, clinical findings, post mortem examination, serological tests and some of the biotechnological tools like PCR-RFLP methods. Differential diagnosis also play an important role in the proper diagnosis of the disease.

Therapy and prevention

As that of other emerging viral diseases this disease also has no effective treatment. Symptomatic treatment is rendered. Vaccination is the only way to prevent the disease.

8. Respiratory Disease Complex in Dog (Kennel Cough)

This infection is prevalent in both the pups and dogs but mostly found in the aged dogs. It is also called as kennel cough.

Aetiology

This disease complex is caused by a group of organism i.e. Canine adenovirus (CAV-2), Parainfluenza virus, Bordetella bronchoseptica and by mycoplsma.

Transmission

Disease is transmitted by inhalation and contact.

Clinical findings

There is presence of cough, bronchitis, weakness, lathargyness and anorexia etc.

Diagnosis

It Includes history, clinical findings, isolation of organisms and virus neutralization test.

Therapy and prevention

For viral involvement no treatment is available for kennel cough. Only symptomatic treatment is rendered. Vaccination is the only way to prevent the viral infection. PCR & RFLP analysis are also helpful

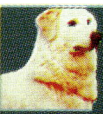

Bacterial infection can be treated with antibiotics like erythromycin, tetracyclines for bordetella infection and chlortetracycline, tetracycline, oxytetracycline for mycoplasmosis.

9. Rotavirus Infection

Rotaviruses are the most common cause of severe diarrhea worldwide. It is a viral disease causing gastrointestinal disorder in young pups. It is also considered to be one of the emerging diseases in the world. Rotavirus paves the way for the protozoal infection like cryptosporidiosis.

Aetiology

Neonatal diarrhea is caused by *Rota virus* a double stranded RNA virus.

Transmission

Rotaviral infection is transmitted by contamination of food material with faeces.

Clinical signs

Rotaviral infection is manifested by gastrointestinal disorders. Rotaviruses cause messy but generally self-limited infections, rare in adults and trivial in consequence, but may kill infants unless properly treated. There are clinical signs like diarrhea, dehydration, yellowish-white faeces and lethargyness etc.

Diagnosis

Diagnosis is based on the history, clinical signs, isolation of the virus, serological tests and RT-PCR method.

Therapy and prevention

No effective treatment is there for Rotaviral infection. Only symptomatic treatment is given to combat diarrhea, dehydration and antibiotic therapy to treat secondary bacterial infections.

B. BACTERIAL DISEASES

Some of the important bacterial diseases of dogs are brucellosis, tetanus, leptospirosis, tuberculosis and listeriosis. Secondary bacterial invasion of wound and gastrointestinal tracts are also encountered.

1. Brucellosis

It is one of the diseases characterized by reproductive failure, abortions and stillbirths. The disease is zoonotic in nature and owners are advised to observe utmost hygiene in handling the patients.

Aetiology

The disease is caused by the infection of *Brucella canis*, which is morphologically different than the smooth cell coccobacilli brucella organisms of other species. Canines are also infected by *Brucella abortus, B. suis* and *B. melitensis* and target organs are as usual reproductive organs causing different reproductive disorders including reproductive failure. Like many other species of brucella the *B. canis* also infects almost all canidae, human and non-human primates.

Transmission

It is a zoonotic disease and human infection occurs due to contact of infected animals. Infection of *B. canis* in human causes mild illness. Therefore, owners are always advised about the hazards of keeping an infected pet in the house. Samples received for the suspected infection of Brucella organism should be handled very carefully in the laboratory. In veterinary hospitals also effective disinfection and hygienic measures should be used specifically after the visit of a brucellosis patient.

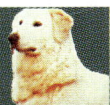

Clinical findings

Pathogenesis of the disease is very slow and clinical signs appear after a long gap. Serious illness in adult dogs is rare. The other symptoms of dry and rough coat, loss of vigour and reduced working efficiency are not specific for the brucellosis. Occurrence of reproductive disorders is suspected for brucellosis in adult dogs. Abortions and stillbirths of usually partially autolysed foetuses are characterized in the bitches in advanced pregnancy. Vaginal discharge following abortion is brown or greenish-gray, which may be excreted for one to six weeks. The other clinical features are the failure of conception, embryonic death and resorption of foetus.

Brucella infection in adult males causes inflammation of genital organs accompanied with the atrophy of one or both the testicles.

Diagnosis

The infection can be diagnosed by serological tests in suspected animals and isolation of organisms. Preventive vaccination against brucella is not in practice.

Therapy

A prolonged course of antibiotic treatment may suppress the infection, however, elimination of the infected animal from the kennel is desirable.

Prevention

Brucella abortus strain 19 is used for vaccinatin.

2. Tetanus

The disease is characterized by severe tetanic spasms starting from face and extending to other parts, and creating lock jaw condition. The symptoms are correlated with the presence of a cut wound or laceration on the body.

Aetiology

The disease is caused by the damaging effect of a neurotoxin secreted during the vegetative multiplication of *Clostridium tetani* in the body of infected animals. It is a motile, anaerobic, non-capsulated, gram positive and spore-forming rod. Despite strain differences the toxins produced are antigenically homogenous. Spores are highly resistant and present in the environment of enzootic areas particularly the dirty, soiled, unused and rusty iron articles and the soil.

Transmission

The disease is transmitted by the entrance of spores through the open wounds and their vegetative multiplication is enhanced by the anaerobic conditions in the inflamed wounds in association with the invasion of other microorganisms. Two types of toxins are secreted by the *C. tetani*, i.e. tetanolysin and tetanospasmin. The tetanolepsin causes haemolysis but it is considered clinically less important than the tetanospasmin. The later enters the body circulation and causes rapid damage of nervous system. The toxins are not absorbed from the healthy intestinal tract and destroyed by the digestive juices. The large molecular weight of toxin prevents its transmission through the placenta.

Clinical findings

The incubation period of disease is 5 to 8 days but may be longer in few cases. The disease is characterized by the development of generalized muscular spasms commonly starting from the temporal muscles and exhibited by convulsions of the third eyelids, stretched upper lids, retracted lips and ears. These are followed by lock jaw syndrome. Localized tetanic spasms are more common in dogs due to relatively higher resistance to intoxication. The dogs with

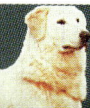

generalized tetanus walk with stiff gait and outstretched or dorsally twisted tail. The animals feel difficulty in standing as well as lying position due to uncontrolled muscular spasm. Rectal temperature is usually elevated due to excessive muscular contraction.

Diagnosis

The history of a recent cut wound by a rusted and soiled article and soiling of open wound alongwith the clinical signs are the primary sources of diagnosis. This is supported by the measurement of serum antibody titers to tetanus toxin.

Therapy

Treatment of tetanus at initial stages in dogs is started with the administration of antitoxin for the neutralization of unbound toxins. This is supported by administration of antibiotics for controlling secondary bacterial infections and treatment of open wounds with topical preparations of penicillin. The supportive treatment includes the use of suitable sedatives and fluid therapy with electrolytes and nutrients. Preventive measures are avoided in dogs for the control of tetanus.

Prevention

Antitoxin and toxoid sera are used for immunization.

3. Leptospirosis

It is a disease of zoonotic importance all over the world and disease is produced by the infection of *Leptospira icterohaemorrhagiae, L. canicola and L . grippotyphosa*. Acute form of disease is febrile and can be treated effectively with the administration of antibiotics. Subclinical infection has been observed to be more harmful, which causes interstitial nephritis and in few cases occurrence of jaundice has been also reported.

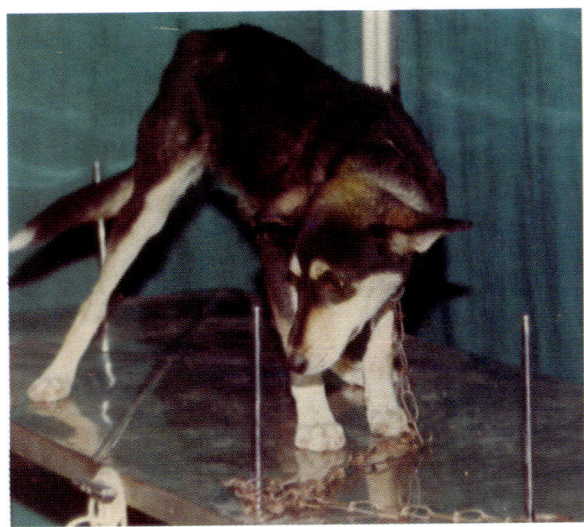

Fig. 126 A Case of Leptospirosis

Aetiology

The causative organisms are *Leptospira icterohaemorrhagial, L. canicola* and *L. grippotyphosa*.

Transmission

The disease is transmitted by direct contact between the infected and healthy dogs. The urine of infected animal is the source of bacteria and ingestion of urine or food and water contaminated with infected urine. The other routes of transmission are bite wounds, placenta and intake of infected meat. Infected dogs become carrier after recovery and continue to shed the organisms intermittently in urine for several months or even for few years. The known reservoirs of leptospira are rat, mouse, vole, dog, pig and cow. Several wild animals have been also found to be carrier of the disease.

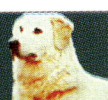

Clinical findings

Various factors like age, immunity, environmental factors and virulence of the infecting serovar affect the infectivity and development of diseased condition. In peracute form there is extensive leptospiremia with high fever (39.5-40°C), shivering, generalized muscle tenderness and death. These symptoms are accompanied with vomiting, rapid dehydration and collapse of peripheral blood vessels. The pulse is rapid and irregular and respiration is also rapid. Blood coagulation system is disturbed. There may be vascular damage and blood may pass in vomitus and faeces. Epistaxis, melena and largely distributed petechial haemorrhage may occur in advanced illness. These are quickly followed by depression, hypothermia, death without renal and hepatic failure.

The common symptoms of subacute illness are fever, inappetance, emesis, dehydration and increased thirst. Inflammation of muscle, meninges and kidneys causes painful stress and dogs do not like to move. Visible mucous membrane are injected and there is occurrence of conjunctivitis, rhinitis and tonsillitis accompanied with coughing and dyspnoea. Further damage of urinary system causes oliguria and anuria. In surviving patients renal function may become normal in 2 to 3 weeks time or may develop into chronic compensatory polyuric renal failure.

Occurrence of jaundice is also common in the sub acute form of infection. The colour of faeces changes to grey due to extensive inflammatory changes causing intrahepatic cholestasis. Chronic hepatitis shows clear signs of hepatic failure exhibited by loss of appetite, decrease in body weight, ascites and hepatoencephalopathy.

In some animals suffering from sub acute leptospirosis there may be occurrence of intestinal intussusception associated with persistent vomiting and diarrhea. The faeces void is scanty and melena type.

Diagnosis

The disease suspected on the appearance of clinical symptoms is confirmed by the isolation of organisms from the blood of recently infected animals and urine of advanced cases.

Treatment

All common antibiotics may be used for the treatment of the disease but streptopenicillin injection has been found to be more effective. The antibiotic treatment is supported by the symptomatic treatment of hepatitis and renal disorders.

4. Tuberculosis

The dogs are more resistant and occurrence of disease condition takes a long course. This situation is very dangerous as an infected pet dog may spread the disease for long time. The development of patho-clinical changes depends on the sources and route of infection.

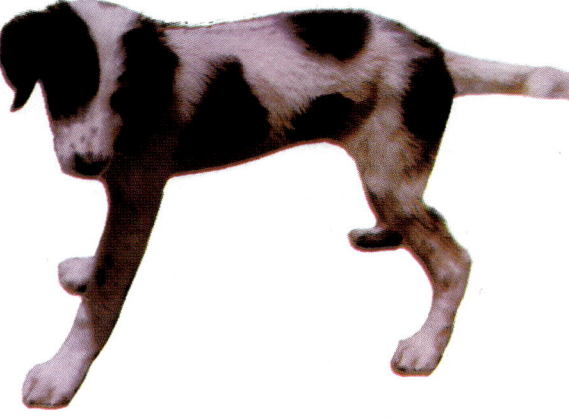

Fig. 127a A Case of Tuberculosis

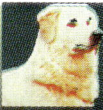

Aetiology

Infection of *Mycobacterium tuberculosis* is the primary cause but dogs are also infected with *M. bovis* and occasionally with *M. avium*.

Transmission

The disease is wide-spread and being more resistant the dogs and cats are potent spreaders of infection.

Clinical findings

The disease in infected dogs remains sub-clinical for a long time. The clinical signs reflect the site of granuloma formation. The dogs suffering from pulmonary tuberculosis suffer from bronchopneumonia and enlarged lymph glands. Those suffering from gastrointestinal tuberculosis show abdominal pain.

The pulmonary tuberculosis is exhibited by pleural and pericardial effusion accompanied with cyanosis, dyspnoea and heart failure.

In extensive diffuse form involving gastrointestinal tract and other organs the symptoms are anaemia, loss of body weight, vomiting and diarrhea. The mesenteric lymph nodes are prominently enlarged. In some animals there may be abdominal oedema and in very advanced cases there may be incidence of diffused calcification of the chronic tubercles in the lungs and other organs. In some animals cutaneous form of tuberculosis is characterized by the formation of non-healing ulcerating abscesses in the region of face, neck and adjoining parts.

Diagnosis

History of the sickness, clinical signs, isolation of acid fast rod shaped bacteria and radiography showing inflammatory masses and enlarged lymph nodes in the thoracic region are quite useful in diagnosis of the disease. Tuber culin test may be also used with reasonable accuracy.

Therapy

The disease can be treated successfully with the administration of the following drugs under the supervision of a veterinary doctor:

1. Streptomycin
2. Isoniazid
3. PAS (Paraamino salicylic acid)
4. Rifampicin
5. Ethumbutal
6. Pyrazinamide

5. Listeriosis

The occurrence of this disease is very rare but it is a dangerous disease characterized by primary encephalitis. The disease may be confused with other infectious diseases like cerebral form of rabies and distemper. However, course of listeriosis is very short and ranges from few hours to 3 or 4 days.

Aetiology

The causative organism is *Listeria monocytogenes*

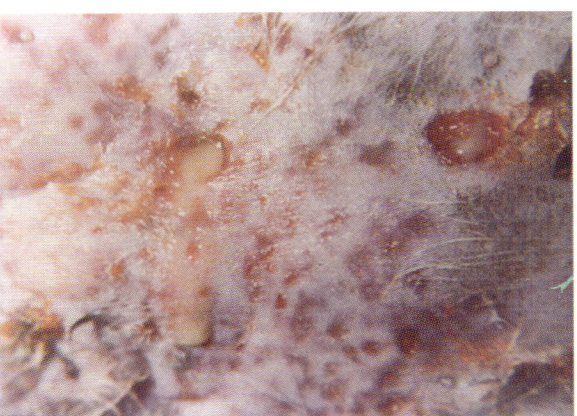

Fig. 127b Cutaneous Lesions on a TB Patient

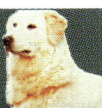

Epidemiology

Almost all species of domestic animals may be infected with the disease.

Clinical findings

On the onset of disease difficulties are often experienced in differentiating this disease from canine distemper and rabies. The common clinical symptoms of listeriosis are the loss of appetite, irritability, depression and pneumonia. There is profuse lacrymation and the pupils are dilated. Chewing of gums, unprovoked barking, lameness, convulsions and stupor are the other symptoms observed during the later stage.

Diagnosis

The clinical signs are differentiated on careful examination and the disease is confirmed by the isolation of organism from the cerebrospinal fluid.

Prevention and therapy

So far there is no effective vaccine and treatment of the disease.

6. Anthrax

This disease is considered to be a very serious infection of herbivorous animals, which is acute in nature. The disease is prevalent all over the world. It is a peracute septicemic disease causing death of livestock.

Aetiology

The causative organism is a bacteria known as *Bacillus anthracis.*

Epidemiology

The disease occurs almost all over the globe. Animals mostly affected are sheep and cattle, even though all the mammals are affected. The disease is important from zoonotic point of view.

Clinical findings

Cattle and buffaloes are affected mostly with the acute form, where there is high rise of temperature, anorexia, depression, development of tympany, and with advancement there is muscle tremor and dyspnoea. On the other hand, sheep are affected with per-acute form manifested by sudden death.

Diagnosis

The diagnosis depends on clinical manifestations which is confirmed by the demonstration of *Bacillus anthracis* in the blood samples. Serological tests are also available. Utmost precaution is required for the handling of suspected cases of anthrax.

Prevention and therapy

In case of early diagnosis of the disease, treatment is effective. The disease can be treated successfully with the administration of the following drugs, viz., Penicillin, Oxytetracycline, Erythromycin, Chloramphenicol and Sulphonamide.

Vaccination: Anthrax spore vaccine, given 1 ml s/c is effective and repeated annually.

7. Salmonellosis

The disease may be acute or chronic in nature and characterised by gastroenteritis. The disease is also important from public health point of view.

Aetiology

Several serotypes of Salmonella have been isolated so far. *Salmonella typhi* and *S. paratyphi* affecting man also be affecting dogs.

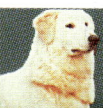

Epidemiology

The disease is cosmopoliton in distribution affecting almost all the species of animals.

Clinical findings

The disease has been classified into two different forms, enteric form, which is manifested clinically by loss of appetite, weakness, depression, increased body temperature and diarrhea. Another form of the disease is septicemic form, in which there is depression, recumbency, increased body temperature and nervous signs.

Diagnosis

Diagnosis is done on the basis of history, clinical signs, isolation of the organism and some of the serological tests.

Prevention and therapy

Several antibiotics used for effective treatment are chloramphenicol, nitrofurazone and also the sulfa drugs.

8. Actinomycosis

Actinomycosis of dogs is a chronic, sporadic, bacterial disease manifested in two principal forms: a localized granulomatous abscess involving the skin and subcutis; and a pyogranulomatous thorax, with suppurative lesions involving the lungs, pericardium and pleura and occasionally the peritoneal cavity.

Aetiology

The gram-positive rod *Actinomyces viscosus* and/or *A. hordeovulneris* (very rarely *A. bovis*) and occasionally unnamed *Actinomyces* are the causes. These actinomycetes occur as commensals in the oral cavity of dogs and cats.

Distribution

Occurrence is probably worldwide. A moderately common infection; seen most often in hunting dogs.

Transmission

Infection is spread by inhalation and via wounds, often from bites and occasionally due to gunshot.

Clinical features

The disease is chronic but rarely disseminated. The course is variable. In the thoracic form abnormal lung and pleural sounds, low fever, dullness, dyspnoea, anorexia, vomiting, abdominal swelling and tenderness, ascites and weight loss are the common symptoms. In the skin form there are pyogranulomatous abscesses and nodules in various locations.

Diagnosis

The disease resembles nocardiosis clinically which is also seen in the two forms mentioned above. Other diseases to be considered are blastomycosis, cryptococcosis, other fungal infections, abscesses due to other causes and various pulmonary and pleural infections. Demonstration of the organism in gram-stained smears, isolation and identification of *A. viscosus* or *A. hordeovulneris* from characteristic lesions are definitive.

Therapy and prevention

Surgical debridement and drainage including placement of a chest tube for pyothorax. Prolonged treatment with penicillin G, amoxicillin, tetracyclines or chloramphenicol is usually effective. However, because there may be a difference between the antimicrobial susceptibility of *A. viscosus* and *A. hordeovulneris*; thus all significant isolates should be subjected

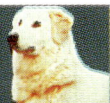

to drug susceptibility tests. Penicillin is not effective in the treatment of nocardiosis. Vaccines are not used in dogs.

9. Botulism

Botulism is a noncontagious, intoxicative disease of animals caused by the neurotoxins of *Clostridium botulinum* and characterized by progressive motor paralysis.

Aetiology

Clostridium botulinum is a large, gram-positive, spore forming, anaerobic rod.

Transmission

Ingestion of food containing the toxin. Botulism is not contagious. Dogs and other carnivores usually develop the disease after consuming carrion or spoiled meat.

Clinical signs

Clinical manifestations depend on severity. The signs are progressive, ascending motor paralysis, weakness, difficulty in chewing and swallowing impaired vision and finally, death due to cardiac or respiratory failure.

Diagnosis

Rabies, pseudorabies, Coonhound paralysis, tick paralysis and other diseases affecting the nervous system should be considered for differentiation. Botulism has been called a catch-all clinical diagnosis. A definitive diagnosis depends on the identification of the type of *C. botulinum* by toxin neutralization tests in mice.

Therapy and prevention

 Botulinum antitoxin of the appropriate type, or a polyvalent product, has been used in treatment with variable success; however, once signs have developed and toxin is fixed to receptors, the efficacy of antitoxins is questionable. The animals are not vaccinated.

10. Tizzers Disease

Tizzer's disease is caused by *Clostridium* species, which is highly fatal in nature.

Aetiology

The disease is caused by *Clostridium piliforme*, a spore forming, gram negative bacterium affecting wide range of animals including dogs.

Transmission

Animals acquire infection by contact with or ingestion of rodent faeces having the spore of bacteria.

Clinical findings

Clinical signs exhibited by the animals are depression, loss of appetite, lethargyness, abdominal pain, enlargement of liver, decrease in body temperature and ultimately death.

Diagnosis

Diagnosis is made mostly by necropsy findings and histological examination, because the disease is fatal in nature and its course is short.

Therapy and prevention

No treatment has been found successfull.

Other bacterial diseases

Few other bacterial diseases of lesser importance or sporadic occurrence encountered in dogs are purulent eye infection and infections caused by Proteus, Pasteurella, Pseudomonas

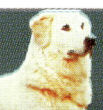

and Escherichia coli etc. Dogs can be infected with *Haemobartonella canis* but clinical disease is rare. Dog can also be affected by pyoderma which may be due to improper treatment of wound.

C. RICKETTSIAL DISEASES

1. Canine Ehrlichiosis

Canine ehrlichiosis is an acute to chronic rickettsial disease characterized by infection of monocytes and lymphocytes.

Aetiology

The cause is a rickettsia, *Ehrlichia canis*.

Transmission

The brown dog tick *Rhipicephalus sanguineus* is the vector and reservoir. Ticks may harbour the organism for as long as five months.

Clinical features

These include recurrent fever, epistaxis, mucopurulent nasal discharge, vomiting, subcutaneous haemorrhages and edema, depression, emaciation, anaemia, splenomegaly, polyarthritis, generalized lymphadenopathy, meningoencephalitis, convulsions, paralysis and loss of weight.

Diagnosis

A clinical diagnosis should be confirmed by laboratory means. Unclotted blood for buffy coat and regular smears. In necropsied dogs, smears are made from the lungs and other organs, stained with Giemsa and fluorescent antibody procedures. A PCR procedure and in situ DNA hybridization have been used in the identification of *E. canis* in tissues.

Therapy and prevention

Oxytetracycline and Doxycycline are found to be effective if the disease is diagnosed early; treatment should be given for at least two weeks. Without antibiotic therapy, dogs may remain carriers for many months.

2. Rocky Mountain Spotted Fever

Rocky mountain spotted fever is a febrile disease, principally of humans. Dogs are susceptible but the disease is usually mild or subclinical; however, some young dogs may catch severe infections.

Etiology

Rocky mountain spotted fever is caused by *Rickettsia rickettsii*.

Transmission

The reservoir of the agent is principally wild rodents, hares, rabbits and the ticks that feed on them. Dogs may bring infected ticks into contact with humans.

Clinical signs

Clinical signs of disease in dogs are general malaise, high rise of temperature, lymphadenopathy and petechial haemorrhages on mucous membranes.

Diagnosis

Because the agent is highly infectious for humans, blood and tissues should be handled with great care. The serologic procedures recommended for canine sera are the microimmunofluorescence test, ELISA and the latex agglutination test. A four-fold increase in IgG titer is considered significant.

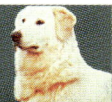

Demonstration of rickettsia in fluorescent antibody - stained preparations of skin biopsies is significant.

Therapy and prevention

Tetracyclines or chloramphenicol for two weeks are effective. Supportive therapy includes fluid replacement also. Prevention in dogs involves tick control in endemic regions. Ticks should be removed daily and destroyed. No vaccine is available.

D. PARASITIC DISEASES

The parasitic diseases have been described separately for endoparasites and ectoparasites. The parasites are more prevalent in the stray dogs but domestic pets also frequently suffer from different kinds of parasitism. Parasites are of two types, viz., endoparasites and ectoparasites.

1. Endoparasitic Diseases

Endoparasites of gastrointestinal tract are more prevalent than those of heart and respiratory tract. The common signs of the presence of gastrointestinal parasites are diarrhea and/or dysentery followed by dehydration, vomiting, anorexia and weakness. The conditions easily diagnosed by the microscopic examination of faeces. The infection of haemoprotozoan and filarial worms causes lack of growth, loss of conditions, anoemic, weakness, alopecia, dermatitis and ulcerative crust formation, thickening of the skin and often pot belly. The conditions are diagnosed by the microscopic examination of blood smears.

There are many other signs which may be suspected for parasitism in dogs, they include cutaneous ulceration, lacrimation, photophobia, coughing, sneezing, nasal discharge, loss of body weight, anorexia, dehydration, haematuria, subcutaneous edema and allergy.

The history is very helpful in the diagnosis of parasites which are further confirmed by the signs, lesions and microscopic examination. Recently some serological tests are also available for specific diagnosis of a few parasitic diseases.

2. Ectoparasitic Diseases

Any laxity in the grooming and management of dogs often leads to serious ectoparasitic infection by the infestation of mites, ticks and lice. The dermatitis caused by ectoparasites is further contaminated by bacterial and fungal infections if left uncared and under unhygienic conditions. Mange is the most serious of all ectoparasites.

Ectoparasitism is manifested by various degrees of alopecia, pruritus, dermatitis and even ulceration in severe cases. The common parasitic dermatitis of dogs are pediculosis, flea bite, mange caused by *Demodex canis*, *Sarcoptes scabiei* and *Cheyltiella* spp. A mite, *Octodectes cynotis* is mainly responsible for the pathogenesis of otitis externa. Infestation of ticks causes pruritus, erythematous nodules formation, itching and alopecia. The diagnosis of parasitic skin infestation is simple and effective treatments have been given for the specific ectoparasite.

The details regarding the various parasites and their treatment are given in the following Tables.

E. MYCOTIC DISEASES

Several fungi are responsible for internal and external disease conditions. The causes of pathogenicity are mostly the toxins produced by the fungi. Mycoses may be described as dermatomycoses responsible for skin lesion. Deep mycoses are responsible for systemic diseases.

The term dermatomycosis denotes the fungal infestation and lesions limited to the cornified

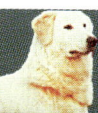

Table 6.1: Endoparasitic Diseases and their Treatment

Organ affected & Aetiology	Main Clinical	Basis of Diagnosis Symptoms	Line of Treatment
1	2	3	4
Small Intestine *Ancylostoma caninum* (Canine hookworm diseases).	Pneumonia, blood loss anaemia, black tarry faeces with diarrhea, anorexia, unthriftiness, hookworm dermatitis.	History, clinical signs, presence of elliptical, thin-shelled egg (65m × 40 m) in the faeces. Blood examination shows Eosinophilia.	**1. Tetramisole Compounds** (a) Ascaris tab(Merucy) orally Pup: 50 mg tab Adult 150 mg tab (b) Decaris tab (Ethonor), orally. **2. Levamisole compounds** (a) Vermisole tab (Khandelwal), orally, **Pup:** 50 mg tab, **Adult:** 150 mg tab (b) Helmonil tab (Alved), orally, 150 mg tab/10 kg B.W. (c) Helmonil injection (Alved): @ 1 ml/5 kg B.W., S/c. (d) Vizole cap. (M.M. Lab), orally 150 mg/tab **3. Disophenol compounds** (a) Ancylol injection: 4.5% (Cyanamid) @ 1 ml/4.5 kg B.W., S/C **4. Pyrantel pamoate compounds** (a) Pyrantel suspension (Dolhin) orally 50 mg/ml @ 10 mg/kg B.W. for 3 days. (b) Expent (Merind) 10 mg/kg body wt as single dose. **5. Buphenium hydroxynaphthoate** (a) Alcopar (B.W.) orally **Pup:** 2-3 g and **Adult:** 3-5 g (b) Hoopar (Cadila) orally **Pup:** 2-3g, **Adult:** 3-5 g **6. Mebendazole Compounds** (a) Wormin (Cadila), orally @ 0.5 mg/kg B.W.

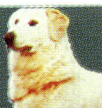

(b) Endazole (Biddle Sawyer), orally, 100 mg tab. 1 tab BID for 3 days.

(c) Mebex (Cipla), orally 100 mg tab 1 tab BID for 3 days.

(d) Eben (GUFIC) orally 100 mg tab 1 tab BID for 5 days.

(e) Zodex powder (Concept), orally, **Pup:** 1/2 TSF **Adult:** 1 TSF

(f) Zodex bolus 500 mg (Concept), orally, **Pup:** 1/2 bolus **Adult:** 1 bolus

(g) Humla (ACI), orally, 5 mg/kg B.W.

(h) Robendole (ITK), orally 100 mg tab, 1 tab BID or TID

7. Albendazole com pounds

(a) ABZ (INDICO) 400 mg tab as a single dose.

(b) Gecare (Glaxo), 400 mg tab as a single dose.

| Small Intestine Toxocara canis, Toxocara leonina (Ascarid worm infection/ Ascaridiasis). | Lack of growth and loss of condition, pot bellied, rough hair coat, respiratory distress, diarrhea vomiting, pneumonia intestinal obstruction, unthriftiness, anaemia, malabsorption, distended abdomen. | History: The infection may be transmitted from mother to foetus: Clinical signs: orally @ 100 mg kg b.w. presence of oval, eggs (75 m x 85 m) in the faeces. | |

1. Piperazine adepate, hydrate and andictrate compounds

(a) piperex (Sarabhai), thick shelled, pitted

(b) Vermex liquid, orally (Pfizer) @ 2.5 ml/10 kg B.W.

(c) Antepar liquid (B.W) orally @ 2.5 ml/ 10 kg B.W.

(d) Piperazine liquid @ 2.5 ml. 10 kg B.W.

(e) Helmacid (4.5%) (Glaxo), orally @ 0.2 ml/kg B.W.

(f) Verban liquid (Cyanamid), orally @ 0.2 ml/kg B.W.

(g) Pipirocid (Arex), orally 2.5 ml/10 kg. B.W.

2. Mebedanzole and levamisole compound may be used in infestatin of Ancylostoma Caricide `

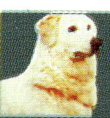

(Cyanamid), orally, 50-70 mg/kg B.W. for 10-20 days.

3. **Tetramisole compounds** at in hook worm disease.

4. **Albendazole and Praziquantal combination** Praziplus (Petcare) orally 1 bolus/10 kg BW.

5. **Fenbendazole compounds**
   (a) Curaminth (Sarabhai) orally 50 mg/kg BW for 3 days.
   (b) F-Zole (Vet India) @ 50 mg/kg BW for dog and 30 mg/kg for cat for 3 days.

6. **Pyrental pamoate compounds:**
   (a) Expent (Merind) orally 5-10 mg/kg BW
   (b) Nemocid (IPCA) orally 5-10 mg/kg BW.

Small Intestine *Strongyloides stercoralis* (thread worm infestation or strongy loidiasis).	Blood streaked mucoid diarrhoea, emaciation, loss of body weight, shallow rapid breathing and little pryexia, verminous pneumonia, consolidation of lung, enteritis with haemorrhage and mucus, dermatitis & diarrhea.	History, clinical signs, presence of small thin walled and rounded eggs or larvae in faeces.	1. Compound containing mebendazole may be used in similar doses and route as indicated vide supra 2. Albendazole compounds 　(a) Albomar (Glaxo) 25-30 mg/kg BW for 3-5 days. 　(b) Combantrin-A (Pfizer) orally, 400 mg as a single dose for adult.
Large intestine *Trichuris vulpis* (whip worm infection)	Loss of body weight, diarrhea, presence of fresh blood in faeces, pot bellied, loss of body condition. Mild form of disease may not show the symptoms	History, clinical signs, eggs (30mx 40 m) yellowish, lemon shaped and plug at pole.	1. Compound containing levamisole and mebendazole as mentioned earlier should be used in a similar manner.

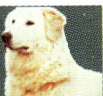

2. Ivermectin compound
   (a) Mectin (Alembic)
       200 mg/kg BW s/c,
   (b) Neomac (Intas,
       200 mg/kg BW s/c.

**1. Compound con
taining Diethyl
carbamazine citrate.**
   (a) Caricide (Cyana
       mid), orally 15 mg/kg
       B.W. for 7 days
   (b) Banocide (B.W.)
       orally. 50 mg tab @ 1
       tab TID for 10 days.
   (c) Hetrazan (Lederle),
       orally 50 mg tab @ 1
       tap TID for 10 days.
   (d) Unicarbamezan
       (Unichem), orally 50 mg TID
       for 10 days.
   (e) Carbamyl syrup (Kopran)
       orally, @ 5 mg/kg/B.W. for
       7-10 days.

2. Disophenol preparation
   (a) Ancylol 4.5% (Cyanamide)
       @ ml 4.5 kg B.W. S/C

3. Levamisole compounds
   (a) Dewormis (Ethnor) Orally,
       150 mg single dose.
   (b) Almizol (Alembic) orally
       7.5 mg/kg BW.

Oesophagus/sto-mach/arteries
Spirocerca lupi
(Oesophageal
worm infestation.
Right ventricle
and adjacent
vessels like
anterior vena cava,
pulmonary
artery and
hepatic vein.

Vomiting,
haemorrhage,
emaciation,
watery or bloody
faeces with putrid
odour, difficulty
in swallowing, dull
depressed, degluti-
nation difficulty.

History, clinical
signs, presence of
thick shelled,
parallel eggs with
blunt side ends
(30 m x 15 m) in the
faeces.

*Dirofilaria
reconditum*,
Dracunculoides
(Heart worm
disease, filariasis
or microfilariasis.

Chronic dyspnoea,
cough, rough body
coat, or dermatitis,
lack of stamina,
easily tired, lack of
interest in exercise,
anaemia, ascites,
hydrothorax, enlar-
ged liver haemoglob-
binuria, some blunt
cut lesions on
tongue.

History, clinical
signs, presence of
microfilaria in
blood (may be seen
hanging blood drop
stained blood smear
or by modified knott
technique), microfi-
laria may also be
recovered from
urine and skin
scrapings.

Preparation containing
Diethyl carbamazine
citrate:
1. Carcide (Cyanamide).
   Orally. 25-40 mg/kg
   B.W. for 30 to 60 days.
2. Banocide (B.W.)
   orally 50 mg tab TID
   for 1 month.
   Worcid (Vets Farma)
   orally, 65.6 mg/kg
   day for 3-4 weeks.

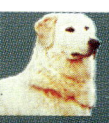

3. Hetrazan (Lederle) orally 50 mg tab @ TID for 1 month.
4. Unicarbazan (Unichem) orally, 50 mg tab @ 1 tab TID for 1 month.
5. Carbamyl syrup (Kopran), orally, @ 5 mg/kg B.W. for 1 month. Antimony preparations like Fouadin (Trivalent antimony compound) given I/V as 6.3% aqueoous solution 2.5 ml daily for 12 days. *Anthiomalin (M and B) @ 0.5 ml in small breeds. @ 1 ml in large breed. I/M for 5 days.
6. Antimosan (Bayer) @ 0.5 ml in small breeds @ 1 ml in large breeds 1/M on alternate days, 4-5 injections.

Others
1. Caparolate sodium diacetate @ 2 ml/kg B.W., I/V.
2. Dithiazanine Iodide, orally @ 50 mg/kg/B.W./day.
3. Capasotate, orally @ 500 mg/kg/B.W. for 1 week or more.

4. Milbemycin oxime Interceptor (Novartis) 0.5 mg/kg BW, Orally. No effective treatment. Only surgical removal of work is useful.
Mebendazole compounds

Kidney *Dictophyma renale (Giant* kidney worm infestation).	Marked loss of body weight, anaemia, haematuria, frequent urination, severe abdominal/	History, clinical signs, presence parasitic eggs in urine, eggs are elliptical, brownish thickshelled, pits	

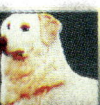

	lumpar pain, pet may cry, stretch, display nervourness and trembling.	on all parts except poles (80 m x 50m) Radiographic examination.	(a) Mebex tab (Cipla) 22 mg/kg BW for 3 days. (b) Mebazole (Torrent) 22 mg/kg BW for 3 days. Injection or inhalations are not very effective. Trephining of the nasal passage and removal of parasites followed by irrigation with antiparasitic or antiseptic drugs is useful.
Nasal and respiratory passage *Linguatula serrata* (Tongue worm infestation).	Severe irritation, sneezing coughing fits and difficult breathing, uneasiness, reslessness, dog rubs its nose with forefeet and snore while sleeping, blood stained mucus discharge from nostrils	Eggs are (90m x 70m) oval, thick shelled, yellowish; eggs may be found in the nasal discharge or in the faeces.	
Duodenal and jejunal mucosa **Trichenella spiralis** (***Trichenella infestation of intestine***)	**Initial stages** (About 24 hours after taking infected meat), gastroenteritis, diarrhoea, nausea, vomition, slight fever and mild abdominal pain & dyspnea.	History, clinical signs; adult worms may occasionally be found in the faeces, larvae may be demonstrted in muscle biopsy, the sample being examined, either pressed between two pieces of glass or after digestion in an acid pepsin (1:1) solution. Haematological examination indicating high percentage of eosionophils (about 25%). Number of immunodiagnostic tests such as complement fixation, haemaglutination etc, are used.	**1. Thiabendazole compounds** are effective against both adult intestinal and larval muscle phases. (i) Thiabendazole premix (Arex), orally, 50 mg/kg B.W., repeat after 3 weeks. (ii) Thiabendole bolus (MSD), orally, 50 mg/ kg B.W. repeat after 3 weeks. **2. Methyridine** is also effective against the muscle stage of the infection. Methyridine is also effective against the muscle stage of the infection. Methyridine product 20 ml S/C.

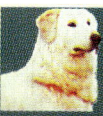

Eyes: **Thelazia coliformensis** *(Eye worm infestation)*.	Corneal opacity, lacrymation, photophobia, severe conjunctivitis.	Larvae and adult worms may be present in the lacrymal ducts and under the eyelids.	Manual removal of parasite by fine forceps in local anaesthetics and antibiotic or sulpha eye drops, piperazine salt 0.5% with sterile normal saline solution for irrigation of eye ethyridine product 20 ml S/C, local application of 3% boric acid, 0.05% mercuric chloride, 0.05% Iodine, 0.5% lysol or 0.5% diethyl carbamazine give good results. Morental citrate (Banminth Tab)- 7.5 mg/kg BW. **Levamisole compounds** (a) Decaris (Ethnor) 50 mg single dose. (b) Dewormis (Ethnor) 50 mg single dose.
Bronchi, trachea: *Cremosoma vulpis (Lung worm infection).*	Bronchitis, pneumonia, coughing, necrotic lesion in lung or liver & difficulty in breathing.	History, clinical signs, presence of eggs in faeces or in the nasal discharge, auscultation of lung.	Fouadin and anthiomaline are effective.
Lung: *Filaroides osleri (F.mildk)* Tracheal worm infestation (Filaroidiasis).	Harsh persistent coughing loss of body weight, anorexia breathing with mouth, ataxia.	Eggs (60mx50m) thin shelled, colourless, larvated.	Preparations containing tetramisole and levamisole as mentioned earlier should be used in a similar manner. **Tetramisole preparation** (a) Vermisol (Khandelwal) 2.5 mg/kg BW, single dose. (b) Nilverm (Glaxo) 2 mg/kg BW for 2-4 days.
Subcutaneous tissue of limbs: *Dracunculus insignis*	Non-healing ulcer and swelling of subcutaneous tissue.	History, clinical signs, presence of adult parasites under the skin of	1. Removal of worms through incision. 2. Diethyl carbamazine

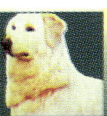

(Dracunculosis).

		the limb larvae may be detected from faeces.	in high doses, EOFIL tab (Fourts) 6.6 mg/kg BW/day for 3-4 weeks. Eggs in urine There is no effective treatment.
Bladder:	Cystitis		
Capillaria plica (Bladder worm infestation)	Cloudy urine, sometimes irritation while urinating	Nearly Colourless, slightly long, wormed, 65mx25m in size.	Surgical removal of worm may be done
Skin Peloderma strongyloides (Peloderma dermititis).	Pustular and erythematous lesion on thorax, abdomen, auxillary inguinal region, upper part of limbs and presence of scabs.	History, clinical signs, and by finding nematodes in skin scraping from the affected area.	Organophosphate local application of antibiotic ointments, provide clean and dry shedding
Blood vessel: Angiostrongylus vasorum Angiostrongylus infection).	Loss of body weight/ and condition, easily tired, lesions found in the right ventricle of the heart and pulmonary arteries, blood coagulation time is increased, oedema.	History, clinical signs, presence of eggs or larvae in the stool.	Preparation contain ing tetramisole and levamisole as men tioned above should be used in a similar manner.
Lung: Paragonimus spp. (Fluke infestation)	Anaemia, jaundice, wasting oedema, cough dysponea.	History, clinical signs, presence of operculated eggs with yellowish colour in the faeces.	1. Trodax (M&B) 0.2 ml/5 kg B.W. S/C repeated after 1 month 2. Flukaphene (Ethicare) orally 0.50-75g/10 kg B.W. 3. Flukin (Arex), orally 100 mg tab 1 tab single dose. -do
Liver: Fasciola hepatica (U.K. and Europe)	Diarrhoea, anaemia, jaundice, weakness, emaciation and loss of appetite, bottle jaw.	-do	**Albendazole Preparation** (a) Alzad (Merind) Orally, 400mg as a single dose. (b) Noworm (Alkem) Orally 400 mg as a single dose. -do-
F. gigantica (Asia, Africa &	Prolonged course and same	1. History 2. Clinical signs	**Oxyclozanide Preparation**

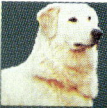

other tropical countries)	as above	3. Immunological study	(a) Distodin tab **(Fascioliasis)** Pfizer 15 mg/kg BW orally.

Small Intestine: *Diphylobothrium latum, Echinococcus granulosus; Spirometra species, Taenia pisiformis, T. taeniaeformis, T. hydatigena,* Unthrifitiness, capracious appetite, intermittent diarrhoea and constipation, anaemia, stunted growth, pot bellied rubbing anus on the ground and attempt to bite the anal region due to irritation in advanced cases; nervous signs, sometimes tape worm segments pass in faeces; skin coat harsh and dry dehydration.

History, clinical signs presence of segments of tapeworm in faeces; presence of tapeworm egg in faeces.

(a) Distodin tab **(Fascioliasis)** Pfizer 15 mg/kg BW orally.

(b) Tolzan-f (Intervet) 15 mg/kg BW orally.

1. Preparation containing niclosamide may be used orally.
   (a) Niclex (Alved) 1 g tab/7.5 kg B.W.
   (b) Niclosan (Biddle Sawyer) 500 mg tab; 3-4 tab.
2. Preparations containing mebendazole may be given in double doses.
3. Preparation like Panacur (Hoechst), containing Fenbendazole may be given @ 50-100 mg/kg B.W for 3 days.

Others:
1. Cestophene (Pearl Chemical), orally 0.2 g/kg B.W.
2. Niltape (Ethicare) orally 2-4 g.
3. Bunamidine orally @ 25 mg/kg B.W.
4. Bithional orally @ 50 mg/kg B.W.
5. Pyrental pamoate preparation
   (a) Nemocid (IPCA) orally, 5 mg/kg B.W.
   (b) Expent (Merind) 5 mg/kg B.W orally.
6. Praziquantal Combinations
   (a) Drontal plus (Bayer) 1 tab/kg orally,
   (b) Plozin (Ranbaxy) 1 tab/kg orally.

Herbal preparation
1. Helmex PW. (Vetmed), orally 4-10 g.

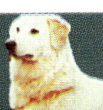

Muscle fibre *Cysticercus cellulosae* (Cysticercosis).	Dog with cysts in brain may show symptoms resembling those of rabies	History, clinical signs, presence of cysts in muscle fibress. Eggs are present in faeces	2. Pulp arecanut, orally 3-5 g. 3. Taenil pw, orally 2-5 g. 4. Krimos orally 20-30 g. As above, but specific treatment is not available.
Small Intestine: *Nanophytus salmincola, Alaria spp.,* (flukes)	Haemorrhagic enteritis, dull, depressed and loss in body condition and difficulty in absorption.	History, clinical symptoms with presence of eggs in faeces.	1. Carbon tetrachloride, Tetrachloro ethylene is used in the fluke infestation. Simultaneously Tetracycline is also used for rickettsial infection.
Small Intestine: *Giardia canis* (Giardiasis).	Blood and mucus pass with stool, excessive straining during defaecation, irregular appetite and diarrhea.	History, clinical signs, presence of cyst in stool, ELISA, Western Blotting.	Preparation containing metronidazole is very useful, duration and severity of the disease. 1. Flagyl (Rhone-Poulenc) 20-50 mg/ kg B.W. Orally in divide dose 2. Unimezol (Unichem), orally 1 tab TID for 7-14 days. 3. Unimezol suspension, orally, 5 ml TID for 7-14 days. 4. Metro (Alkem), orally 1 tab TID for 7-14 days. 5. Metrogyl (Unique), oraly 1 tab TID for 7-14 days. **Metronidazole Combination** (a) Amedol-F (Vetchem) 3-5 ml orally. (b) Dependal -M (S & B) 1 tab TID orally.
Large instestine: *Entamoeba histolytica* (Amoebiasis).	Chronic diarrhea with, or sometimes without blood or mucus, mild to severe haemorrh-	History, clinical signs, presence of aemoeba cysts in stool.	Same as Giardiasis, Ornidazole compounds (a) Dazolic (Sun Pharma) 500 mg bid for 5 days orally.

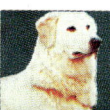

Intestine

Eimeria canis, Isospora canis, I bigemina and I. revolta (Coccidiosis).

agic enteritis and ulcer in intestinal mucosa. Pain in abdominal region. Dysentery, loss of appetite weakness, anaemia, dehydration, stool may also be passed with blood and mucus, loss of body weight.

History, clinical signs presence of oocyst in the faeces.

(b) ONIZ (Stadmed) 500 mg bid for 5-10 days orally.

I. Preparations containing sulphonamides
are choice of drugs.

1. Sulpha bolus (Sarabhai), orally @ 1 g/5 kg B.W. daily for for 5 days.
2. Sulphadmidine (Arex) orally. 150 mg/kg B.W. followed by half dose for 5 days.
3. Diadin (Pfizer), ½ Tab/10 kg followed by ¼ Tab/10 kg B.W. for 5 days.
4. Coccil liquid (Akelvi) orally 150 mg/kg B.W. on first day followed by 75 mg/kg B.W. for 5 days.
5. Hamidin (HAL) orally, 200 mg/kg followed by half dose for 5 days.
6. Oriprim tab (Cadila), orally. 1 tab first day followed by half tab for 5 days.
7. Robatran Vet. Granuless (ITK) orally 15 g on first day followed by 7.5 g for 5 days.

II. Preparations containing nitrofurazone

1. Neftin (SKF). 1 tab TID for 4-5 days.
2. Enterovioform (Ciba), orally 1 tab TID.
3. Entobax, orally 1   tab TID.

Preparations containing triple sulpha

1. Pyrimethamine (Daraprim), orally @ 2.2 mg/kg B.W.

Whole Body:

Toxoplasma gondi (Toxoplasmosis).

Coughing, pneumonia, dyspnea, discharge from nose and eyes, haemorrhagic

History, clinical signs, presence of bradyzoides and Tachyzoides in faeces by

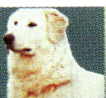

	enteritis, anaemia, enlargement of lymph nodes, increased body temperature nervous signs like convulsions, paralysis and chorea and signs of anaemia.	serological test, viz., haema glutination test.	followed by half the dose daily for 2-3 weeks. 2. Trinamide (M&S) orally, @ 1 g/7 B.W. daily for 2 weeks. 3. Equal parts of sulphadimidine, sulphadiazine and sulphapyridine may be mixed and given in same manner as above preparations.
Skin *Leishmania tropica, L. donovoni (Leishmaniasis).*	**Cutaneous form:** Dry or wet ulcer covered with thick brown scabs, boundary of lesions is red and hairless, itching. **Visceral form:** Anaemia, emaciation, debility, kerato-conjunctivites, enlarged spleen and liver, epistasis, lameness and diarrhea.	History, clinical signs, presence of the parasites in blood or lymphnode smear, serological test.	There is no specific treatment. Preparations containing **antimony compound** may be used, Lithimony (Indian Immonologicals) 6% W/V, 1-2.5 ml on alternate days i/ml
Blood: *Haemobartnella canis (Haemobartonellosis)*	High temperature, anaemia, dull, depressed, pale mucous membrane, urine dark brown and contains bilirubin, enlarged spleen and lymphnodes para central necrosis.	History, clinical signs, presence of cocoid, oval ring, or rod-shaped organisms in enlarged spleen anaemia.	Broad spectrum antibiotics like oxytetracycline, tetracyclin, Chlorotetracycline and Chloramphenicol @ 5 mg/kg B.W. I/M may be used. Five injections should be given. Berenil (Hoechst). @ 0.1 g/10 kg B.W., I/M or S/C.
Blood: *Trypanosoma evansi, T. cruzi*	Enlarged lymphnode, intermittent	History, clinical signs, presence of trypanosoma in	1. Berenil (Hoechst), similar dose as in babesiosis.

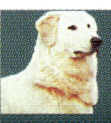

T. brucei T. rangeli (Trypanosomiasis).	fever, anaemia, subcutaneous oedema, keratoconjuncti-vitis, weakness and convulsions.	blood smear, serological tests.	2. Babesan (ICI) doses similar as for babesiosis. 3. Corridan (HAL). 1 g PW should be mixed in 5 ml water @ 0.025 to 0.040 ml/kg B.W. S/C, single injection. 4. Nilbery (Intas) 1 ml/ 10-20 kg BW i/m. 5. **Suramin compound:** Naganol injection (Bayer) 30-50 mg/kg B.W, i/vly. Preparations containing 4, 4 diaminodiazo amino benzene diaceturate is the best drug for babesiosis. Berenil (Hoechst), @ 0.8-1.6 g/100 kg B.W. S/C or I/M.
Blood: *Babesia canis, B gibsoni, B. vogeli (Babesiosis)*	High temperature, increased pulse and respiration, haemoglobinuri a, anaemia jaundice, acute from is mostly fatal.	History, clinical signs, presence of babesia organism in blood smear, serological tests.	* Berenil (Intervet) 5-10 ml/100 kg BW, I/M. * Berenil RTU (Hoechst) 1 Ml/20 kg or 3.5 mg/kg B.W, I/M. Babesan (Quinuronium sulphate B-vet.C) (ICI) @ 0.2 ml of 0.5% solution 4.5 kg B.W. S/C injection. Trypan blue B. vet. C. (Ethicare), orally 20-150 mg according to size and severity of disease, slow I/V, injection.

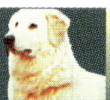

Table 6.2: Ectoparasitic Diseases and Their Treatment			
Ectoparasitic diseases(s) and its Aetiology	**Main clinical symptoms**	**Diagnosis**	**Treatment**
1	2	3	4
Ear mange/ Otitis/Canker *Otodectes sp.*	Dog shakes its head, stretches the ears, brown to blackish waxy powdery deposit in ear.	History, clinical signs, by removing parasite from waxy powdery deposit of the infected ear.	1. Use insecticide spray in the ear to kill the mite. 2. If there is more wax then clear by putting lukewarm water containing a pinch of washing soda. If there is any sign of pus, blood or a foul smell, consult a veterinarian. 3. **Decusates:** Topical ear wax softener, put 5-10 drops & let the animal lie down for 5-10 mins. Before using this, the internal ear should be cleaned properly with H_2O_2.
Cheletiella mite infection *Cheletiella sp.*	Itching of the body, mostly involves neck and back.	History, clinical signs presence of reddish colour mite in the skin scraping.	**Insecticide spray** * Amitraz: Taktik 5% (Intervet) 50 mg/ ml, 6-10 ml/lit of H_2O and give bath.
Scabies *Sarcoptes scabiei*	Highly contagious skin disease thickenings of skin, intense irritation, alopecia, bare patches on the skin, hyperkeratitis thickened and folded appearance of skin.	History, clinical sign, presence of mites in the skin scraping examination 10% NaOH or 10% KOH should be mixed in skin scraping to separate the mites.	Remove the hair, insecticide spray may be used 1% solution sevin, kilex carbaryl, 1:500 solution of asuntol 16% liquid. Ascabiol (M&B), Scabitex (Ballotun) Gamma BHC. Scarab (Aristo), Emscap (MM Lab),

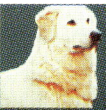

Fig. 129 A Dog Suffering from Otitis

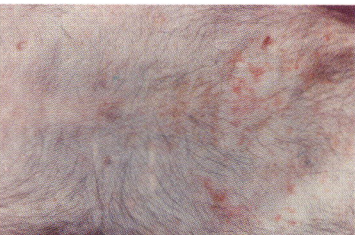

Fig. 130a A Case of Scabies in Dog

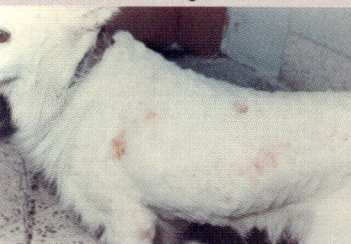

Fig. 130b A Case of Scabies in Dog

Demodectic mange or follicular mange
Demodex canis D. folliculorum

These mites live in hair follicles and sebaceous glands. Loss of hair, thickening of the skin is found.

Squamous form:
Scaly wrinkled often resembling ringworm infection, seborrhea, Pustules hyper and secondary bacterial infection may develop, occasional itching.

History, clinical signs, presence of cigar shaped mites in the skin scraping.

Lorexane (ICI) GAB (Guffic), Ethnoscab (Ethnor). Scabinidon (Indopharma).

Herbal preparations
Haranj oil – 50 ml
Turmeric powder 10 g
Lemon extract 4 ml
Onion extract 20 ml
Mix and apply BID
for 5-10 days.
Other herbal drugs
are Himax.
* Amitraz: Ridd
(PetCare) 3-4 ml/lit
or water, Advice for bath.
* Ivermectin: Ivomec
(Glaxo) 200 mcg/kg BW s/c.

Clip the hair, bathe with antiseptic solution like Savlon, Dettol or Piripol. *Tetmosol Solution (ICI) 5% V/V, for bath.

* Blaze Shampoo (IHO 200 ml liquid, for bath.
Give broad- spectrum antibiotic treatment to check bacterial infection and antihistaminic drugs like Avil, Phenargan. Above mentioned insecticides, acaricides, and Benzyl benzoate and gamma BHC preparation may be given. Supportive therapy with vitamin B complex and fluid

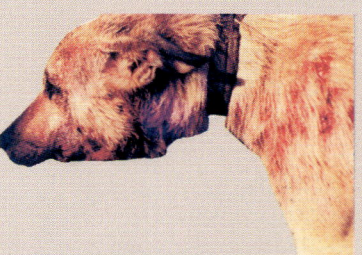

Fig. 131 A Case of Demodectic Mange in Dog

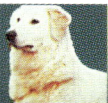

therapy, advanced cases euthanasia is the only course.
*Amitraz and Ivermectin same as above.
* Melathion compound: Cython, 10 ml/lit and advice for bath.
* Doramectin compound: Dectomax, 200 mcg/kg BW s/c.

Pediculosis (louse infection/) *Linognathus setosus,* *Trichodectes canis,* *Heterodoxux*	Blood sucking or biting lice causing pruritis, dermal irritation dog scratches, rubs or bites infected area, rough dry hair coat and small wounds are seen.	History, clinical signs and lice seen on hair and body coat.	1. Clip the hair insecticide spray as in scabies or by spraying rotenone in 1% or malathion in 2% dilution or in talcum powder, lorexane lotion or cream (ICI). Ethnoscab cream (Tthnor) Same spray advocated for ticks may be used. Gamma Benzene

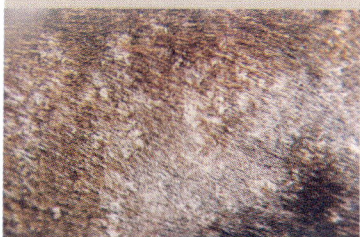

Fig. 132 A Case of Pediculosis in Dog

Hexachloride Compounds:
(a) GAB (Gufic) 1% solution apply to the scalp and hair, repeat after 1 wk if required.
(b) Ascabiol (Rhone Poulenc) GBH com pound + Cetrimide, 1% lotion.

Tick Infestation (Acariasis) *Hyalomma sp.,* *Dermacentor andersoni,* *Rhipicephalus*	Local inflammation, worry of the host, dermatitis, irritation, occasionally paralysis may	By seeing the ticks on the body including inner of the ear. Ticks may also be seen near bedding or	Spray of Sevin 0.5-1% Malathion 0.5-1% Lindane 0.03% Toxaphene 0.5% Sumithion 1% Asuntol 0.5%

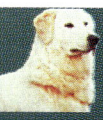

sanguineous	develop due to tick toxins, anaemia, scratching of the body.	kennel.	Chlordane 0.1% Ectozide dusting powder (Balloun) Herboticks powder (Herbolab). Canifur liquid (Cadila) 120 gm for bath. Anti tick vaccine may also be given if available.
			Cypermethrin compounds (a) EctOut (Prima Vetcare). (b) Cisaflux (Ranbaxy) 1 ml/lit for spray. Ivermectin: Endact inj (Sam browne/ Workhardt) 200 mcg/ kg BW, s/c.
Flea Infestation *Ctenocephalides canis* 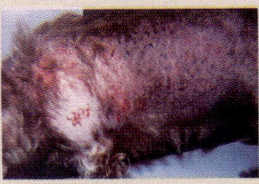 Fig. 133 Flea Infestation in a Dog	Dirty skin due to heavy infestation, dog becomes puzzled, itching, hypersensitization corrugated appearance looking like skin of rhiocerous, allergic dermatitis due to hypersesitivity to the flea, loss of condition.	Presence of flea; allergic sensitivity test with flea antigen.	Same spray as used for tick infestation. Flea repellant may be tied on the collar or around the neck, care being taken to ensure that the dog does not eat the flea repellant. For allergic reaction, antihistaminic drugs should be given. *Seledruff (PetCare) 2.5% solution, for bath. *Notix TALC (PetCare) 5% W/W, apply on the body surface.
Flies Infestation (Myiasis) Common housefly	Irritation by biting, larval stage of fly may produce maggot wounds which may become	Presence of larva in the wound.	Use fly repellant, like turpentine oil or Sevin powder in the wound along with topical and

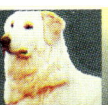

septic, sometimes causing very deep wounds in the skin.

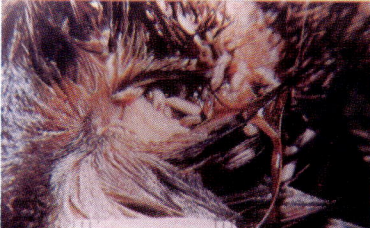

Fig. 134 A Case of Myiasis in a Dog

| Mosquito Infestation **Common mosquitoes like Anopheles, Culex etc.** | Irritation by biting, causing restlessness. | Presence of mosquitoes in the dogs' house or nearby places. | parenteral antibiotic therapy to check secondary bacterial infection. For control of flies, dog house or kennel should be cleaned properly and sprayed with insecticides like DDT, gamma BHC, Seven 50% wp @ 0.5 to 1% spray in 2 months. Asuntol 0.25%-0.5% Mosquitoes may be controlled by providing mosquito net fencing (Wire) or doors, windows, by insecticides spray by avoding dampness and humidity. |

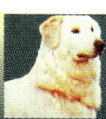

layer of the skin. Dermatophytes prevalent in the dermatophytosis of dogs are *Microsporum canis*, *M. gypseum* and *Trichophyton mentagrophytes*, *T. rubrum* and other species of these fungi. The lesions are ring like, with development of alopecia and pruritis giving the common name ringworm. The disease is diagnosed by the presence of hyphae and spores in the skin scrapings.

The subcutaneous mycoses are more severe conditions produce by the penetration of the fungi, which include different species of *Sporothrix, Zygomycetes, Actinomyces, Nocardia, Streptomyces, Curvularia and Aspergillus.* The subcutaneous mycoses are mostly characterized by the swelling and ulceration of superficial lymph nodes, raised and granulomatous lesions often associated with fistulous tracts and a thick exudate. In aspergillosis in addition to subcutaneous tissues, respiratory tract and gastrointestinal tracts are also involved. It produces pneumonia and enteritis respectively.

The systemic mycoses are caused by the infection of *Blastomyces dermatitis, Histoplasma capsulatum, Cryptococcus neoformans* and *Coccidioides immitis.* These fungi mostly produce pathogenesis in the respiratory tract, which is manifested by pyrexia, anorexia, dyspnoea, coughing and unthriftiness. Sometimes central nervous system, nasal sinuses and facial sinuses are also involved. The defects of various mycotic conditions are given in the form of a table.

F. ZOONOTIC DISEASES

The term zoonosis means intercommunicable diseases from animals to man and viceversa. Since dog is the most popular pet which usually lives within the house in close contact with humanbeings, it is essential to have an adequate knowledge about the zoonotic diseases. This will be helpful in adopting preventive measures and precautions in the routine management and handling of the pets. The zoonosis has been classified into the following four categories:

Direct (ortho) zoonosis: From vertebrate host to man by direct contact or by a mechanical vector (no development in vector) e.g. Rabies, Trichomoniasis and Brucellosis.

Metazoonosis: Transmitted by invertebrate vector, e.g. Plague, Arbovirus infection and Schistosomiasis.

Saprozoonosis: Have both vertebrate and a non-animal development site (like organic matter, soil and plants) e.g. Larva migrans and Mycotic infection.

Anthropozoonosis: The term *anthropozoonosis* has been widely used for the diseases transmissible from animal products, consumption of tissues or products of diseased animals, and consumption of animal products contaminated during processing, storage or delivery.

The zoonotic diseases of bacterial, viral, rickettsial, mycotic and parasitic nature have been tabulated as follows.

Precautions to Avoid Zoonotic Diseases

1. Diseased dog should be kept away from healthy dogs and human beings, especially children.
2. Kissing a pet should be avoided because it can potentiate danger of worm infection and rabies, if the dog is suffering from these conditions.
3. Dogs should not be permitted to lick your face, hands, legs and other body parts as this may transmit some disease.
4. Regular and periodical deworming and vaccination of pet is absolutely necessary to prevent the transmission of zoonotic diseases.
5. Regular spraying of insecticide to check ectoparasitic infestation.

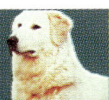

6. Proper bathing using suitable soap should be done at regular intervals.

7. Hair should be clipped and groomed regularly. This is necessary for the cleanliness of dog.

8. Use protective gloves, spectacles, dangri and gumboots while handling a rabid dog.

9. Shoes and clothes used for handling a dog, suffering with zoonotic diseases should be properly washed and kept separately.

10. After handling a dog hands and feet should be washed properly with soap or antiseptic solution.

11. Children must not be allowed to play with a sick dog or pup.

12. Utensils for a dog should be kept separately and cleaned properly with soap or detergent.

13. Children should not be allowed to play with the utensils of dogs.

14. A pregnant lady should take precautions while gardening or working near the dog house as the soil may be contaminated with the faeces of dog which may have *Toxoplasma gondii oocyst.* It is a very dangerous disease and may be transmitted to foetus while in the womb.

15. Regular and proper cleaning of dog house or kennel and premises must be done with disinfectant but avoid the use of carbolic containing compound.

16. Place of defaecation and urination should be away from the public places. In case dog defaecates or urinates in the house, excreta should be disposed properly.

17. Pup or dog should not be allowed to mix with stray dogs and wild animals.

18. Raw meat or meat from diseased animals and offal should not be given to the dogs.

19. Notification of infectious and communicable diseases should be recorded immediately. Information must be relayed throughout the country through media such as radio, television, and newspaper.

20. Quarantine of New arrivals: Pet(s) at the house or dog kennel specially from other states and countries where some diseases are zoonotic should be kept in isolation ward to observe the signs of any infectious diseases as per the quarantine rules.

21. Sick pets especially when suffering with zoonotic disease must be kept isolated from healthy pets and human beings.

22. All hygienic measures such as cleaning of pet, house, utensils and other belongings of pet should be maintained to minimize the infections.

23. Wild animals like fox, dog and jackals are mainly responsible for spreading the infectious diseases like rabies in human population. Therefore, destruction of the wild animals and stray dogs is important to control disease like rabies.

24. The carcass of animals which have died of rabies, brucellosis and other such diseases should not be kept open, but immediately disposed off by burning or burial. Burial should be at least 1.8 meters deep with layers of lime sprinkled over the carcass.

25. Disinfection is the important preventive measure for control of infectious diseases. This can be achieved by using U.V. rays, heat, chemicals like soda bicarbonate, mercuric chloride, bleaching powder, copper sulphate, sodium carbonate, lime and gases like HCN, sulphur dioxide and formaldehyde.

26. During breeding season the pet should not be allowed to mate with stray dogs where it can pick up some infection.

27. If any person is suspected for zoonotic illness, he should contact a doctor immediately and the pet should be taken to a veterinary doctor.

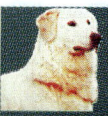

Common zoonotic diseases			
Name of disease	Causative agent	Host	Mode of infection to man
1	2	3	4
1. Bacterial Diseases			
Brucellosis (Common)	*Brucella canis*	Dog	Contact, ingestion of infected secretions.
Tuberculosis (common)	*Mycobacterium Tuberculosis Var. hominis*	Dog	Contaminated secretions, water and aerosol.
Salmonellosis (Common) Hemolytic diseases	*Salmonella typhi murium*	Dog	Infected meat, contaminated food and water etc.
(i) Scarlet fever	*Streptococcus pyogenes*	Dog	Through contact
(ii) Sore throat	*Streptococcus epidermidis*	Dog	Through contact
Leptospirosis (rare)	*Leptospira pomona*	Dog	Contact and exposure
Anthrax (rare)	*Bacillus anthracis*	Dog	Contact with hair and Contamination of food Contact
Diphtheria (rare)	*Corynebacterium diphtheriae*	Dog	Contamination of food and water
Pasteurellosis	*Pasteurella multocida*	Dog	Bite, contact, contamination etc.
2. Viral Diseases			
Rabies (common)	Neurotrophic virus	Dog, Cat, Wild Animals	Animal bite, abrasion
Aujeszky's disease/ Pseudorabies (rare)	Virus	Dog	Contaminated secretions
Lymphocytic choriomeningitis	Virus	Dog	Ingestion
Meningitis	Virus	Dog	By contact with a carrier dog
Mumps	Virus	Dog	Contact
3. Parasitic Zoonosis (a) Protozoan Diseases			
Toxoplasmosis	*Toxoplasma gondii*	Dog	Ingestion and contact
Chagas diseases (not in India)	*Trypanosoma cruzi*	Dog	Faecal material of bug
Leishmaniasis, visceral (kala-azar)	*Leishmania donovani*	Dog	Sandfly bite

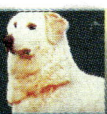

Balantidiasis	*Balantidium coli*	Dog	Contaminated food and water
Amoebic dysentery	*Entamoeba histolytica*	Dog	Contaminated food and water
Giardiasis	*Giardia spp.*	Dog	Contaminated food and water

(b) Helminthic (Infesticision)

Ascariasis	*Toxocara canis*	Dog	Contaminated food and water
Hydatid diseases	*Echinococcus granulosus*	Dog	Swallowing parasitic eggs through contamination with dog faeces
Dracunculosis	*Dracunculus medinensis*	Dog	Drinking infected pond water
Filariasis	*Dirofilaria immitis*	Dog	Mosquito
Trichuriasis	*Trichuris vulpis*	Dog	Infection of larvae
Schistosomiasis	*Schistosoma japonicum*	Dog	Mosquito (through skin)
Fasciolopsiasis	*Fasciolopsis buski*	Dog	Eating infected snails
Echinostomiasis	*Echinostoma*	Dog	Raw aquatic plants
Hookworms and related infections	*Ancylostoma ceytanicum*	Dog	Through broken skin
Strongyloidiosis	*Strongyloides stercolaris*	Dog	Through skin
Larva immigrans	*Bunostomum spp., Ancylostomum spp. and Toxocara canis*	Dog	Through broken skin
Diphylobothriasis	*Diphylobothrium latum, Dipylidium caninum*	Dog	Evading raw fish
Gnathostomiasis	*Gnathostomum spp.*	Dog	Eating infected fish

(c) Mites

Scabies (mange)	*Sarcoptic scabiei*	Dog	Contact
Follicular mange	*Demodex canis*	Dog	Contact
Cheleticlar scabies	*Cheyletiella yasguri*	Dog	Contact
	Cheyletiella bakei	Dog	Contact
Flea allergy and dermatitis	*Ctenocephalides canis*	Dog	Flea bite

4. Fungal and Rickettsial zoonosis Mycotic Diseases

Ringworm	*Trichophyton spp.*	Dog	Contact

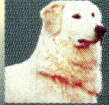

Coccidioidomycosis	*Coccidioides immitis*	Dog	Inhalation and through wounds
Histoplasmosis	*Histoplasma capsulatum*	Dog	Inhalation of dust and ingestion
Cutaneous streptothricosis	*Dermatophilus congolensis*	Dog	Contact
Nocardiosis	*Nocardia asteriodes*	Dog	Contact
Candidiasis	*Candida albicans*	Dog	Endogenous in nature usually
Blastomycosis	*Blastomyces spp.*	Dog	Injury, trauma, wound and inhalation
Sporotrichosis	*Sporotrichum spp.*	Dog	injury

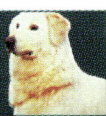

Fungal diseases and aetiology

Fungal diseases and aetiology	Clinical signs	Diagnosis	Treatment
1	2	3	4
Dermatomycosis (Ringworm) *Microsporum canis* M. andovini M. distortum M. vanbre M. cookie M. gypseum *mentagrophytes* T. verrucosum T. schoenleinii T. rubrum T. equinum T. gallinae	Scattered lesions on the body, loss of hair and discrete circular areas of hair loss with scaling and sometimes inflammed borders are common. Crust may also develop in severe cases, heavy crusted areas of widespread hair loss, hair scaling and erythema, itching and irritation. Lesions always spread from centre to periphery indicating recovery from centre showing ring like lesions.	History, clinical signs, direct examination of skin in 10% KOH mount showing mycelium and chain of arthrospores examination in 10% KOH showing sheath of small spores (2.8m) in mosaic, completely surrounding the hair at the base, easily separated from hair in preparation mycelium running within the hair, parallel to its length, wood's light examination may give bright yellow, green fluorescence in infected hair in some cases.	Griseofulvin 25-50 mg/kg B.W. generally treatment is given for 1 month but depending on the severity of the disease, it may be reduced or increased. Preparations of Griseofulvin Fulvi (Indica), 125 mg tab Grisovin FP (Glaxo), 125 mg tab, Idifulvin (IPPL), 125 mg tab, Mycorl (Plazma), 125 mg tab Walavin FP (Carter Wallace) 125 mg tab. preparations for local application. Captan (1:200 sol), 2.5% boric acid, potassium permanganate (1:5,000), bezoic acid 6%, sulphur, salicylic acid, resposcinol 10% Phenol 10%, Iodine 2.5% (Tincture or ointment) of 1% Sevin 50% wp, 1% chlorophos, 0.2% thimerosal solution, 1% kilex carbaryl 50% w.p. Tinaderm (Full Ford), Apply twice daily. Jadit oitmentro Jadit solution or Jadit H (Hoechst). Apply twice daily. Mycostatin ointment (Sarabhai); apply twice daily. Kanaderm ointment

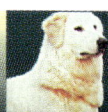

Fig. 137a A Case of Ringworm Infection

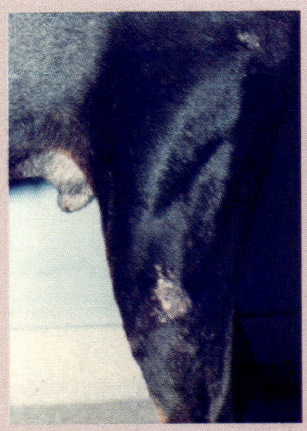
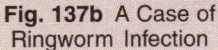

Fig. 137b A Case of Ringworm Infection

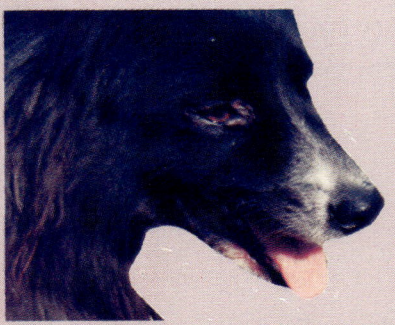

Fig. 137c A Case of Ringworm Infection

(Sarabhai) apply 2-3 times daily. Himax (Indian Herbs) apply 2-3 times daily Quardriderm (Fulford) apply twice daily. Pentaderm (Mercury Laboratories),apply twice daily.

Tolnafate Compounds:
(a) Tinaderm (Fulford) 1% W/W, solution apply daily bid, for 2-3 weeks.
(b) Tinavate (Dabut) 1% W/W, Solution apply daily bid, for 2-3 weeks.

Terbinafine compound:
(a) Fungotek cream (FDC) 1% W/W, apply once or bid for 2-3 weeks.
(b) Lamisil cream (Novartis) 1% W/W, apply once or bid for 2-3 weeks. Ichgon wash (Glaxo) 100 ml for bath.

Histoplasmosis
Histoplasma capsulatum (Fungus invades the reticulo endothelial system in various tissues or organs).

Chronic cough, persistent diarrhoea, fluid faeces darker than normal, enlarged mesenteric lymph nodes, often palpable, loss of weight, dehydration, photophobia, ophthalmitis, iris swollen and pupil constricted, anaemia, temperature fluctuating from 102.5°F - 105.5°F.

History, clinical signs, demonstration of organism in tissue or culture examination includes buffy coat peripheral blood biopsy specimens from enlarged lymph node, secretion and exudate from respiratory tract and mouth ulcer.

Amphotericin B-50 mg. Mix with 10 ml sterile water added to 5% dextrose in water to make final volume of 230 ml. Give this solution @ 1-1.25 mg kg B.W. I/V. After a day's rest, give second dose of 1.5-2 ml/kg. B.W. Followed by another day's rest third and subsequent doses are continued on alternate days until 12 I/V, injections are completed. Supportive therapy includes sodium bicarbonate for keeping urine alkaline. Avoid vitamin B and analgesics and corticosteroids.

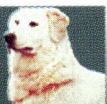

*Amphotericin-B compounds
Amfocare (Criticare) injection, 5 mg in 500 ml, 5% Dextrose infused over 4-6 hrs followed by 5-10 mg over 6 hrs.

* Kitoconazole compounds
(a) Fungicide-200 (Torrent) 200 mg BID orally.
(b) Kenazole (PCI) 200 mg BID orally.

Blastomycosis
Blastomyces dermatidis (may infect organs like lung, eyes, skin muscle)

Pulmonary form
Persistent non-productive cough, bronchial rales, loss of weight, fever, nasal exudate, neutrophilia.
Ocular form
Aqueous humour becomes cloudy, iris swollen, pupil constricted and photophobia.
Cutaneous form
Small papules, scaly ulcerated lesions, small abscesses, bone lesions involve long bone, and mostly soft tissue over bone lesions is swollen and very sensitive to touch.

History, clinical signs, serological test like CFT. Exudate from S/c abscesses should be mounted in a drop of 10% NaOH for 15 minutes and examined under microscope for round, thick walled usually single budding yeast (size 8.20 m), Sabourod's agar media.

- do -
*Amphocit inj (Criticare) 5 mg in 500 ml 5% Dextrose infused over 4-6 hrs followed by 5-10 mg over 6 hrs.

Cryptococcosis
Cryptococcus neoformans involved are skin, lungs, CNS, oro nasal and foot)

Irritability lameness, blindness, ulcerated soft tissue, swelling with clear and brown exudate from skin lesions, focal granulations

History, clinical signs, by seeding the fungus in tissues or in culture by serological tests.

Same as in histoplasmosis by Amphotericin B.
*Fluconazole compounds
(a) Cazole (Synokem) tab.
(b) Consize (Indico) tab. 300 mg followed

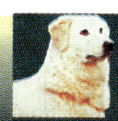

	in lung, thickened gelatinous meninges.		by 100 mg/day for 14 days.
Coccidiomycosis *Coccidia immitis*	Dyspnea cough, exudate from nose, poor appetite, intermittent diarrhea, loss of weight, enlarged joints, temperature 102°F - 104°F. Nasal and occular discharge.	History, clinical signs presence of fungus in nose discharges, serological tests.	Same as in histoplasmosis by Amphotericin B. ***Itraconazole compounds** (a) Canditral (Glenmark), (b) Flucovar (Saga labs) 100-400 mg/kg for upto 6 months orally.
Nocardiosis *Nocardia asterioides*	*Dyspnea, coughing anorexia nasal and ocular discharge, diarrhea, temperature 102°-102°F*	History, clinical, signs direct, microscopic examination, by culture examination	Sulphonamides orally are the drugs of choice in canine, dose rate is 1-2 g daily (4-6 weeks). Penicillin alone or in combination with sulphonamide is also used.
Actinomycosis *Actinomyces bandeti*	More common in older and hunting dogs, coetaneous actinomycosis is more prevalent in dogs. Chronic granulomatous pruritus, subcutaneous lesions like abscess, fistulous tracts.	History, clinical signs and definite diagnosis can be made by identification of organism from culture.	Potassium or sodium iodide 0.5 g daily until signs of iodism appear or the visible lesions are markedly reduced in size. Penicillin is effective.
Candidiasis *Candida albicans*	General debility, favour the development of diabetes mellitus, diarrhea anorexia dehydration.	History, clinical signs and definite diagnosis can be made by identification of organism from culture.	Amphotericin B. **Fluconazole compounds** (a) Flucan (Bombay), (b) Flucos (Cosme) 200 mg followed by 100 mg/day 14 days.
Aspergillosis *Aspergillus fumigatus A. glaucus*	Formation of yellowish caseous nodules in most of the organs of the	-do-	No effective treatment exists. ***Amphotericin-B compound**

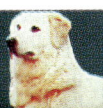

A. niger	body, pneumonia,		Fungizone (I.V) (SPPL)
A. nidulans	elevated		0.6 to 1 mg/kg/day.
	temperature,		***Itraconazole**
	mucoprurulent		**compound**
	discharge,		Sporanox (Johnson &
	conjunctivitis and		Johnson) tab, 100-
	coughing.		400 mg for upto 6
			months orally.

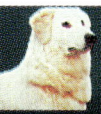

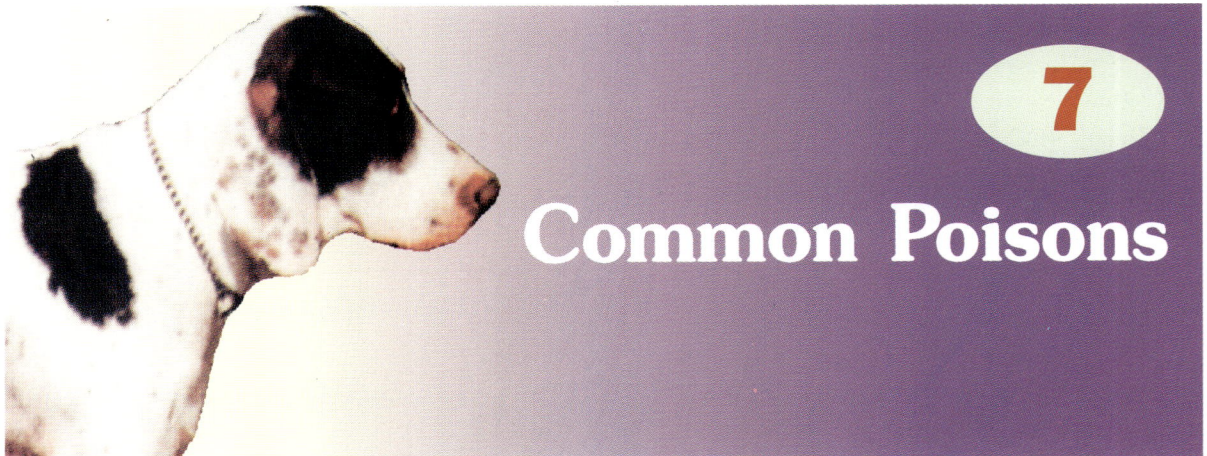

Common Poisons

It is difficult to define precisely a poison. Misuse of most of the things may be poisonous. In day-to-day life pets are exposed to small amounts of different harmful substances but body detoxifies and eliminates them regularly. The toxic effect depends upon the quantity of the poison induced in the body, the nature of the compound, and age and body condition of the dog. Young pups and aged dogs are more susceptible.

Almost all toxic substances are chemicals but they may be natural chemicals, synthetic chemicals or biochemicals synthesized in plant and animal tissues and organs. The hazardous toxic substances are insecticides, pesticides, rodenticides, fertilizers, petroleum products, plant toxins, and poisonous animals like snake, scorpion, bee, wasp and lizard.

Over-dosing of some drugs, minerals and vitamins may also be toxic. The non-judicious use of chloroform, atropine, barbiturates, aspirin, formaldehyde, phenol, morphine, digitalis and some antibiotics may cause serious illness and often result in death. The brief information about the source and signs of poisoning and its diagnosis and treatment are given in the tabular form for easy understanding.

EMERGENCY KIT

Arrangements must be there at clinics for handling the emergency cases for providing first-aid to facilitate safe transfer of the patient to a nursing home. A list of medicines and appliances is given as follows:

Medicines

1.	Analgesics	Baralgan, novalgin, pethidin etc.
2.	Antibiotics	Penicillins tetracyclines etc.
3.	Antiseptics	Ointments, lotions and dusting powder
4.	Antihistaminics	Avil, phenargan etc.
5.	Antispasmodics	Atropine sulphate
6.	Febrifuse	Paracetamol etc.
7.	Therapeutic fluid	Physiological saline
8.	Tranquilizers	Largactil, siquil etc.

If possible some of the drugs may also be included in the kit box i.e., Tincture iodine, Tr. Benzoin, potassium permanganate, dettol, spirit, liquid paraffin, adrenaline, corarmine and corticosteroids etc.

Instruments

Clinical thermometer, stethoscope, syringes and needles, dressing material, sutures and suturing needles, stomach tube, muzzle, catheters, scissors, forceps, scalpel and blades, artery forceps and glove etc.

GENERAL MANAGEMENT OF EMERGENCY CASES

The handling of patient in emergency depends on the type of damage or diseased condition, which are variable, viz., a patient of heat stroke requires immediate application of ice cold pack while that of a shock should be provided warmth. The various measures required for handling different kinds of emergency are listed as follows:

1. Immediate consultation with a veterinarian.
2. Handling of patients as necessary, viz., Immobilization in cases of trauma and fracture, and also first-aid for controlling bleeding.
3. Application of tape or other kind of available muzzle.
4. Administration of sedative, if required.
5. Wrapping in the rug in case of shivering and shock.
6. Gentle handling and movement of patients of shock and coma etc.
7. Administration of need-based therapeutic fluid.
8. Foreign body, if any, should be removed as early as possible.
9. Surgical intervention, if necessary.
10. Heart rate, respiration rate and temperature should be monitored.
11. Need-based palatable diet should be fed. Tube feeding or parenteral fluid administration may be needed in problems associated with ingestion and digestive disorders.

Suggestions for Indoor Patients

1. Clear instructions should be given in writing on the patient's history sheet with the signature of the veterinarian attending the patient.
2. Instructions may be revised on according to conditions of the patient.
3. Previous instructions should be cancelled if not required to be followed before recording the new instructions.
4. Treatment schedule should be clearly recorded.
5. Chart of cardinal signs, viz., pulse, respiration and temperature should be maintained.

Suggestion to the owners

For outdoor patients and also for patients released after indoor treatments necessary instructions to owners should be given in writing for the various steps to be taken for the administration of drugs and management of the patient. All suggestions should be recorded on the standard patient slip or health record book with date and signature of the consultant veterinarian.

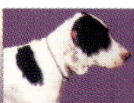

Common Poisoning and their Treatment

Type of poison	Source of poison	Main symptoms	Line of treatment
1.	2.	3.	4.
Acid (Sulphuric acid, nitric acid and hydrochloric acid)	Contaminated feed by accident, due to change of gastric pH (indigestion) or infection etc. mistakenly in therapeutic preparation	Vomiting, abdominal pain, diarrhoea, convulsion, staggering gait, restlessness, dyspnoea, tympany, corrosion of the mucous membrane of the upper digestive tract, severe colic & visible damage to the membrane of the orophrynx.	1. Chalk or kaolin 15-30 g orally. 2. Sodium bicarbonate 5-20 g orally. 3. Sodium bicarbonate, limewater followed by sedative and stimulants. In case of burn, first flood with water, then with dilute alkali. 4. Other weak alkalies, milk and water. 5. Magnesium carbonate or magnesium oxide 1-5g orally 6. Magnesium hydroxide (milk of Mg) 1-15 ml orally.
Alkalies (Caustic soda, other weak alkalies like ammonium carbonate)	Contaminated feed by accident due to change of gastric pH (indigestion or infection etc.)	More or less same as in acid poisons.	1. 5% acetic acid/ citric acid/citric potash and caustic acid/glacial acetic acid. Give according to body weight and severity of poison (normally 20-200 ml orally). 2. Weak acids like acetic acid, citric acid, glacial acetic acid, hydrochloric acid 1-5 ml in 1 litre of water, orally. 3. Vinegar, 20-50 ml diluted in water, orally. 4. Sour wine 10-30 ml diluted in water orally. 5. Milk demulcents and oil. 6. Tannic acid 200-500 mg in 30-60 ml of water orally.

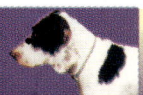

Type of poison	Source of poison	Main symptoms	Line of treatment
1.	2.	3.	4.
			7. **Sedative and Analgesic:** Megatil (Intas) 1-2 mg/kg BW i/m or 3 mg BW orally. Novalgin (intervet) 0.5-2.5 g orally, i/mly.
Ammonia (Ammonium phosphate and ammonium carbonate)	Contaminated feed, excessive dose in therapy.	Dyspnea, convulsions, pulmonary oedema results in forced rapid breathing, severe colic, staggering, marked thumping pulse, violent struggle and death.	As stated in alkali poisoning. When air passage is affected, inhalation of diluted acetic or citric acid and hot water vapour inhalation should be given.
Arsenic	Feed contaminated with arsenic spray, accidental use of arsenic preparation, concentrated arsenic dipper, spraying at animal to control the ectoparasites, use of arsenic preparations as weed killer, insect poison and wood preservative.	Intense abdominal pain, staggering gait, paralysis, excessive salivation, trembling vomition, rice gruel like diarrhea and prostration.	1. Gastric lavage with lukewarm water or oil or saline purgation. 2. Prompt emetic. 3. Precipitated iron oxide in emergency. Add a solution of ferric chloride and washing soda. Filter through muslin or thin cloth. Wash precipitate. Administer in large quantity as lukewarm water at 5-10 minutes intervals or mix 3 parts of solution per chloride of iron with 17 parts of water, add calcinated magnesia (1:17) in water, dose 1-5 ml every 5-10 minutes. 4. Sodium thiosulphate 0.5-1g as 15% solution I/V, 5g orally in 0.5 litre of water in a day. 5. Dimercaprol (BAL) 3-5 mg/kg B.W., I/M. Repeat every 4 hours

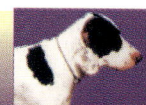

Type of poison	Source of poison	Main symptoms	Line of treatment
1.	2.	3.	4.
			for first 2 days, 4. times on 3rd day and twice daily upto 10 days.
Antimony (Tartar emetic)	Contaminated feed, miscellaneous use in therapy.	Same as in arsenic poisoning.	1. Gastric lavage and purgative. 2. Strong tea, tannic acid, milk demulcents, small dose of washing soda and diluted acids. 3. Patient should be warmed and treated with some stimulants. 4. Dimercaprol (BAL) same as in arsenic. 5. Milk of magnesia and limewater of calcium hydroxide.
Carbon monoxide	Coal gas due to fume in closed house.	Asphyxia and dyspnea, intermittent heart beat, coma and death. Visible showing pink colour, blood becomes cherry red.	1. Treat with pure oxygen containing 5% carbon dioxide. 2. In severe cases or in coma give respiratory mucous membrane analeptic such as nikethamide or leptazole.
Cyanide	By enemity/ cyanogenic fodder feeding, cyanide containing fumigants, fertilizers.	Excessive salivation jerky movement of the eyeball, convulsions, paralysis, stoppage of respiration even before that of heart-beat, bright red colour of blood, death within few seconds.	Sodium nitrite (1%), 16 mg/kg B.W. I.V. sodium thiosulphate (20%) 30-40 mg/kg B.W. I.V. Inhalation of Amyl Nitrate 5-8 drops.
Copper	By feed contami-nated with copper sulphate, due to rich copper contain-ing soil which causes chronic	**Acute cases** Excessive salivation, nausea, vomition, purgation, abdominal pain, convulsions,	1. In acute poisoning animal should be handled as in irritant poison such as by using purgative, emetics and gastric

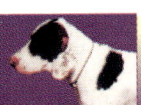

Type of poison	Source of poison	Main symptoms	Line of treatment
1.	**2.**	**3.**	**4.**
	poisoning, due to heavy dose of copper sulphate used for snail control, treatment of foot and mouth disease, foot rot, parasitic infestation and while being used as a spray or dip.	paralysis of body parts and death.	lavage, BAL may also be used. 2. Chronic cases may be treated with 15-70 mg of ammonium molybdate and 50-60 mg sodium sulphate daily for 20 days by adding the molybdate in diet. 3. Lavage with egg and milk sodium bicarbonate, morphine, saline purgatives are also useful. 4. Ferrocyanide (sodium salt) 0.3-0.5g oral. 5. D-Penicillamine 40 mg/kg BW orally.
Carbolic acid (Phenols and cresols)	By heavy use as disinfectant, by contaminated feed, by accidental use, used as wood preservative, by licking of wood	Nausea, vomiting, convulsions, staggering gait, restlessness, weakness, jaundice and anaemia	1. Emetics, enema, epsom or glauber's salt, white of eggs, milk and stimulants. In case of dermatitis treat with soap and water or alcohol. 2. For emetics, use strong salt solution or large crystal or washing soda or mustard and water. 3. In small animals Apomorphine hydro-chloride, 0.9 mg/kg B.W. S/C or I/M. Sodium bicarbonate, kaolin, bismuth orally and glycerine over the affected skin is very useful.
Iodine	Prolonged use of iodine preparations as a therapeutic	Lacrimation, nasal catarrh, scruffiness, skin rashes of	1. Stop use of iodine. Give milk and starch mucilase as

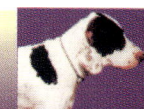

Type of poison	Source of poison	Main symptoms	Line of treatment
1.	2.	3.	4.
	agent, accidental use.	variable character anorexia, heavy and prolonged treatment of iodine may cause atrophy of testicles, blind ness, paralysis, palpitation of heart and sweating.	demulcents. Nikethamide or leptazol may also be given. Sodium bicarbonate is orally given.
Iron	Ingestion of high dose of iron salts, iron-carbohydrate complexes when injected.	Laboured breathing cyanosis, staggering gait, weakness bloody diarrhea, prostration and shock.	1. Desferrioxamine 1-2g I/M. 2. Milk of magnesia orally. 3. Ascorbic acid. 4. Corticosteroids. 5. Emetics. 6. Oxygen therapy. 7. Antihistaminics.
Fluorine	Excessive fluorine in water. Intake of amount of soluble fluorine compounds. Feeding of fluorine in excessive qunatity in plants in some areas. (Bone sink).	**Acute:** Gastroenteritis, diarrhea, vomiting abdominal pain, muscular weakness, and death. **Chronic:** Lameness, bone abnormalities, presence of dental lesions with dark pigment deposit in defective enamel and pitted teeth.	Aluminium sulphate or chloride 0.25-1 g daily, orally. Calcium borogluconate, 60-150 ml I/V.
Lead	By licking of lead paints, lead pipes. By ingestion contaminated feed, water with lead spray, spray on fruit. Used as in therapy (lead acetate white lotion) and storage batteries.	**Acute poisoning:** Staggering gait, muscles of head and neck showing tremor, rolling eye and frothing mouth, muscular spasm and tetany, during convulsions animal may become blind, and sometimes try	1. Wash the stomach and give saline purgative and emetics. 2. Give sedative such as siquil or largactil. Milk, white portion of eggs or tannic acid should be given. Sodium sulphate or magnesium sulphate or both. Sodium

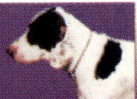

Type of poison	Source of poison	Main symptoms	Line of treatment
1.	2.	3.	4.
		to climb a wall or a tree. In severe poisoning, abdominal pain intermittent circling directions, constipation followed by diarrhea. **Chronic poisoning:** No tremor and excitement, animals lying in recumbent form.	calcium EDTA is the drug of choice, dose 30-50 mg/kg B.W. daily for 5 days I/V as 100% solution. 3. Calcium salt and vitamins or BAL may also be given @ 2-3 mg/kg BW i/m.
Mercury	By contaminated feed. By accidental use. While as fungicide on grains and also by industrial effluents.	Severe gastrenteritis, diarrhoea, stomatitis, patient shows signs of acute nephritis. Difficulty in breathing, coughing, nasal discharge, colic and subnormal temperature.	Remove all the material from stomach. Give white raw egg followed by purgative. BAL same as in arsenic poisoning. Sodium thiosulfate 2-10 ml 20% solution, I/V.
Urea	Accidental use of urea and excessive urea treated feed.	Acute pain, shivering, staggering gait, rapid breathing, jugular pulse, neuromuscular and death.	1. Give 50-200 ml of 5% acetic acid. 2. Inject adrenergic blocking agent. 3. Give calborol 50 ml orally. 4. Sedative and tranquilizers to treat neuromuscular manifestations.
Strychnine (Nux Vomica)	By accidental ingestion; by enemity, poisoning may also be caused due to ingestion of rat or mice which died due to Nux Vomica poisoning	Nervousness, restlessness, twitching of muscle, stiffness of the neck, and spinal cord, convulsion is developed by slightest external	1. Check disturbance and external stimuli. 2. Emetics such as morphine or apomorphine may be given instead of stomach tube to empty the stomach when convulsions

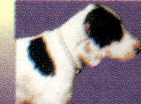

Type of poison	Source of poison	Main symptoms	Line of treatment
1.	2.	3.	4.
		stimulus such as touching, talking or sudden noise. Pupil is dilated and death occurs due to asphyxiation or respiratory paralysis.	have alreay appeared. Apomorphine HCl may be given 3-6 mg S/C or by dropping a prepared tablet into the conjunctival sac. 3. (a) Pentobarbital-Na is good for controlling convulsion. The dose is half of an anaesthetic dose (10-15 mg/kg B.W.) I/V. (b) Gardenal (Phenobarbitone tab), 30-300 mg according to B.W. (c) Thiopentone sodium 4. Gastric lavage using warm hypertonic saline solution or $KMnO_4$ 1:1000 or strong tea or 2% tannic acid solution can be attempted. High enema with warm saline may be advantageous.
Datura Stramonium (Contains alkaloids atropine, hyoscyamine and hyoscine)	By enemity	Nausea, vertigo thirst, dilated pupil, terminal convulsion and quick death.	1. Gastric lavage, kaolin or tannic acid per os. 2. Respiratory stimulants should be given. 3. Cardiac stimulants (i) Aminophyline, 5-7 mg/kg B.W. TID (ii) Calcium gluconate 20% sol. 10-15 ml/kg B.W. I/V until the heart rate is normal. (iii) Digoxin tablets; the total digitalization dose for the dog is 0.075 mg/kg B.W. orally for equal dose

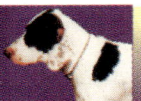

Type of poison	Source of poison	Main symptoms	Line of treatment
1.	2.	3.	4.
			over 2 days. (iv) Epinephirn sol. 1:1,000, 0.1 to 1.0 ml S/C or 0.01 ml I/V.
Mycotoxicosis, aflatoxicosis (Aflatoxins)	By ingestion of infected food due to *Aspergillus flavum* fungi, and *A. parasiticus.*	In all animals the first sign is an outbreak, reduced growth, loss of condition and inappetance. After 7-14 days or before death icterus and haemorrhagic enteritis may be seen. calcium	Any food containing fungus or even suspected for fungal infection and spoiled food should not be given to the pet. Activated charcoal orally, stanzolol 2 mg/ kg BW I/M single dose can be given. Hydrated sodium alluminosillicate orally is the choice of treatment.
Mouldy corn toxicosis	Due to consumption of diet containing mouldy feed corn (maize)	Gross icterus and tissue haemorrhage. In acute case, massive haemorrhages are observed in most of the tissues. In chronic cases extensive icterus and cachexia are prominent. Other Symptoms include depression and anorexia.	No treatment, only prevention by avoiding mouldy corn.
Aspergillosis	*Aspergillus spp.* through dog meal.	Hepatitis, diagnosis can be made on the basis of history and clinical symptoms,	Food contaminated with fungus should not be used. Antifungal drugs and symptomatic treatment.
Snake bite Venomous snake can be divided into two classes. 1. Elpine snakes	Dogs are frequently bitten on their legs but the most common site is probably the shoulder and thigh	Venoms from viperine snakes may produce prolonged intense pain, impaired	1. First-aid should be given immediately. Animal should be placed at rest and hair should be clipped

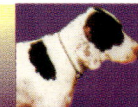

Type of poison	Source of poison	Main symptoms	Line of treatment
1.	2.	3.	4.
include cobra, mamba, and 2. Coral snakes. Elpine snakes (i) True vipers putt adder Russel's viper. (ii) Pit viper, e.g. Rattlesnakes, Cottonmouth moccasin, Fexdelane etc. Elpine snake has short fangs and chew their victim. Their venom is neurotoxic and kills by paralyzing the respiratory centre. Viperine have long hinged fangs. They strike once and withdrawn and venom is mainly haemotoxic. However, all snake venoms contain both neurotoxic and haemotoxic factors.	next in order. The presence of hair may hide the typical fang marks, though a close examination should reveal the point of entry of the venom.	vision, muscular weakness, nausea, paralysis, oedema, shock, cyanosis, haemolytic anaemia; necrosis of the tissue and the bleeding tendencies. The venom of rattle snake causes an almost immediate reaction in the form of extensive swelling around the wound. When dog is bitten on face and submaxillary region becomes grossly swollen, causing dyspnea, sloughing of the skin in the region of the wound. Shock is severe in snakebite. If a dog has been exercising violently as is frequently the cases and if the venom is deposited in a highly vascular area death occurs commonly in 5-10 mins.	from the wound. If bite is on limb, a wide tourniquet should be placed 5 cm above the bite. It should not be tight as to arrest arterial circulation. 2. In case of a bite from a dangerous snake such as rattlesnake, the fang wound should be enlarged with linear incision. Rubber tube or any other such material should be applied to remove the venom by sucking it out as early as possible. 3. Polyvalent antivenom should be given as early as possible, the initial dose per day may be as high as 100 ml 1-5 ampoule (10 ml) should be administered. All antivenom should be given I/V a little antivenom may also be injected at the site of bite. Anti-snake venom polyvalent (10 ml Haffkine) is available. 4. Corticosteroids prolong the survival time. 5. Broad spectrum antibiotic should be administered. 6. Blood transfusion or infusion of isotonic saline or dextrose

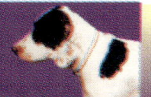

Type of poison	Source of poison	Main symptoms	Line of treatment
1.	2.	3.	4.
			solution is beneficial.
			7. Incision wound should be kept open and draining should be continued until the animal shows improvement.
			8. Tetanus anti toxoid should be given in the prophylactic doses.
			9. If antivenom is not available and if the animal is seen by the veterinarian with in an hour and if the bite is located in the area where tourni quet cannot be applied, then excision of an area of skin 5-6 cm in diameter, including the associated S/C tissue may be life saving in the course of a bite by a viper or pit viper.
			10. Excessive heat or cold is contraindicated.
			11. Some cobras are capable of spitting their venom at the eyes of their victim from a distance of several feet, causing severe pain and temporary blindness. For this the eyes should be washed with water or diluted serum.
Bee sting and wasp sting	By biting of bee and wasp	Bee and wasp stings produce severe local swelling in the form of urticarial	1. Remove stings as early as possible. 2. Affected area of the body should be washed with washing

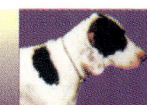

Type of poison	Source of poison	Main symptoms	Line of treatment
1.	2.	3.	4.
		weals on the skin, pain, irritation due to deposition of the formic acid on the skin by stings which is responsible for irritation, there is presence of local pain erythema and edema, restlessness and excitement. In case of attack on head dyspnea and difficulty in feeding. Severe bites may sometimes result in death.	soda (30 gm in one litre of water). 3. Antihistaminic preparations (Avil, 0.5-1 ml I/M Phenargan, 0.5-1 ml I/M should be given. 4. Pet should not be disturbed and proper management and feeding helps in recovery. 5. Apply weak acids (Vinegar) locally.
Tick paralysis (Neurotoxin)	Caused by *Dermacentor* (wood tick)	Varying degree of paralysis, tick paralysis occurs commonly in U.S. Animal becomes week and then suffers a complete ascending flaccid paralysis.	Either spray insecticide over the dog or dip it into the solution, or remove manually. Recovery usually takes place in 1 to 3 days.
Lizard poisoning	Mexican beaded lizard (*Heloderma horridum)* and the Gila monster *(Heloderma suspecturm)* vomiting, shock and poisonous, mostly found in USA. Accidental ingestion of lizard such as in milk also causes poisoning.	Venom transmitted through bite wounds infected by the lizard's upper teeth, animal starts some antiseptic and death.	Immediately give purgative, antihistaminic drug and supportive therapy for wound. Apply antibiotics therapy.
Insecticides (a) Organophosphorus insecticides	Ingestion by accident. By spray on animals and crops.	Acute poisoning: Lacrimation, weakness of	In case of oral poisoning give saline purgative, 5% dex-

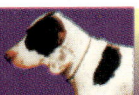

Type of poison 1.	Source of poison 2.	Main symptoms 3.	Line of treatment 4.
like thimet, TEPP, VP Parathion, malathion, ciordin, diazinon, cythion carbophernotheion vos, dimethoate, trichlorophon, disulphoton		voluntary muscles and muscular twitching. Excessive salivation, difficulty in breathing, constriction of pupil, abdominal pain, along with protrusion of tongue, animal shows watery discharge from nose and diarrhea, bronchial secretion and spasm, irregular violent contractions.	trose I/V. Phenobar bital 30-300 mg according to B.W. Inject acetyl cholinesterase reactivator (Praliodoxime, 5 mg/dichlor-kg B.W.) Atropine sulphate 4 mg/kg Later B.W. 1/3, I/V remainder S/C or I/V. The dosage may be re peated. 2PAM: Hydroxyiminomethyl-N-methyl pyridinium is of practical value 20 mg/kg B.W. S/C, TMB-4 is also considered very good.
		Chronic poisoning: Hypermotility of the gastrointestinal tract and excessive secretion. Twitching of the muscular part of the body and later on death due to respiratory failure.	Artificial respiration and administration of oxygen is advanta geous. Tranquilizer should be avoided at least for one week.
(b) Organochlorine, insecticides like chlorinated hydrocarbon, BHC, DDT, aldrin	Taken by accident. By spray on animals.	Acute poisoning: Animal shows symptoms within 24 hours. Hypersensitiviy and hyperexcita-bility, spasms of facial and cervical forequarter and hindquarter muscles. Concurrently there may be increased salivation with chewing movement	1. Give only saline, not oil purgatives to remove the poison in oral intake. 2. Phenobarbitone sodium. 3. Calcium borogluconate, 15-75 ml I/V. 4. If due to spraying, wash the body and remove poison. 5. Anticonvulsant drug, i.e. methadone is effective in all

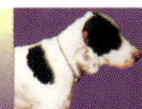

Type of poison	Source of poison	Main symptoms	Line of treatment
1.	2.	3.	4.
		of the jaw which adheres to the lips. Later on inco-ordination, staggering, jumping on imaginary objects and movement in a circle. Abdominal posture, fever, grinding teeth, coma, death. Chronic poisoning: Usually similar as in acute poisoning but tremors in muscles of neck and head are observed which extend to other muscles of body convulsions, depression, respiratory failure and death.	animals except toxophene toxicity in dogs. Riboflavin in DDT poisoning. 6. Dioxyanthraquinone @0.1 mg/kg in the form of aqueous suspension in 2 daily doses and glucose therapy. 7. Barbiturates: Gardenal (Rhone Poulenc), Luminal (Bayer), 2.2-6.6 mg/kg BW orally.
Rodenticides Warfarin 3-(d-acetonylbenzyl hydroxy coumarin)	1. Warfarin can be added as act of maliciousness to meat or other bait palatable to dogs and cats. 2. Poisoning in dog and cat by ingestion of rat or mice that died from warfarin poisoning.	Haemorrhage is a prominent symptom. The haemorrhage may be internal but is usually manifested by loss of blood externally as in vomitus or finally fatal haemorrhage from the body opening. Other symptoms are pale or cyanosed mucous membrane, rapid and weak pulse, shock, sub-normal temperature, prostration and collapse leading to death.	The emulsion of Vitamin K should be injected I/V for prompt therapeutic effect. If blood is not available immediately then glucose and saline solution may be substituted. Vitamin K @ 5-6 mg/kg BW i/m, and Oxygen therapy is also required.

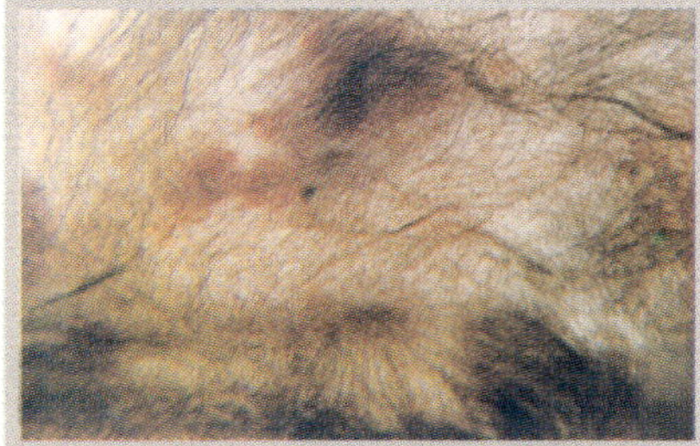

Fig. 136 A Case of Warfarin Poisoning

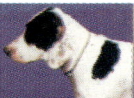

Type of poison	Source of poison	Main symptoms	Line of treatment
1.	2.	3.	4.
Alfanaphthyl thiourea (ANTU)	(i) By accidental ingestion. (ii) By enemity. (iii) Poisoning may also be caused due to ingestion of rat or mice which died due to ANTU poisoning.	Dyspnoea, pulmonary edema, vomition, foaming in the airways.	Stomach is promptly emptied. Silicone aerosal (10%) is administered to prevent the fatal foaming in the airways associated with pulmonary edema.
Zinc phosphide (Zn_3P_2)	By eating large number of rats which died due to zinc phosphide poisoning which is commonly used for killing rats. By enemity By accidental ingestion	Repeated administration of small quantities of zinc phosphide results in death which may occur immediately after ingestion, chronic poisoning of high quantity so the symptoms are frequently not observed. The symptoms are not diagnostic. Rapid deep breathing that often becomes wheezy follows anorexia and lethargy or stertorous, vomiting with presence of dark blood in vomitus, weak-ness, finally animal gasps for breath. Hyperesthesia or convulsion may occur. Lesions, acute congestion and liver necrosis, dark colour blood, enlargement of	Stomach is promptly emptied. In chronic cases symptomatic treatment may be beneficial but in acute poisoning treatment is not so effective. Gastric lavage with a 5% solution of sodium carbonate zinc phosphide should be given to clear the entire gastrointestinal tract, calcium gluconate 1/6 M sodium lactate may help in counteracting the acidosis. Sodium thiosulphate (10% sol). Liver tonic agent and dextrose may check the liver damage.

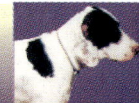

Type of poison	Source of poison	Main symptoms	Line of treatment
1.	2.	3.	4.
		heart, odour of carbide (acetylene) in the stomach contents. It is due to liberation of phosphene from zinc phosphide.	

Drug Poisoning Due to Overdose or Given by Mistake/Accident

	Drugs	Antidotes
1.	Alcohol or methylated spirit	Sodium bicarbonate or sodium citrate (1%) use as gastric lavage or give 100 mg/kg B.W./ day orally
2.	Arecholine	Atropine sulphate @ 0.2–0.5 mg/kg B.W. I/V, S/C or I/M
3.	Aspirin	Alkalinization of urine above pH 8 by giving sodium bicarbonate, emetics, respiratory stimulants like coramine
4.	Barbiturate	Amphetamine sulphate @ 0.5–1.0 mg/kg B.W., S/C, I/V, I/P, Doxapram @ 3–5 mg/kg B.W. I/V. Leptazol, glucose is also useful.
5.	Barium	Magnesium sulphate
6.	Belladona	Tannic acid 200–500 mg in 20–60 water orally
7.	Benzyl acid	Sedative like siquil, largectil and also use dextrose
8.	Benzyl benzoate	Washing with soap or detergent, tranquilizer, dextrose
9.	Bromide	Chlorides (sodium or ammonium salts) @ 0.5–1 g/day orally.
10.	Camphor	Sedative like siquil, largectil and saline diuretics
11.	Castor oil	Gastric lavage, atropine sulphate, tranquilizers
12.	Ephedrine	Gastric lavage, emetics
13.	Chloroform	Oxygen, coramine, calcium borogluconate I/V
14.	Formaldehyde	Gastric lavage with sodium and ammonium carbonate (1%) solution
15.	Morphine	Nalorphine 5–10 mg I/V
16.	Digitalis	Propranolol 0.5 mg/kg B.W. gastric lavage, I/M Sodium sulphate or magnesium sulphate
17.	Coumarine anti-coagulants	Vitamin K or Menadione @ 1 mg/kg B.W. orally
18.	Analeptic	Pentylene tetrazol (10% solution) @ 10–20 mg/kg B.W. I/V
19.	Narcotic analgesic	Demerol @ 15 mg/kg B.W. S/C
20.	Iron toxicosis	Desferrioxamine @ 20 mg/kg B.W.
21.	Inorganic phosphorus	Copper sulphate 0.2–0.4% solution 20–100 ml orally

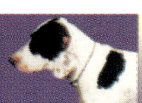

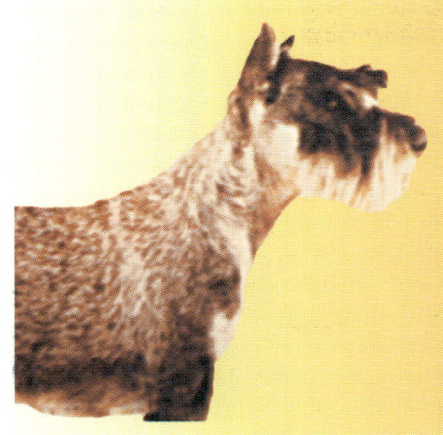

Appendices

Appendix I: NORMAL BLOOD VALUES IN DOGS

Blood constituent	Values
Haemoglobin (g/100 ml)/g/dl	11–13
Packed cell volume (%)	35–45
Ertyhrocyte count (million/cmm)[1]	5.8–6.2
Leukocyte count in thousand/cmm[2]	10–12
Neutrophils	68–70
Lymphocyte	18–25
Eosinophils differential	2–10
Basophils count (%)	0–2
Monocytes	1–4
Platelet count in thousands/cmm	145–155
Mean corpuscular Volume (Cubic microns)	65–67
Mean corpuscular Haemoglobin (Micro-Micro gram)	20-24
*Mean corpuscular Haemoglobin concentration (%)	31–33
Mean corpuscular diameter (microns)	4.0–4.1
pH of blood	7.32–7.68
Specific gravity of whole blood	1.054–1.062
Relative viscosity of whole blood	4.0

[1] Can also be expressed as $X\text{-}10^6/\mu l$ or $10^{12}/l$.
[2] $X\text{-}10^3/\mu l$.

Clotting time (mts.)	1–5
Erythrocyte fragility (NaCl)	0.45–0.36
Erythrocyte sedimentation rate (mm/hr)	5–13
Myeloid/Erythroid ratio	0.7–2.4/1
Blood volume (% body wt.)	8–9
Blood pressure	80–110
Icterus index (unit)	2–6
Proximal thromboplastin time (seconds)	18–25
Prothrombin (seconds)	8–13
Thrombinginal (second)	7–2
Fibrinogen degradation product (mg/ml)	up to 64

Appendix II: NORMAL BIOCHEMICAL VALUES IN DOGS	
Blood constituent	**Values**
Bicarbonate (mmol/lts)	18–24
PCO_2 (mmHg)	29–42
TCO_2 (mmol/l)	17–24
Cholesterol ester (mg/dl)	135–270
Createnine (mg/dl)	0.5–1.5
Fibrinogen (mg/dl)	200–400
Glucose (mg/dl)	65–118
Total protein (g/dl)	5.4–7.1
Albumin (g/dl)	2.6–3.3
Globulin (g/dl)	2.7–4.4
a	–
a_1	0.2–0.5
a_2	0.3–1.1
b_1	0.7–1.3
b_2	0.6–1.4
g	–
g_1	0.5–1.3
g_2	0.4–0.9
Calcium (Ca) mg/dl	9.0–11.3
Chloride (Cl) meq/l	114
Copper (Cu) mg/dl	100–200
Cobalt (Co) µg/dl	–
Iodine (I) mg/dl	5–20
Iron (Fe) (mg/dl)	30–180
Lead (Pb) (mg/dl)	–

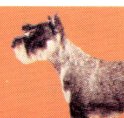

Blood constituent	Values
Magnesium (mg/dl)	1.8–2.4
Manganese (µg/dl)	3–15
Inorganic phosphate (mg/dl)	2.6–6.2
Potassium (mmol/l)	4.3–5.3
Phosphorus (mg%)	2.2–4.0
Sodium (mmol/l)	107
Sulfate (meq/l)	2.0
Zinc (µg/dl)	150–350
Acetylcholinesterase (µl)	270
AST (I.U.)	21–100
Amylase (mg maltase/ml plasma)	12.5
Arginase	185–700
Aspartate Amino Transferase (I.U.)	22–66
Butyryl cholinesterase (U/l)	1210–3020
Glutamate dehydrogenase(U/l)	3
Glutamyl transferase (U/l)	1.2–6.4
Glutathione (GSH) mmol/l	2.07
Glutathione reductase (µ/100ghb)	137
Isocitrate dehydrogenase (U/L)	2–10
Lactate dehydrogenase	0.4–7.3
Malate dehydrogenase	45–233
Phosphatase alkaline	199
Sorbitol dehydrogenase	20–156
Bile acid (total) µmol/l	2.9–8.2
Bilirubin (mg/dl)	0–5
Total Bilirubin	0.06–0.12
Cortisol (µg/dl)	0.1–0.5
Icterus index	0.96–6.8
Insulin (µg/ml)	2–5
Total Iron Binding capacity (µg/dl)	12
Thyroxine (µg/dl)	165–418
Triidothyronine (µg/dl)	3.53
Urea mmol/l	82–138
Urea nitrogen mg/dl	1.6–3.3
Vitamin A (Carotene) µg/dl	10–28
Retinol mg/dl	35–90

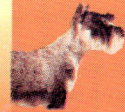

Appendix III: PROFORMA USED IN CLINICAL DIAGNOSIS

PROFORMA FOR PRESCRIPTION WRITING

Name of institute/Vety. Hospital Clinics _____

Clinic No. _____   Species _____

Owner _____   Breed _____

Clinician Dr. _____   Age and Sex _____

Diagnosis _____

Rx

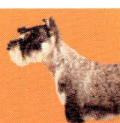

Appendix IV: PROFORMA FOR HAEMATOLOGICAL EXAMINATION

Name of institute/Vety. Hospital/Clinics _____

_____

_____

BLOOD EXAMINATION REQUEST/REPORT

Clinic No. _____   Species _____

Date _____   Breed _____

Owner _____   Age and Sex _____

Referred by Dr. _____

History:

CHECK TEST(S) DESIRED
Haemogram

1. Haemoglobin _____ g/dl

2. E.S.R. _____ mm/hr

3. P.C.V. _____ %

4. R.B.C. Count _____ X 10^6 µl\

5. Reticulocyte Count _____ %

6. W.B.C. Count _____ X 10^3/µl

7. Differential Count _____

8. Blood Parasites:

    Protozoa _____

    Microfilariae _____

9. Bacteria _____

10. Blood picture:

    Neutrophils changes: _____

    Leukaemic changes _____

    Myelo _____ %

    Juv _____ %

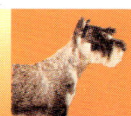

Stab _____ %

Seg _____ %

Lymphocytes _____ %

Monocytes _____ %

Eosinophils _____ %

Basophils _____ %

HAEMOSTASIS TESTS

1. Platelet count _____ X $10^3/\mu l$

2. Bleeding time _____ / minute

3. Coagulation time _____ /minute

4. Prothrombin time _____ /second

_____ Officer-in-charge

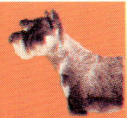

Appendix V: PROFORMA FOR BLOOD CHEMISTRY EXAMINATION

Name of institute/Vety. Hospital/Clinics _____

_____

_____

BLOOD EXAMINATION REQUEST/REPORT

Clinic No. _____ Species _____

Date _____ Breed _____

Owner _____ Age and Sex _____

Referred by Dr. _____

History:

CHECK TEST(S) DESIRED

Blood sugar _____

(Use sodium fluoride as anticoagulant) _____ mg%

Serum cholesterol _____ mg%

SGOT _____ unit

SGPT _____ unit

Bilirubin _____ mg%

BSP (Clearance test) _____ % Ret./45 minutes

B.U.N. _____ mg%

Others _____

Miscellaneous test _____ Check test(s) desired Cerebrospinal fluid

Total cell count _____

Synovial fluid _____ Pandy's protein

Coagulation _____

Differential count _____

Bacteria _____

Officer-in-charge

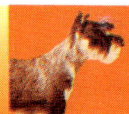

Appendix VI: PROFORMA FOR FAECAL EXAMINATION

Name of institute/Vety. Hospital/Clinics _____
_____
_____

BLOOD EXAMINATION REQUEST/ REPORT

Clinic No. _____   Species _____

Date _____   Breed _____

Owner _____   Age and Sex _____

Referred by Dr. _____

History:

CHECK TEST(S) DESIRED

Faecal Examination Result

Eggs

Ciliates _____

Protozoans _____

E.P.G. _____

Nasal washing

Eggs _____

Spores _____

Officer-in-charge

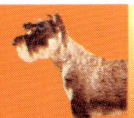

Appendix VII: PROFORMA FOR URINE EXAMINATION

Name of institute/Vety. Hospital/Clinics _____

_____

_____

URINE EXAMINATION REQUEST/REPORT

Clinic No. _____   Species _____

Date _____   Breed _____

Owner _____   Age and Sex _____

Referred by Dr. _____

History:

CHECK TEST(S) DESIRED

Colour _____   Bile _____

Sp. gravity _____   Bile pigments _____

Consistency _____   Occult blood _____

Reaction _____   Urobilinogen _____

Protein _____   Calcium _____

Sugar _____   Others _____

Ketone bodies _____

Microscopic Examination:

R.B.C. _____   Epithelial cells _____

W.B.C. _____   Crystals _____

Casts _____

Officer-in-charge

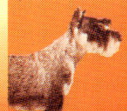

Appendix VIII: PROFORMA FOR SKIN SCRAPING EXAMINATION

Name of institute/Vety. Hospital/Clinics _____

_____

_____

SKIN SCRAPING EXAMINATION REQUEST/REPORT

Clinic No. _____ Species _____

Date _____ Breed _____

Owner _____ Age and Sex _____

Referred by Dr. _____

History:

CHECK TEST(S) DESIRED

Skin Scraping Examination Result

Ectoparasites _____

Mites _____

Fungus _____

Bacteria _____

Officer-in-charge

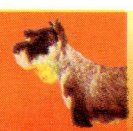

Appendix IX: PROFORMA FOR INDOOR-OUTDOOR PATIENT RECORD

Name of institute/Vety. Hospital/Clinics _____

_____

_____

Case Sheet

Case No. _____ In/Out patient _____

Date of admission _____ Date of discharge _____

Clinician Dr. _____ student _____

History and Duration of illness:

DESCRIPTION OF THE PATIENT AND CONDITION ON ADMISSION

Colour _____ Breed _____ Sex _____ Age _____

General condition ____ Temp. _____ Heart _____ Lungs _____

Skin _____ Limbs _____ Abdomen _____

Tentative Diagnosis _____

Final Diagnosis _____

Secondary complications if any after final diagnosis:

Result   C   D   Dd   I   NI   R   DC   A

Note: C-cured; Dd-Died; NI-Not important; DC-discontinued; D-Discharged; I-Improved; A-Advised.

INVESTIGATION

Blood   Urine   Faeces   Skin scraping   X-ray   Elctrocardiogram

Explanation in detail of abnormality of system(s)

Treatment:

           Rx

Surgical details

Pre-operative diagnosis   Assistant(s)   Date of operation

Post-operative diagnosis   1.   Type of Procedure

Surgery   2.

Anaesthesia   3.   Minor   Major

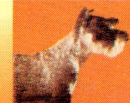

Findings

Procedure

Details in (special sheet)

Treatment:

      Rx

Discharge summary

Admitted on _____   Discharged on _____

1. Presenting   4. Investigation   7. Final diagnosis

2. Physical   5. Operative   8. Condition at discharge

3. Clinical   6. Treatment   9. Recommendation

                                                Signature of Doctor-in-charge

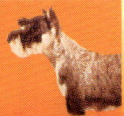

Appendix X: PROFORMA FOR ELCTROCARDIOGRAM

Name of institute/Vety. Hospital/Clinics _____

_____

_____

URINE EXAMINATION REQUEST/REPORT

Clinic No. _____ Species _____

Date _____ Breed _____

Owner _____ Age and Sex _____

Referred by Dr._____

History:

Results/Interpretation

Treatment:
        Rx

I   a VR

II   a V

III   a VF

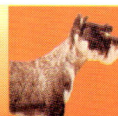

Appendix XI: PROFORMA FOR REPRODUCTIVE PERFORMANCE

Name of institute / Vety. Hospital/Clinics _____

Name of the place _____   Date _____   Name of Veterinary Surgeon _____

Species and breed	General condition: Excellent A V. Good B Good C Fair D Poor E	Identity	Owner's name and address	Age/ date of birth Y/M/D	No. of pregnancy /whelping (indicate abortion, stillbirth)	Date of last whelping	No. of heats after whelping	Date of last mating	Investigation of sexual organs: ovaries uterus cervix vagina and vulva	Remarks

Name and Signature of the Vet. Doctor with Seal

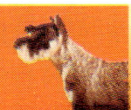

Appendix XII: PROTO TYPE OF REPORT

This is to certify that I have today personally examined at the request of Mr/Mrs _____
S/O, D/O, Shri _____ resident of the _____
animal/carcass answering the descriptions given below and found the under-mentioned injuries/lesions/
laboratory findings on its body/carcass.

Description of Animal:

1. Species _____

2. Breed _____

3. Sex: Male/ Female _____

4. Colour _____

5. Identification mark _____

6. Size _____

7. Weight _____

8. Birthmark _____

9. Registration number _____

10. Insurance number _____

11. Pedigree _____

Injuries/Lesion/Lab finding:

1. _____

2. _____

3. _____

4. _____

Opinion:
In my opinion the lesions/injuries (1), (2), (3) etc. are simple/serious and seem to have been caused
by sharp/blunt/external violence/accident/poisoning.

Date:

Signature of Veterinary Surgeon Seal

Signature of person to whom
the report was issued

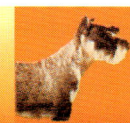

Appendix XIII: THE DETAILS OF THE ANIMAL INCLUDING IDENTIFICATION CHARACTERISTICS

Owner's Name and Address _____

Animal Name _____

Reg. No. (if any) _____

Species _____

Breed _____

Sex _____

Age _____

Colour _____

Identification mark _____

Birthmark _____

Insurance No. (if any) _____

Pedigree i. Sire – GS – GGS _____

          ii. Dam – GD – GGD _____

    (GS = Grand sire, GD = Grand dam, GGS = Great grand sire, GGD = Great grand dam.)

Language used with the animal:

Feeding system followed:

I _____sign this certificate on this day of _____ month
Year _____ (in words).

Date:

Signature of Veterinary Surgeon with Seal

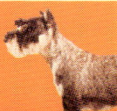

Appendix XIV: CERTIFICATE OF SOUNDNESS

This is to certify that I have examined the animal the details of which are given below belong to Mr./Ms_____ S/o, D/o Mr. _____
resident of _____to the best my capabilities and skill for soundness.

Description of animal:

Owner's Name and address _____

Animal's name _____

Reg. No. (if any) _____

Species _____

Breed _____

Sex _____

Age _____

Colour _____

Identification mark _____

Birthmark _____

Insurance No. (if any) _____

Pedigree i. Sire – GS – GGS _____
          ii. Dam – GD – GGD _____

Language used with the animal:
Feeding system followed:

1. The general health status of the animal is excellent, very good, good, fair, poor.

2. The animal is fit/not fit for keeping.

3. The animal has temporary defect, which may or may not lead to unsoundness, therefore a further examination is needed on date_____

4. The animal is suffering from _____(disease).

In my opinion the health and general condition of the animal is good/bad at the time of examination. The animal described above is sound/unsound.

I _____ sign this certificate on this day of month _____
_____Year _____ (in words).

Date: _____

Signature of Veterinary Surgeon with Seal

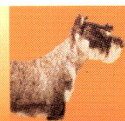

Appendix XV: CERTIFICATE OF SICKNESS

This is to certify that I have examined the following animal (details given below) at the request of Mr./Ms_____ S/o, D/o Mr. _____ resident of _____in detail.

Description of pet:

Owner's name and address _____

Animal's name _____

Reg. No. (if any) _____

Species _____

Breed _____

Sex _____

Age _____

Colour _____

Identification mark _____

Birthmark _____

Insurance No. (if any) _____

Pedigree i. Sire – GS – GGS _____

          ii. Dam – GD – GGD _____

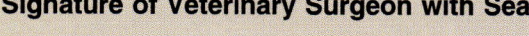

Signature of Veterinary Surgeon with Seal

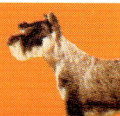

Appendix XVI: CERTIFICATE OF QUARANTINE

This is to certify that the animal described below was kept in quarantine for 10 days/1 months/2 months/3 months/6 months under direct observation of a qualified veterinarian.

Dr. _____

The animal was vaccinated against

(i) _____   (ii) _____

(iii) _____   (iv) _____

1. The animal was found negative for diseases

    (i) _____   (ii) _____

    (iii) _____ on testing at the time of examination (notifiable and schedule diseases).

2. The animal was suitably treated against ecto-and endo-parasites during _____ quarantine period.

3. The animal was accompanied with valid health certificate by a qualified veterinarian of the government of _____ (country).

4. The animal is not liable for detention in quarantine.

Description of animals:

Owner's name and address : _____

Animal's name _____

Reg. No. (if any) _____

Species _____

Breed _____

Sex _____

Age _____

Colour _____

Identification mark _____

Birth mark _____

Insurance No. (if any) _____

Body weight _____

Height _____

Pedigree: (i) Sire–GS–GGS _____

             (ii) Dam–GD–GGD _____

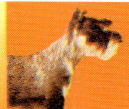

Language used with animal _____

Feeding system followed _____

Country from which imported _____

Date: _____

Signature of Veterinary officer

Name and Seal

Countersigned by Chief Vety. Officer

(Quarantine Officer)

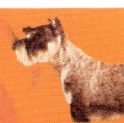

Appendix XVII: RISK NOTE FOR EUTHANASIA BY OWNER

I _____ s/o/D/o Shri _____ resident of _____ hereby undertake that the animal _____ (species, breed, sex, age, colour, identification mark) belongs to me. The animal is suffering from _____ as declared by _____ (Veterinary Officer). I, as owner, give full authority to Veterinary Officer or his authorized representative to destroy. Kill the animal (or euthanasia) in all manner the Veterinary Officer deems fit.

I am willingly giving my consent for the destruction of the animal and the veterinary surgeon/ any authority shall not be responsible for the said euthanasia (killing).

This is further certified that the animal has bitten/not bitten any animal/person(s) during last 15 days and to the best of my knowledge is not suffering from rabies.

Date

Signature

Place

Name of the Owner

Address

Countersigned by Veterinary

Assistant Surgeon Seal

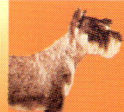

Appendix XVIII: CERTIFICATE OF FITNESS FOR DESTRUCTION OR EUTHANASIA

Certified that the following pet has been thoroughly examined by me. The animal is more than 15 years of age. It has become permanently unfit and/or unserviceable. The animal is suffering from _____ (incurable/infections/contagious disease(s)).

The animal may be destroyed in the manner the veterinary surgeon deems fit. This is also certified that the animal is suffering/not suffering from rabies.

Description of animal:

Owner's name and address _____

Animal name _____

Reg. No. (if any) _____

Species _____

Breed _____

Sex _____

Age _____

Colour _____

Identification mark _____

Birth mark _____

Insurance No. (if any) _____

Body weight _____

Height _____

Pedigree : (i) Sire–GS–GGS _____

            (ii) Dam–GD–GGD _____

Language used with animal _____

Feeding system followed_____ _____

Consent of the owner has already been obtained.

I Dr. _____sign this certificate on this day of _____

month _____ year (in words).

Date: _____

Signature of Veterinary Surgeon with Seal

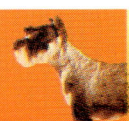

Appendix XIX: DOG SHOW

The beauty of a dog lies in its purity of breed, good health, clean coat and intelligence. All over India, various dog shows are conducted to judge these essential qualities in a dog. Knowledge about various qualities of each pure breed of dog is necessary to prepare a dog for the show. The kennel clubs of India have formulated a class rule of dogs as per their specifications.

Registration of a Dog

Before a dog can be shown at any dog show held under Kennel Club of India (KCI) rules it must be registered at Kennel Club of India. The pet owner must enter in the registered form accompanying all schedules in respect of the dog show, the particulars of the dog be proposes to show. Without registration a pet or change of ownership may lead to disqualification.

Preparation for Show

The preparation of a dog for the show requires considerable experience and expertise. An expert should be trimmed the dogs. It should be clean and in good optimum health. Ideal condition for any particular breed is best understood by observing the winning exhibits at various dog shows. Generally, a dog show should have a little fat on it in keeping with the correct scales provided to that particular breed. Cleanliness is essential for giving an overall good appearance to a dog. The breeds possessing hard coat should be seldom given bath and the last bath should be given two or three days before the show. In certain breeds, it is better for a dog to wear a light coat during the period between the final bath and the show to prevent it from becoming dirty again. The breeds where hard coat is not a necessity, there may be given a bath the evening before the show. All white coated dogs should have dry cleaner (dog cleaning powder) well, rubbed into their coats on the morning of the show.

Trimming and Grooming

The dog may be trimmed by an expert. Several breeds are groomed before the show but the

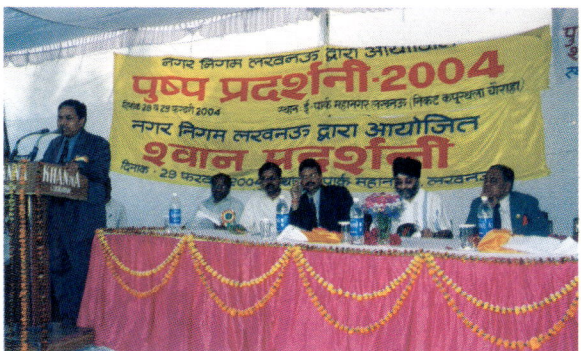

Fig. 137a Dog Show

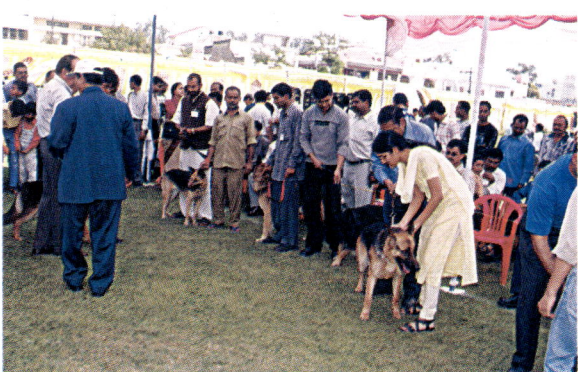

Fig. 137b Dog Show

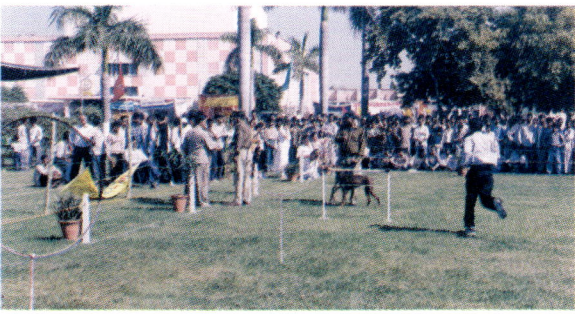

Fig. 137c Dog Show

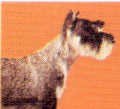

most extensive work is carried out on the Terrier species.

Generally, the old coat is easily removed in the early summer and in the late autumn. The new coming through thick and close will prevent the dog from feeling the cold in the coming winter.

During trimming only the finger and thumb should be employed, pulling the hair in the direction of the lay of the coat. The use of a knife results in the cutting of hair, whereas the finger and thumb method ensures the removal of only dead hair and the final appearance is greatly enhanced. The use of clippers should not be permitted, except in French Poodle. The fingers may be rubbed with powered resin or ordinary household whitening powder. Efforts should be made to pluck evenly and to avoid patchiness. The dog should not be trimmed to closely. Every effort should be made to maintain the smart appearance by attention during the regular grooming. Show-dogs need considerable more attention in this way than do other dogs.

The object of trimming and grooming is to display the outline of a dog to perfection, and to accentuate certain features that are thought to be desirable.

Transportation of Dog for Show

Before dispatching the dog by rail, the route and time of arrival should be enquired, if the journey is long, water may be made available enroute.

The larger breeds may be sent loose with collar, chain and muzzle. For the smaller breeds a strong travelling box with peaked roof and air-holes in the top and on each side should be used. The box should have a stout guardrail by round standing from the side about an inch and a half (4 cm); this proves useful when the box is carried, and prevents the piling up of luggage tight against the box. Painted upon the box in large letters should be the words "Valuable live dog". The journey may preferably be arranged in the night. Aggressive dog may be mildly tranquilized. Dog may also be transported by ship, plane, bus and taxi.

Veterinary Examination at Show

Clinical examination of the dog is conducted by the qualified veterinarians at the show to rule out any infectious disease, and ectoparasitism. Dogs with ectoparasites, eczema etc. are refused entry at the show. The dog may get infection at the show as the overcrowding during examination may help to disseminate infection. For this reason, it is better to reach for the show well in advance to avoid rush during examination. It is advisable to give bath to all the dogs with antiseptic soap after show.

In the Ring

It is important to train the dog for show in a lively, alert manner and in a way to disguise any faults. The dog should be regularly taught to walk in a wide circle and to stand in the position which will show him off to the best advantage. A lead of 3 ft. (*90 cm) or so should be used, and held loose enough to maintain gentle control of the dog.

The best time for the training is just prior to the principal meal. The trainer should provide himself with tit-bits to induce and to reward good behaviour; small pieces of hard-boiled goat or sheep liver or dog biscuits (containing meat extract) are ideal for this purpose.

To prevent the dog from getting nervous when handled by strangers, the service of friends should be enlisted. The aim should be to get the dog interested in his work and train him in such a way that its attention is on his master and he behaves well.

The exhibitor, in-turn, must play well and concentrate his attention solely on the judge and

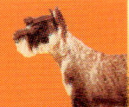

on his own dog. After the judge has examined the dog, the exhibitor should allow the dog to stand at ease but while the judge is examining him and during the parades, the dog should be "on his toes".

Toy dogs, which usually suffer from slight stomach trouble after a show, may be given a few doses of a mild laxative.

Procedure to Conduct a Dog Show

Entry fees: It is charged as per Kennel Club Rules.

Address of Kennel Club who is conducting the dog-show must be given in full.

Eligibility

Only dogs registered with K.C.I. may compete. Monorchid and cryptorchid dogs will not be allowed to compete. Bitches in season shall be allowed to participate in the breed shows only.

Rules

The decision of the Dog Show Committee is final, subject to appeal only to the K.C.I. should arise the objection which are not provided for in the rules, the decision of the committee will be final. Any breach of the rules and/or K.C.I. Regulations will render the exhibitor liable to disciplinary action by the committee. Exhibitors are also liable for any damage done by them, or their servants or their dogs. The committee reserves the right to refuse or accept any entry without assigning any reason.

Veterinary Examination

All dogs must be passed by the veterinary doctor present at the gate and certified fit by him before admission into the dog show.

Objections

Only after depositing prescribed fee may be entertained.

Precautions

Exhibitors shall make themselves familiar with the K.C.I. rules and regulations for shows, copies of which may be obtained from the secretary, K.C.I. on payment of the stamp or cash.

Penalty

All willful misrepresentations regarding ownership, age, name, pedigree etc. of dogs entered and prepared for exhibition in contravention of the K.C.I. regulations will be liable to disciplinary action by the committee.

Dogs that are not present in the ring when their classes judged, will be deemed to have been absent.

Various Classes of Dog Show

(a) Puppy Class: In this only dogs of 4 months and not exceeding one year on the first day of the show can compete; date of birth, sire, dam must be shown on the entry form.

(b) Junior Class: In this only dogs of 9 months and under 18 months on the first day of the show can compete. Date of birth, sire, dam must be shown on the entry form.

(c) Maiden Class: In this no dog which has won any prize in any class at any dog show can compete.

(d) Novice Class: In this no dog which has won a first prize in any class other than puppy can compete.

Maiden limit at a championship or open shows.

(e) Limit Class: In this no dog which has won first prizes in all open and Limit Classes at championship open shows can compete.

(f) Special limit Class: This is similar to an open class, say that no dog, which has won three challenged certificates, can compete.

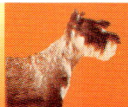

(g) Bred in India Class: This is a class in which only dogs bred and begotten in India shall be eligible. Dogs begotten abroad and born in India or on the voyage out or imported dogs under regulations for registration are not considered.

(h) Open Class: This competition is confined to a breed or to a variety of a breed classified as such by K.C.I. All dogs of that breed or variety of breed may compete in this show.

(i) Brace: In this class two exhibits of the same breed or a variety of a breed (either sex or both) being the property of the same owner can compete, provided such exhibits can be entered in one or more of their breed classes.

(j) Team: Team class is one in which three or more exhibits of the same breed or variety of a breed (either sex or both) being the property of the same owner can compete, provided such exhibits can be entered in one or more of their breed classes.

(k) Variety Class: In this class more than one variety of a breed are entered for competition.

(l) Litter Class: Puppies not less than two in number, of one of the same litter being not less than 45 days not more than 4 calendar months

Type of Breed and Obedience Classes for Dog Show (Classification shown by letters)		
Dogs	**Bitches**	**Obedience classes**
A Puppy	I Puppy	C-1 Pre-beginners
B Junior	J Junior	C-2 Beginners
C Maiden	K Maiden	C-3 Novice
D Novice	L Novice	C-4 Class A–Under-graduate
E Limit	M Limit	C-5 Class B Graduate
F Special Limit	N Special Limit	C-6 Class C Open
G Bred in India	O Bred in India	C-D Companion Dog
H Open	P Open	

List of Variety Classes	
A.V.1 Any Variety Litter	A.V.12 Any Variety Imported
A.V.2 Any Variety Puppy (4-6 months)	A.V.13 Any Variety Brace
A.V.3 Any Variety Puppy (6-12 months)	A.V.14 Any Variety Bred by the exhibitor
A.V.4 Any Variety Junior (9-18 months)	A.V.15 Any Variety Handled by a lady
A.V.5 Any Variety Bred in India	A.V.16 Any Variety Team
A.V.6 Any Variety Open	A.V.17 Any Variety Veteran–7 years or above
A.V.7 Any Variety Sporting	A.V.18 Any Variety Indian Breed
A.V.8 Any Variety Non-Sporting (Other than Toy)	A.V.19 Any Variety Hound Group
A.V.9 Any Variety Toys	A.V.20 Hound Group
A.V.10 Any Variety Terrier	A.V.21 Any Variety
A.V.11 Any Variety Gun Dogs	

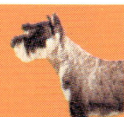

of age on the first day of the dog show. A litter shall be exhibited by one breeder only and not more than one entry can be made for one class.

(m) Champion Class: In this class dogs which have qualified for the title champion with accordance with the regulations can compete.

(n) Field Trial Class: For this class only dogs that have won a prize or certificate or diploma or merit in actual competition at a recognized field trial may compete.

(o) Veteran: In this class only dogs not less than 7 years old on the first day of the show can compete.

Important Points to be kept in mind by owners and/or Organizers

(i) No dog shall be eligible to compete in a variety class unless it is entered and competes in at least one of its breed classes.

(ii) A dog imported from abroad shall not be eligible to be entered in any class except open junior and puppy.

(iii) A dog may be entered in Obedience classes only, without being entered in any Breed classes.

(iv) **Best in show:** All exhibits that have been awarded a.c.c. or reserve c.c. at this show shall be eligible to compete for best in show.

(v) A dog, which is entered in obedience classes only shall not be eligible to compete for best in show.

Should any judge or judges be prevented from fulfilling his engagement, the committee has the right to appoint substitutes.

(vi) No refund of the fees will be made if a dog entered for a show is prevented from being exhibited at the show due to any cause whatsoever.

(vii) **In obedience:** The same dog can not compete in more than two tests. Dog

entered in class 'C' may not compete in any other class. One handler can only handle one dog per class.

(viii)**Reserve challenge certificates:** Not withstanding rights to award challenge certificates the right to award reserve challenge certificates shall also be given in such cases where a challenge certificate has already been awarded to a dog/Bitch or to both. The dog/bitch in that respective breed classes beaten by the dog /bitch awarded the challenge. Certificate shall also be called in for a reserve challenge certificate.

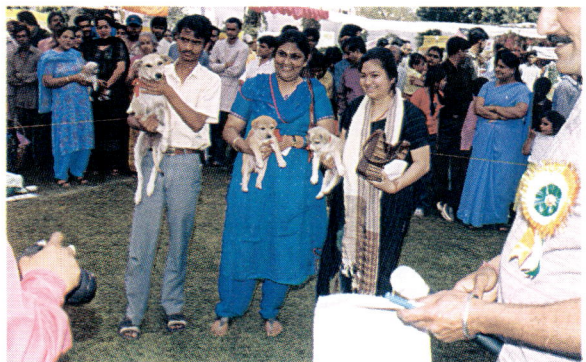

Fig. 138 Care of Stray and Abandoned Dogs by Welfare Organization Brought at Dog Show

RULES OF THE KENNEL CLUB OF INDIA

The Kennel Club of India is affiliated to the Kennel Club , London, 1900, and following are the regulations for registered kennel clubs in India which is essential for each club.

1. No dog club or society shall be recognized by the Kennel club of India until it has been registered in the books of the Kennel Club of India.

2. Application for registration shall be made to the committee of the Kennel Club of India accompanied by the following:

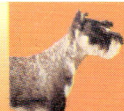

(i) Copy of the notice or advertisement calling a meeting for the purpose of forming the club.

(ii) Copy of the proceedings of such meeting signed by the Chairman and Secretary, together with a list of members present at the meeting:

  (a) In the case of All India Specialist Clubs, a list of members who have agreed to join the club.

(iii) Copy of the proposed rules of the club for approval.

(iv) A list of the official and committee with their addresses.

3. The prescribed fee for registration of a club must accompany the application. No name or title of a club shall be accepted for registration which is similar to a name or title already registered, or which is a colorable imitation thereof, or is calculated to mislead. The club shall notify on all printed matter below its own name or title "Registered under K.C.I. Regulations".

4. The application, if received by the Kennel Club of India, not later than the 15th of any month, shall be published in the Indian Kennel Gazette for that month, if later for the following month; and it shall be submitted to the committee for approval together with the objections, if any, received with regard to same.

5. Registration of a club shall only be granted, if the rules of the club recognize. The kennel club of India is the ruling body for kennel affairs in India and the final court of appeal as provided in K.C.I. show regulations. All proposed alterations and amendments to the rules shall be subject to the approval of the K.C.I. Committee.

6. A copy of the K.C.I. Regulations for registered clubs, shall be printed and bound in the rules of every registered club, and every registered club shall supply a copy of the rules to each of its members on joining; and at any time thereafter on payment of a fee to be fixed by each club. **Note:** If desired the K.C.I. Committee will supply standard size copies of these regulations for binding up in club rules, at the actual cost of printing.

7. All challenge cups and trophies donated to any club or show, and all other assets shall be deemed to be held in trust by such registered club or show for the benefit of exhibitors, and shall be vested in the committee of the Kennel Club of India, and shall be made over to the K.C.I. Committee, in the event of the club or show ceasing to function. The K.C.I. Committee shall in each eventually, hold all such assets in trust for any future club or show that may be instituted having the same or similar objects.

8. The K.C.I. Committee shall not sanction the registration of a second club, in any area (such as the presidency towns or any provincial area), or in any breed, without first referring any application to the existing club in such area or breed. This regulation shall not, however, make it illegal for the Kennel Club of India to allow the formation and registration of a new club, in the interest of dog owner, breeders and exhibitors, in any area or breed, should be existing Club in such area or breed be struck off the register of the kennel club of India .

9. Every Registered club shall publish annually a complete list of members either in its annual show catalogue, or where no show is held, in the annual report; such list shall be circulated to all members of the club concerned and submitted to the Kennel Club of India with the maintenance fee.

10. The rules of the Club, together with a list of the officers and committee and a copy of the accounts for the last completed year,

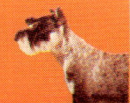

must be supplied to the Kennel Club of India in each year, not later than 60 days after the close of the club's official year. These shall be accompanied by a certificate signed by the Chairman and Secretary of the club showing.

(a) The number of members on its books at the close of the year; and if required a list of members with their addresses at any time.

(b) The name of the bank and branch in which the funds at credit of the club are deposited.

(c) The name of the firm in whose care the challenge cups and trophies owned by the club care deposited for safe custody.

(d) The place where the club's show gear and other property is stored.

11. Every registered club shall pay to the Kennel Club of India an annual maintenance fee as prescribed for every 50 members or part of 50 members. The payment of such maintenance fee shall then entitle club to nominate one delegate on the committee, who shall have power to act and vote on all matters arising out of or in connection with K.C.I. Regulations. Every such delegate shall be deemed to officially represent the club by which he/she has been nominated.

12. The delegate shall be elected by the vote of Members at a General meeting of the club, or as provided in the club rules for the election of the officers of the club, and shall be recorded in the minutes, a copy of which signed by the Secretary and the Chairman, shall be forwarded to the Kennel Club of India.

13. The term of office of a delegate shall be one year. In the event of a vacancy occurring during a delegate's term of office, a successor may be similarly elected for the unex-

pired period of the term. All delegates so elected shall be subjected to the approval of the committee of the Kennel Club of India.

14. A registered club shall be completely autonomous in the management of its affairs and shall act generally as co-trustee with the committee of the Kennel Club of India for the exhibiting public in its area or breed; it may organize or hold dog shows and dog trials with the sanction of the Kennel Club of India and award their such prizes and special prizes, as the members may decide.

15. A registered club may receive and adjudicate upon all complaints and charges as between member in respect of exhibitions at its shows, in accordance with its own rules and the K.C.I. Regulations; provided that in all cases, an appeal against the decision of any club shall lie in the committee of the Kennel Club of India, if posted within 30 days. A copy of the proceedings in respect of any complaint, or charge or objection, shall be immediately forwarded to the Kennel Club of India together with any other information that may be required.

16. All cases under K.C.I. show regulation No. 12 (Disqualification), or No. 17 (suspensions), or any disqualification or expulsion or suspension of a member or an exhibitor for any fraudulent or discreditable conduct, or any irregular conduct in connection with dogs. Dog shows or trials must be immediately reported by the Secretary of such club to the committee of the Kennel Club of India, with full particulars of the case, and a copy of the proceedings in respect of the same.

17. Any person   against whom a decision is given by any club or show committee shall be served by such club or show Secretary

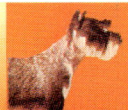

with a copy of such decision and shall be informed that he/she has the right of appeal to the committee of the Kennel Club of India provided the same is posted within 30 days accompanied by a prescribed fee as laid down in K.C.I. show regulations. No disqualification or suspension shall have effect unless and until confirmed by the committee of the Kennel Club of India.

18. No person disqualified or suspended under K.C.I. regulations may be elected or remain a member of any registered club, should any such person be retained on the list of members of any registered club, the officials of such club shall be liable to be proceeded against under regulation 17 of the K.C.I. Regulations for shows.

19. Registered clubs and shows may report to the Kennel Club of India the name of defaulters or any person indebted to the club to the show; and no person who is indebted to the Kennel Club of India, or to any registered clubs or show, shall be eligible to judge or compete or win a prize at, or take any parting a show, or dog trials, held under permission of the Kennel Club of India. The K.C.I. committee shall have the power to punish the names of owners and addresses and description of such defaulters, as provided in K.C.I. show regulations.

20. All official communication from the Kennel Club of India shall be recorded by the club for future guidance. Copies of all members' circulars and of important proceedings of the club shall be sent to the Kennel Club of India for record.

21. Any club which fails to comply with the K.C.I. rules and regulations, or whose returns under these regulations are not submitted by due date may be struck off the register, unless good cause be shown for such failure or delay. All officers and members of any registered club struck off the register of The Kennel Club of India continuing as officers or members of such club, and all officers and members of any Dog Club Society, or Association, which is not registered by the Kennel Club of India shall be disqualified from judging, competing, winning a prize, making an objection, or taking any part at a show or dog trial held under the permission of the Kennel Club of India. Such qualifications shall also apply to all dogs registered in the name of, or owned by any person disqualified under this regulation.

(a) The K.C.I. Committee shall have power to remove any disqualification under this regulation.

(b) The K.C.I. Committee shall have power to reinstate any club struck off the register.

22. In the event of a Club or show being wound up, a final statement of the accounts with a report as to the disposal of all property and assets of such club or show shall be rendered to the kennel club of India for record. The Committee of the Kennel Club of India shall be empowered under these regulations to take over and to sue for and recover any challenge cups, Trophies and other assets of any Registered Club or Show whose committee may have ceased to function, or which may be struck off the register.

23. An amendment made by the club from time to time should be obtained and followed.

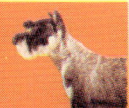

ENTRY PROFORMA FOR REGISTRATION IN A DOG SHOW

Closing Date _____

Name of Kennel Club:
Read the schedule and K.C.I. Regulations for show carefully.
Address: (Registered Under Kennel Club of India Regulations)
Note: Form should be typed or written in BLOCK LETTERS.

Name of Dog and No.	K.C.I. Registration No.	Breed	Sex	Sire	Dam	Date of Birth with	Name of Breeder Address	Imported or Bred in India	Breed No.	Breed Classes Litters	Entered in Class Variety Classes	Anyother Obedience Classes	Description Information

DECLARATION BY OWNERS:

N.B. Sec's for office use only

Brought Forward   Dogs   Entries   Fees
On this Form
Carried Forward
Fees–Remitted with this form:
Entry   Fees Rs. _____
     Total Rs. _____

Remitted by (DD/Money Order/Indian Postal Orders/Cash)
I/We hereby certify that the dog(s) entered above is/are my/our bonafide property and I/We enter them at my/our own risk and that the dog(s) entered on this form is/are registered in India only with the Kennel Club of India.
I/We undertake to abide by the Rules and Regulations and Bye-laws of the Kennel Club of India and of this Show and I/We declare that the dog(s) entered has/have not suffered from or been exposed to the risk of Distemper or any contagious or infectious disease for the six weeks prior to exhibition and I/We will not show them if they incur such risk between now and the day of the show or if they have been inoculated within fourteen days prior to the show.

Signature _____   Dated _____
Name Mr./Mrs. _____
Address _____

NOTES FOR EXHIBITORS:

1. All dogs must be first with the Kennel Club of India.
2. If a Registration Certificate has been lost a Certified Copy may be obtained.
3. Transfer of ownership must also be registered.
4. Entries cannot be accepted unless accompanied by Entry Fees in full.
5. For definition of classes, Puppy, Novice, Limit and open, etc. See K.C.I. Reg. In Schedule.

Receipt No. _____   Dated _____

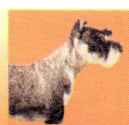

THE KENNEL CLUB OF INDIA   **APPLICATION FOR REGISTRATION OF A SINGLE DOG**

K.C.I. Form C/I

(Founded 1896-Affilliated to the Kennel Club, 1990) (See Regulations 11, 12 (a), 16 and 17 of K.C.I. Regulation for Registn.)

Please write in BLOCK LETTERS or TYPE ALL NAMES and read the NOTES on reverse VERY CAREFULLY before filling in the form

FOR OFFICE USE ONLY

Regn. No. _____

Regd. No. _____

Breed or Variety _____   Sex _____

Fees Rs. _____ by _____

Paid on _____

Receipt No. _____

N.B.: The dog may be registered in the first name applied for, if available but owners must add two alternatives in case it is not or the application may be returned. In the event of names applied for being inadmissible the K.C.I. will select a name, if the applicant marks X in the square of the right and such name shall be the { } registered name.

Name Applied (1) _____ (2) _____ (3) _____

Date of Birth _____

Colour and Markings _____

Sire _____ K.C.I. No. _____   G. Sire _____ K.C.I. No. _____

Owner of Sire _____   G. Dam _____ K.C.I. No. _____

Dam _____ K.C.I. No. _____   G. Sire _____ K.C.I. No. _____

Owner of Dam _____   G. Dam _____ K.C.I. No. _____

Breeder Mr/Mrs/Miss _____

Breeder's Address _____

* Breeder means the person who in the owner of the dam at the time of its whelping, unless a registration varying this definition has been effected Under regulation No. 25 (Loan of bitch for breeding purposes). "Breed in India" means that a dog is bred and begotten in India. Pups begotten abroad and born in India or on the voyage out, shall be deemed to be "Imported".

Breed in India or Imported from _____

1. IMPORTED DOGS: Only in the case of an imported dog please fill in the particular required and mark X in box against (a) or (b) whichever is applicable and strike out has the other (See Regulation 16 and Note 1 (iii) on reverse).

[ ] (a) Certified Pedigree No. .... dated .... issued by the .... Kennel Club sent in original to be returned/photostat copy (to be retained) attached.

2. PROVISIONAL REGISTRATION : If the dog is to be registered provisionally mark X in the box on the left. (See Regulation 17 and Note 1 (iv) on reverse.)

DECLARATION TO BE SIGNED BY OWNER/S (SEE NOTE 5 ON REVERSE)

I/We hereby declare that the above dog is solely and unconditionally my/our property and that the particulars given are true to the best of my/our knowledge and belief. I/We further decalare that I/We are not suspended or disqualified or indebted to the Kennel Club of India or any Registered Club of Dog Show or Dog Trial or Working Trial of Field Trial. In making this application I/We agree to be bound by the Kennel Club of India rules and regulations and bye-laws as may be amended and in force from time-to-time and I/We do hereby acknowledge the jurisdiction of the committee of the Kennel Club of India as the governing body for canine affaris in India and the final Court of Appeal or Umpire, on all questions or disputes or complaints or reports of any kind whatsoever arising in respect of registered clubs. Dog Shows, Dog Trials, Working Trials and Field Trials and of the Registration or Transfer of name of any dog or dogs and of any transaction in respect of breeding or sale or pedigree of any dog or dogs, and I/We hereby expressly agree that the decision of the Committee upon any question or dispute or complaint or report shall be final and binding on me/us. The dog has not been previously registered in India.

Date _____

Name/s Mr./ Mrs/Miss _____

Address Reply for _____

9. Balar Kalvi Nilayam Avenue,
Off. Ritherdan Road,
Madras–600007

Signature/s of Owner/s _____

this form duly completed and signed, should be sent together with the requisite fee to

Secretary:
The Kennel Club of India

Note :- All the particulars required should be entered on the form. When any particulars cannot be given the word "UNKNOWN" must be written, If the Registration Certificate is to be sent by Regd. Post, please add Rs. 10/- to your Remittance.

Name of Kennel Club:
Address:

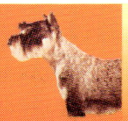

PLEASE READ THE FOLLOWING NOTES VERY CAREFULLY BEFORE FILLING IN THIS FORM

The application for Registration form, K.C.I. Form C/1, should be used in the following cases:

1. For registration of a Single Dog from a litter {Reg. 12 (a)}.

2. For Registration of a dog whose breeding (Sire, Dam, Date of Birth etc.) is partly or fully.

A CERTIFICATE OF OPINION in the prescribed form (K.C.I. Form B) duly filled in and signed by the owner and by a judge whose name is on the panel of judges of the K.C.I. of competent to judge the breed, or by a person who is authorized in the behalf by the committee of secretary of the K.C.I. or in the absence of a certificate of opinion a Certified Photograph of the dog must accompany the application. A separate application form and a certificate of opinion or certified Photograph must be submitted for each dog. (Reg.11).

3. For registration of a Dog imported from abroad either of the following documents must accompany the application, if the dog is registered abroad a Certified Pedigree (Export Pedigree) issued by the Kennel Club of the country of export in original which will be returned with a Photostat copy of the same, which will be retained. A separate application must be submitted for each imported dog. The particulars required should be retained. A separate application must be submitted for each imported dog. The particulars required should be filled in on the form (See item 1 (a) and (b) below the column bred in India or imported from on reverse). (Reg. 16).

4. For registration of a dog Provisionally the owner should mark X in the appropriate box on reverse. (See item 2 below the column bred. In India or imported from _____ (Reg. 17).

5. For the registration permanently of a dog previous registered provisionally. The applicant should indicate on the top of the form the provisional registration number granted to the dog and returned the provisional registration certificate along with the form.

If there are More than one Dog from One and the same litter to be registered in the name/s of the same person (i.e. Sire, Dam, Date of Birth of the Dogs to be Registered and the names of the persons identical) or if a litter of puppies is to be registered by the breeder at the reduced fee of Rs. 10/- per puppy. K.C.I. Form C_2, pink form. Application of registration of more than one dog from the same litter obtainable free on application to the Secretary K.C.I. Form, pink form. Application for registration of more than one dog from the same litter obtainable free on application to the Secretary K.C.I. should be used (Reg. 12 (b) and 15).

REGISTRATION FEE

(i) The fee for registration of a dog bred in India is Rs./- if both parents are registered with K.C.I. or if only one are neither parent is registered or unknown for fee is Rs. 25/-

(ii) The fee for registration of a dog imported from abroad is Rs. 20/- provided the documents required under Regulation 16 are submitted (See Note 1 (iii) above). In all other cases the Fee will be Rs. 25/-

(iii) The fee for registration of a dog – imported or bred in India provisionally is Rs. 20/-

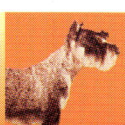

(iv)   The fee for registration permanently of a dog previously registered provisionally is the same as in item (i) or (ii) whichever is applicable.

NAMING FOR THE DOG

Before choosing the name for the dog to be registered the owner is requested to note carefully the following conditions and to give two alternative Names in addition to the first choice, so that incase the first name applied for is inadmissible, the dog may be registered in one of the two alternative names given.

(i)   A dog need not be registered in its pet of house name or in the name by which it is called. The pet or house name or the name to which the dog responds has no connection whatsoever with its registered name, which should be, used in pedigrees and other documents and when the dog is entered at a Dog Show or Dog Trial etc.

(ii)   The names of notable persons, titles, kennels, countries, large towns, common names well known dogs abroad, or numbers in figures or words should not be selected.{Reg. 13(c)}.

(iii)   A name or names excluding a registered prefix/Affix shall not exceed twenty four letters except that in the case of an imported dog registered abroad the same shall be registered in its original name {Reg.13 (e) and (g)}.

(iv)   A word or words shall not be used in the name of more than one dog unless the same is registered as a prefix/affix Reg.13 (b) if the owner has already used a particular word or words in the name of a dog registered by him previously, he cannot use the same word or words again unless he registers the word or words as his prefix/affix (Reg.14). The main advantages of registering a word or words as a prefix/affix are (a) it serves as an indication that the dog has been bred and or registered by a particular person, (b) it can not be used by any other person except by the registered owner thereof, and names becomes more easy.

(v)   Application for registration of Prefix/Affix must be made in the prescribed form and the Fee for registration of a prefix/affix is Rs. 250/- and is for life.

The dog mentioned on reverse must be solely and unconditionally the property of the applicant, and the declaration must be signed by him. In case of joint ownership the names of all the owners must be given and the declaration must be signed by all the owners.

This form duly filled in and the declaration signed with date should be sent along with the requisite fee (Rs.20/-or 25/-as the case may be –(See 3 above) by I.P.O. or M.O. (the M.O. postal receipt should be attached to the Application form for reference) or to The Secretary, Kennel Club of India, 9, alar Kalvi Nilayam Avenu, Off, Ritherdan Road, Madras- 600 007.

The registration of a dog will be published in the issue of the Indian Kennel Gazette for the month following the month of registration or in later issue. If the owner is not a regular subscriber and wishes to have a copy of the I.K.G. in which the registration of his dog will appear, he may remit Rs. 4/- extra towards the cost of the same along with the fee for registration of the dog.

The annual subscription to Indian Kennel Gazette is Rs. 45 /- which includes the annual number issue which is an enlarged and pictorial edition and priced Rs. 20.00 for non-subscribers.

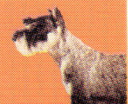

Subscriptions may commence from any month. All communications and remittance regarding the journal should be addressed to the Secretary, K.C.I.

POPULAR DOG SHOWS IN INDIA

Dog shows are organized in different states mostly in big cities and most of the people living at remote places are usually unaware with such activities. The dog is a beautiful creature and owners feel proud when their pets are listed in winners. A brief information about some important clubs organizing dog shows is given for the convenience of dog lovers.

1. Andhra Pradesh Kennel Club
   Mr. R.K. Bakshi
   Hony. Secretary, Andhra Pradesh Kennel Club
   1/2 Vallabhadas Building, Nampa
   Hyderabad-500 001.

2. Bihar Kennel Club
   Mr. K.B. Sinha
   Hony. Secretary, Bihar Kennel Club
   Tata Iron & Steel Co., Ltd.
   Jamshedpur-831 001.

3. Bombay Presidency Kennel Club
   Mrs. Sheila Naharwar
   Hony. Secretary
   Bombay Presidency Kennel Club
   1-B-1, Giriraj Anstey Road
   Mumbai-400 026.

4. Calcutta Canine Club
   Mr. Partha Sekhar Chatterjee
   Hony. Secretary, Calcutta Canine Club
   92, Garpar Road
   Kolkata, Phone-355 724

5. Calcutta Kennel Club
   Mr. Dulal Chandra Banerjee
   Hony. Secretary, Calcutta Kennel Club.
   18/12, Raja Raj Ballabh Street
   Kolkata-700 007.

6. Calicut Kennel Club
   Mr. T.A. Rajagopal
   Hony. Secretary
   Raj Kamal, Calicut-4.

7. Chandigarh Kennel Club
   Major Trilochan Singh
   Hony. Secretary-Chandigarh Kennel Club
   1156, Sector 33-G, Chandigarh.

8. Coimbatore Kennel Club
   Mr. M. Udaychander
   Hony. Secretary, Coimbatore Kennel Club
   699, Ananashi Road
   Coimbatore-144 003

9. Delhi Kennel Club
   Mr. P.S. Sandilya
   Hony. Secretary, Delhi Kennel Club
   3500, Kucha Lalman
   Delhi Gate, Delhi-110 006.

10. Doon Valley Kennel Club
    Dr. A.K. Aggarwal
    Hony. Secretary
    Doon Valley Kennel Club
    11/1, Lytton Road
    Dehradun-248 001

11. Gujarat Kennel Club
    Dr. R.S. Gaekwad
    Hony. Secretary
    Gujarat Kennel Club
    Adhav Bagh, Makarpura Road
    Vadodra-390 009.

12. Haryana Kennel Club
    Dr. K.K. Saxena
    Hony. Secretary
    Haryana Kennel Club
    Shop 3G/34, New Market
    Near Police Post No. 3
    N.I.T., Faridabad.

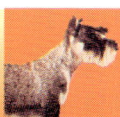

13. Kanpur Kennel Club
Mr. P. Shukla
Hony. Secretary
Flat No. 21, IInd Floor
Naveen Market
Kanpur-308 001.

14. Kohinoor Kennel Club
Major V.P. Singh
Hony. Secretary
Kohinoor Kennel Club
14, Model Town, Jalandhar-144 003.

15. Madras Canine Club
Mr. C.V. Sudarsan
Hony. Secretary
Madras Canine Club

16. Mukathal Street,
Madras-600 007.

17. Mysore Kennel Club
Mrs. A. Gopinath
Hony. Secretary
Mysore Kennel Club
3/1, Cornwell Road, Langford Garden
Bangaluru-560 025.

18. Noida Kennel Club
Mr. R. Shanker Rao
1472, Arun Vihar, Sector 37
NOIDA-201 303 (U.P.).

19. North of India Kennel Club
The Secretary
North of India Kennel Club
H/9, Green Park Extension
New Delhi-110 016.

20. Orissa Kennel Club
Dr. S.K. Ray
Hony. Secretary, Orissa Kennel Club

Qr. No. 3R–33, Agriculture Colony
Bhubaneshwar- 751 003

21. Oudh Kennel Club
Mr. Awadh Narain Srivastava
Hony. Secretary Oudh Kennel Club
Room no. 501, Carlton Hotel
Shahnajaf road, Lucknow-226 001.

22. Palghat Kennel Club
Mr. K. Mohanchandran
Hony. Secretary, Palghat Kennel Club
c/o Instrumentation Ltd., Palghat-678
623.

23. Poona Kennel Club
Captain Sunny Jacob
Hony. Secretary, Poona Kennel Club
B-6, Hermes Park Society (R)
Bund Garden Road, Pune-411 001.

24. South of India Kennel Club
The Hony. Secretary
South of India Kennel Club
Oak End, Ootacamund – 643 001
Nilgris.

25. Tristar Kennel Club
Mr. Rajinder Malhotra
Hony. Secretary Tristar Kennel Club
87, Maharana Pratap Marg
Ambala Cantt- 133 001. Phone: 21231
and 22677.

26. Vishakapatnam Kennel Club
Dr. Narsimha Prasad
Hony. Secretary
Vishakhapatnam Kennel 0Club
49-46-4C Devi Nilayam , Akhayyaapahlam
Vishakhapatnam-530 016.

APPENDIX XX: PET-HEALTH CARD

Owner's name _____

Telephone No. _____

Name of pet _____

Clinician's Name & Add. _____

_____

Telephone No. _____

Species _____

Breed _____

Sex _____   Date of Birth _____

Place of Birth _____

Identification mark _____

Birth mark _____

Registration No. (if any) _____   Insurance No. (if any) _____

Pedigree _____   Dam _____

Sire _____

Language used with pet _____

Feeding system followed _____

HEALTH STATUS

Date of check up	General appearance	Behaviour	Clinical status	Sign. of Vet.

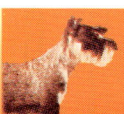

VACCINATION SCHEDULE (For Details See Below)

Sl. No.	Date	Nature	Batch No.	Administration	Next due date	Sign. of Vet.

DEWORMING

Sl. No.	Date of deworming	Dewormer used	Administration	Next due date	Sign. of Vet.

ECTOPARASITICIDAL SPRAY

Sl. No.	Date of Spray	Drug used	Concentration of drug	Next due date	Sign. of Vet.

THERAPEUTIC REGIMEN

Date	Disease	Treatment	Progress	Remarks and Signature of Vet.

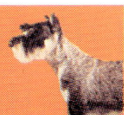

LABORATORY INVESTIGATION
(Punch Laboratory Investigation Report)

A Haemato-biochemical profile	**B** Urine analysis
C Faecal examination	**D** Skin scraping examination
E Electrocardiogram	**F** X-ray
G Microbiological examination	**H** Others

WEIGHT AND HEIGHT RECORD

Sl. No.	Date	Weight (kg)	Height (cm)	Increase Wt.(kg)	Increase Ht.(cm)	Decrease Wt.(kg)	Decrease Ht.(cm)	Remarks & Sign. of Vet.

BREEDING RECORD OF BITCH

Sl. No.	Name of sire	Date of covering I	II	III	Date of whelping	Pup born M	F	Pup died M	F	Remarks & Sign. of Vet.

BREEDING RECORD OF MALE DOG

Sl. No.	Name of dam	Date of mating I	II	III	Pup born Date	M	F	Pup died Date	M	F	Remarks & Sign. of Vet.

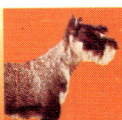

DISTINGUISH WORKS? AWARDS		
Date	Type of work /award	Place

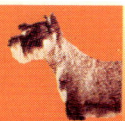

Appendix XXI: BREEDING GUIDE TO BITCH

Sl. No.	Average values of breeding behaviour	Bitch
1.	Age of puberty	6–12 months
2.	Age of breeding	12–18 months
3.	Type of oestrus cycle	Monoestrus (but usually 2 oestrus cycles per year)
4.	Length of oestrus cycle	6 months
5.	Length of oestrus (heat)	6–13 days
6.	Gestation period	55–75 days (63 days)
7.	Time of ovulation	48–60 hours after the receptive phase
8.	Proper time of AI	2–3 days after onset of true oestrus
9.	Breeding season	Biannual: August to September, February to March
10.	Return of heat after parturition	16–20 weeks
11.	Recurrence after non conception	Twice yearly
12.	Age of weaning	4–6 weeks
13.	Time of fertilized ova entering uterus	5–6 days post coitus
14.	Time of implantation begins	15 days post coitus
15.	Type of placenta	Endothallochorial
16.	Expulsion of placenta	Immediately after each foetus
17.	Average pup/born	4–8 pups
18.	Birth weight	65–500 g
19.	Breeding span	7–8 years
20.	Life span	10–15 years (Record is 32 years)

Characteristics of semen and artificial Insemination

Entities	Values
Volume	0.3-23 ml
pH	5.9-7.2
Average concentration of sperms	1.428 million/ejaculate
Collection of semen for AI purpose	2-3 times a week
Site for semen deposition in bitch for AI	Cervix
Volume of diluted semen required for AI	1.5 ml
Minimum number of sperms required for AI	15 million
Rate of semen dilution for AI purpose	1:10
Extenders used for dilution	Egg yolk citrate or heat treated milk
Life span of diluted semen	6 days at 4°C
Life span of fresh/ neat semen	18 hours

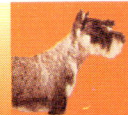

Appendix XXII: VACCINATION SCHEDULE FOR THE DOGS				
Diseases	Vaccine	Inoculations		
		First	Second	Booster
Rabies	(i) Flury (LEP freeze dried) Rabies vaccine	4th to 6th month (freeze dried)	6 months after first inoculation	Annual
	(ii) Rabies vaccine	4th week of life	1 year after Ist	Biennial inoculation
	Commercial Rabies Vaccines:			
	(i) Candur-R Inactivated rabies virus grown in chicken embryo	7 weeks of age	4-6 week after	Annual
	(ii) Nobivac-R Rabies virus grown on BHK21 cell line and inactivated	3 months of age	–	Annual
	(iii) Rabigen Inactivated & adjuvinated fixed strain	3 months and	–	Annual
	(iv) Raksharab (Indian Immunologicals) Inactivated tissue culture rabies virus with aluminium hydroxide	3 months of age above	After 3 months of primary one	Annual
Canine distemper	Modified live virus vaccine	Before 9th week of life	12th week of life	16th week of life
	Canine Distemper vaccine (Megavac-D) Reze dried live attenuated vaccine	6 week	–	Annual
Parvovirus	Parvovirus vaccine	6th to 8th week of life	After 12th week of life	Annual

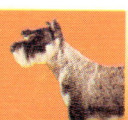

Nobivac-P	Inactivated vaccine	9th to 12th	2-4 weeks later	Annual
Megavac-P	Do-	8th to 9th week	–	Annual
Rabies, canine distemper, leptospirosis and canine hepatitis	Pentadog vaccine	7th to 10th week of life	11th week of life	After 1 year of second injection
Canine distemper, hepatitis	Candur DHLP vaccine	7th to 9th week	12th to 14th week	Annually
leptospirosis and parvovirus	Caniffa vaccine DHL	7th to 9th week	12th to 14th week	Annually
C.D; Adenovirus type-2, hepatitis, parainfluenza, parvovirus, leptospira canicola and icterohaemorrhagica	Adenomune-7	7th to 9th week	12th to 14th week	Annually
Canine distemper, leptospira canicola and icterohaemorrhagica, parvovirus and hepatitis contageiosa canis virus.	Candur-DHL+ P	7th to 9th week	12th to 14th week	Annually
Canine distemper, Canine hepatitis, Canine parvovirus and Canine parainfluenza virus	Nobivac-DHPPi	7th to 12th week		Annually
Canine distemper, Infectious canine Hepatitis, canine parvovirus and leptospira canicola and icterohaemorrhagica	Megavac-6	8th to 9th week	12th week	Annual
Canine distemper, canine adenovirus type-II, parainfluenza virus icterohaemorrhagics, and canine parvovirus	Duramune DA$_2$P + PV	12 weeks	2 to 3 weeks later	Annual

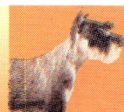

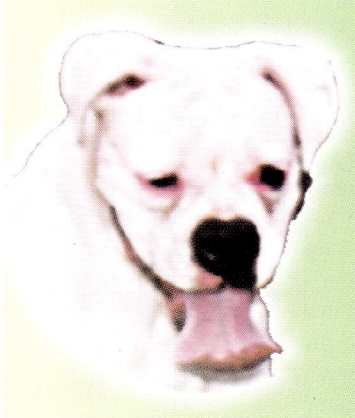

Index

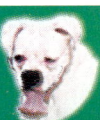

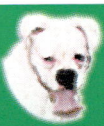

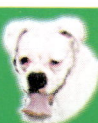

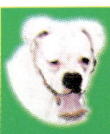

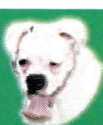

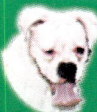